International Handbook of Neuropsychological Rehabilitation

CRITICAL ISSUES IN NEUROPSYCHOLOGY

Series Editors

Antonio E. Puente
University of North Carolina, Wilmington

Cecil R. Reynolds
Texas A&M University

Current Volumes in this Series

International Handbook of Neuropsychological Rehabilitation

Edited by

Anne-Lise Christensen, Ph.D.

Center for Rehabilitation of Brain Injury (CRBI)
University of Copenhagen
Copenhagen, Denmark

and

B. P. Uzzell, Ph.D.

Memorial Neurological Association
Houston, Texas

Springer Science+Business Media, LLC

DOI 10.1007/978-1-4757-5569-5

Originally published by Kluwer Academic / Plenum Publishers, New York in 2000
MyCopy version of the original edition 2000

10 9 8 7 6 5 4 3 2 1

A C.I.P. record for this book is available from the Library of Congress.

Contributors

Yehuda Ben-Yishay • Brain Injury Day Treatment Program, New York University Medical Center, New York, New York 10016

Dmitri Bougakov • The Graduate School and University Center, City University of New York, New York, New York 10036

Lúcia Willadino Braga • The SARAH Network of Hospitals for the Locomotor System, 70.330-150 Brasilia, Brazil

Sheila Bremner • The Oliver Zangwill Center, The Princess of Wales Hospital, Ely, Cambs CB6 1DN, United Kingdom

Sue Brentnall • The Oliver Zangwill Center, The Princess of Wales Hospital, Ely, Cambs CB6 1DN, United Kingdom

Carla Caetano • Center for Rehabilitation of Brain Injury, University of Copenhagen, 2300 Copenhagen S, Denmark

Aloysio Campos da Paz, Jr. • The SARAH Network of Hospitals for the Locomotor System, 70.330-150 Brasilia, Brazil

Raffaella Cattelani • Neuropsychology and Neurorehabilitation Unit, Institute of Neurology, University of Parma, 43100 Parma, Italy

Sabina Cavatorta • Neuropsychology and Neurorehabilitation Unit, Institute of Neurology, University of Parma, 43100 Parma, Italy

Anne-Lise Christensen • Center for Rehabilitation of Brain Injury, University of Copenhagen, 2300 Copenhagen S, Denmark

Giuliana Contini • Trauma Association of Parma, 43100 Parma, Italy

Ellen Daniels-Zide • Brain Injury Day Treatment Program, New York University Medical Center, New York, New York 10016

Georges Dellatolas • INSERM U169, F-94807 Villejuif Cedex, France

Gérard Deloche • CIRLEP and INSERM U472, F-51096 Reims Cedex, France

Georg Deutsch • Department of Radiology, University of Alabama at Birmingham, Birmingham, Alabama 35233

Leonard Diller • Rusk Institute of Rehabilitation Medicine, New York University Medical Center, New York, New York 10016

Rebecca Eberle • Center for Neuropsychological Rehabilitation, Indianapolis, Indiana 46260

Jonathan Evans • The Oliver Zangwill Center, The Princess of Wales Hospital, Ely, Cambs CB6 1DN, United Kingdom

Elkhonon Goldberg • New York University School of Medicine, and the Fielding Institute, New York, New York 10019

Steven W. Henderson • Adult Day Hospital for Neurological Rehabilitation, St. Joseph's Hospital and Medical Center/Barrow Neurological Institute, Phoenix, Arizona 85013-4496

Marja-Liisa Kaipio • Käpylä Rehabilitation Center, Department of Clinical Neuropsychology, 00610 Helsinki, Finland

Clare Keohane • The Oliver Zangwill Center, The Princess of Wales Hospital, Ely, Cambs CB6 1DN, United Kingdom

Pamela S. Klonoff • Adult Day Hospital for Neurological Rehabilitation, St. Joseph's Hospital and Medical Center/Barrow Neurological Institute, Phoenix, Arizona 85013-4496

Carsten Kock-Jensen • Department of Neurosurgery, Aalborg Hospital, DK-9100 Aalborg, Denmark

Sanna Koskinen • Käpylä Rehabilitation Center, Department of Clinical Neuropsychology, 00610 Helsinki, Finland

David G. Lamb • Adult Day Hospital for Neurological Rehabilitation, St. Joseph's Hospital and Medical Center/Barrow Neurological Institute, Phoenix, Arizona 85013-4496

Muriel D. Lezak • Department of Neurology, Oregon Health Sciences University, Portland, Oregon 97201

Anna Mazzucchi • Neuropsychology and Neurorehabilitation Unit, Institute of Neurology, University of Parma, 43100 Parma, Italy

Paul Millemann • The Mulhouse Center for Readaptation, 68093 Mulhouse, Cedex, France

James M. Mountz • Department of Radiology, University of Alabama at Birmingham, Birmingham, Alabama 35233

Pierre North • The Mulhouse Center for Readaptation, 68093 Mulhouse, Cedex, France

Mario Parma • Neuropsychology and Neurorehabilitation Unit, Institute of Neurology, University of Parma, 43100 Parma, Italy

Anne Passadori • The Mulhouse Center for Readaptation, 68093 Mulhouse, Cedex, France

Mugge Pinner • Center for Rehabilitation of Brain Injury, University of Copenhagen, 2300 Copenhagen S, Denmark

George P. Prigatano • Section of Clinical Neuropsychology, Barrow Neurological Institute, St. Joseph's Hospital and Medical Center, Phoenix, Arizona 85013

Marie V. Reichert • Adult Day Hospital for Neurological Rehabilitation, St. Joseph's Hospital and Medical Center/Barrow Neurological Institute, Phoenix, Arizona 85013-4496

Jaana Sarajuuri • Käpylä Rehabilitation Center, Department of Clinical Neuropsychology, 00610 Helsinki, Finland

Paul W. Schönle • A. R. Lurija-Institute for Rehabilitation Sciences and Health Research, University of Constance, Kliniken Schmieder, D-78473 Allensbach, Germany

Donald G. Stein • Brain Research Laboratory, Department of Neurology, Emory University School of Medicine, Atlanta, Georgia 30322

Graham M. Teasdale • Department of Neurosurgery, Institute of Neurological Sciences, The Southern General Hospital, Glasgow G51 4TF, Scotland, United Kingdom

Lance E. Trexler • Center for Neuropsychological Rehabilitation, Indianapolis, Indiana 46260

Susan L. Tully • Adult Day Hospital for Neurological Rehabilitation, St. Joseph's Hospital and Medical Center/Barrow Neurological Institute, Phoenix, Arizona 85013-4496

B. P. Uzzell • Memorial Neurological Association, Houston, Texas 77074

Anna Veneri • Trauma Association of Parma, 43100 Parma, Italy

Huw Williams • The Oliver Zangwill Center, The Princess of Wales Hospital, Ely, Cambs CB6 1DN, United Kingdom

Barbara A. Wilson • MRC Cognition and Brain Sciences Unit, Addenbrooke's Hospital, Cambridge CB2 2QQ, and The Oliver Zangwill Center, The Princess of Wales Hospital, Ely, Cambs CB6 1DN, United Kingdom

Giuseppe Zappalá • Division of Neurology, Garibaldi Hospital, Catania, Italy

Foreword

I am extraordinarily pleased to have been asked by Drs. Christensen and Uzzell to write the foreword for this handbook. This handbook is the result of the most recent of a series of conferences held in Copenhagen, Denmark, at five-year intervals over the past 15 years, under the guidance and leadership of Dr. Anne-Lise Christensen, and under the sponsorship of the Egmont Foundation, which must be acknowledged as well for its constant support of this international effort.

The participants in these conferences are all internationally renowned clinicians and scientists. These experts represent not only the area of neuropsychology, but disciplines ranging from fundamental neurophysiology and neuroanatomy, to medical and financial perspectives on neurological injury and recovery. The participants have, to a significant extent, remained remarkably constant over this period, and this has allowed increasing intimacy among them both professionally and personally. One felicitous result of this camaraderie has been that the conferences have evolved with an increased focus on topics of the broadest interest across disciplines. One aspect of such a continuing dialogue across disciplines is that specific areas of mutual interest are explored in depth, allowing cross-fertilization of ideas to occur. For example, the neuroplasticity and recovery concepts presented by Donald Stein (based upon his work and others) have provided not only a conceptual and physiological basis for the effects of neuropsychological rehabilitation efforts in humans, but have also raised specific intriguing questions for clinicians, for instance, the suggestion that gender specific, and associated hormonal specific, differential recovery paths in animals have relevance to human clinical care.

This handbook is derived from the papers and discussions held at the latest meeting in June, 1997. As such, it represents state-of-the-art updates on the various topics addressed. It is apparent that the science behind the contributions in this book has evolved from an earlier basic description of fundamentals (in previous editions), towards current, more elaborate, and formally scientific discussions. More methodologically sound approaches have been developed and more population-based approaches and studies are represented herein. All of this is to be applauded. Yet, the area of neuropsychological rehabilitation (and affiliated neurorehabilitation topics) obviously require much more of the same effort and analytical thinking reflected in this book. This handbook must, therefore, be seen as a progress report of this overall effort. It will undoubtedly raise as many questions for its readers as it answers. Certain obvious areas remain to be addressed. Very salient (given the general economic constraints emerging upon "health care" in general and being felt across international boundaries) is the need for better analyses and discussion of cost/benefit and cost/effectiveness issues of neuropsychological, as well as other neurorehabilitative technologies and methods. This deficiency certainly reflects not a lack of concern for this issue by the authors, but rather a reflection of the methodological difficulty in performing such analyses. Therefore, one would hope that this process of five-year international revisits of neuropsychological issues, as well as an increasing focus on their economic aspects, continues in the future.

In summary, this handbook represents an excellent and valid international compendium of current thinking in what is a rapidly evolving area.

D. Nathan Cope, M.D.
Paradigm Health Corporation
Concord, California

Preface

Behavioral observations suggestive of brain functioning have always been made, but with advances in neuroscience and neuroimaging during the last decade, public interest as well as the number of neuropsychologists have both increased. As Professor Donald Stein, a neuroscientist and author stated, "We have learned more about the brain in the last ten years than in the last ten centuries."

Much of the effort in neuropsychology has been directed toward assessment, which is beneficial in diagnosing the presence or absence of brain damage. With the appearance of neuroimaging techniques, there has been less need for such diagnoses. Nevertheless, assessment still remains important in documenting and understanding functional losses, and in providing treatment recommendations based on cognitive strengths and weaknesses. In addition to assessment, neuropsychological treatment has been evolving in response to an increasing need, so that time spent on assessment and treatment activities is equally divided for most clinical neuropsychologists. It is this treatment aspect of neuropsychology that we focus upon in this book.

When we completed our first book on the topic of neuropsychological rehabilitation in 1988, interest in this area was present, but not like the explosion of interest and activity that now exists 11 years later as this volume is completed. At different times in different countries throughout the world, more and more neuropsychological rehabilitation is appearing, as knowledge accumulates from pioneering work, new developments, research, and clinical studies. We have much more to contribute than we did a decade ago. This volume contains chapters from programs in Europe, the United States, and South America, covering topics such as neuroscience, acute and chronic brain injury, assessment for neuropsychological rehabilitation, treatment ideologies, and specific treatment programs.

Due to the increased activity and interest in neuropsychological rehabilitation, it has been a challenge and a pleasure to edit chapters for the *International Handbook of Neuropsychological Rehabilitation.* We did not do this alone, but with the aid of our colleagues, whom we want to thank for their time and efforts exerted in writing chapters. We are thankful for the support of the Danish Egmont Foundation given to the Center for the Rehabilitation of Brain Injury (CRBI) at the University of Copenhagen, specifically for a conference on neuropsychological rehabilitation in Copenhagen during June 1997, and for the editorial work in completing this book. We are specifically thankful to the individuals at the CRBI, and particularly to its secretary, Lise Lambek, a valuable collaborator throughout the editorial process.

We hope this book will provide inspiration and direction to our colleagues, particularly to young neuropsychologists entering the field, who will continue to offer services to those with brain injuries who have benefited greatly in the past from this type of treatment.

Anne-Lise Christensen
B. P. Uzzell

Contents

I

Acute Care Management and Brain Recovery

1

Guidelines for Acute Head Injury Management

CARSTEN KOCK-JENSEN AND GRAHAM M. TEASDALE

Quality Improvement in Care of Head-Injured Patients

A head injury can result from many causes and is often complicated by extracranial lesions; discussion of the management of traumatic brain injury needs to be extended to include the general problems of trauma. If the management of the victim is to be most effective, a chain of care needs to be activated as soon as possible after an injury. This chain involves contributions from many different components, starting with the very early phase of prehospital management throughout hospital care and rehabilitation. In the last 10 years, physicians and health care planners have increasingly understood the need to have flexible but organized and integrated systems of trauma care, reflecting the widening appreciation of the importance of quality assurance in health care services.

Priorities need to be set: Which investments in resources, energies and activities are likely to yield the greatest benefits, not only for individuals, but throughout the community. If this processs is going to be justified, reliable and valid performance measures are required.

The complexity of trauma and the difficulties in measuring efficiency and effectivness of treatment have hindered widespread recognition of the scale of the trauma "epidemic" and inhibited proponents of the speciality from using rigorous statistical arguments in support of ways in which the problem might best be approached. In most medical specialities, the delivery of care is dictated and constrained by our knowledge of the disease processes involved and the cost of training and the purchase of equipment and facilities. The care of injured patients is different. In the management of trauma it is the way that these various components are put together that is vital in achieving quality improvement.

"Measuring" the process of trauma care is an aid to the development of optimal systems. This can be achieved only if the input and output are known and well described. The effects of

---

CARSTEN KOCK-JENSEN • Department of Neurosurgery, Aalborg Hospital, DK-9100, Aalborg, Denmark. **GRAHAM M. TEASDALE** • Department of Neurosurgery, Institute of Neurological Sciences, The Southern General Hospital, Glasgow G51 4TF, Scotland, United Kingdom.

International Handbook of Neuropsychological Rehabilitation, edited by Christensen and Uzzell.
Kluwer Academic/ Plenum Publishers, New York, 2000.

injury have been defined widely in terms of the anatomical components and the physiological response on the input side and through mortality on the output side. Current methods often use only survival or death as an outcome measure and the assessment of morbidity has been largely neglected until recently. This is an important omission, because it is estimated that there are at least two seriously and permanently impaired survivors for each person who dies from an injury. Nevertheless, the concept of clinical audit by case analysis and assessment of institutions on the basis of these statistics has generally been well received.

Different methods have been developed and used in assessing trauma care in North America, Australia, and many countries in Europe (Boyd, Tolson, & Copes, 1987; Champoun, Copes, & Sacco, 1990; Baker, O'Neil, & Leng, 1987). As these systems become more robust and reliable, they should be valuable in measuring with confidence the effectiveness of care provided by different systems. Nevertheless, the use of this information to improve care may be achieved only if trauma systems are organized at national or at least regional levels.

Guidelines for the practice of clinical medicine are recommendations for processes of care that are developed by a formal process that incorporates the best scientific evidence with expert opinions. They can be defined as systematically developed statements to assist practitioner and patient about decisions for appropriate care for specific clinical circumstances. One of the crucial key words is the concept of systematic development.

General guidelines for management of trauma have been developed and disseminated during the last decade. In United States, the Amercian College of Surgeons Committee on Trauma developed educational programs based on the concept of advanced trauma life support (ATLS) (Committee on Trauma, 1993a) and, with the American College of Emergency Physicians, established criteria defining the minimal requirements for a trauma center and the components necessary to deal with injury in a comprehensive system.

Implementation of systems of care for the injured patient has been slow, even though trauma systems have been reported to reduce preventable death, to improve outcome, and to be cost-effective. In the United States, in 1990, the "Trauma Care System and Development Act" developed a model (Committee on Trauma, 1993b) that described the formation of an inclusive trauma system into which each care provider and facility was incorporated. This model provides a template and supports the development of a health care plan encompassing hospital, personal, and public services. Every patient is cared for at that specific level that is important for the patient's need. The goal is to match the level of facilities with a patient's medical requirement so that optimal and cost-effective care is achieved. This development is only possible if participants in the system develop and follow widely accepted guidelines. Accurate identification of the level of care which is needed, early triage to bring the patient to the appropriate facility, and coordination of support and rehabilitative services to reintegrate the patient into the community are crucial factors in quality improvement.

Guidelines for Management of Head Injury

Guidelines for the acute care of head-injured victims have emerged from different sources throughout the world. Unfortunately, these were not developed through the same fundamental processes. The sources of published guidelines range from empirical, literature-based reviews to expert opinion. Nevertheless, guidelines are often referred to as standards of care, but this term should be reserved for statements that define an organization, management, clinical, and support services' capacity to provide quality care. A standard is an internationally accepted measure that should be adhered to at all times. The complexity of medicine and the situation in acute stage where one often is dealing with "problems" rather than specific diagnoses, however, means that sometimes nothing seems to be absolute. In this situation "standards" may be too restrictive and guidelines or clinical policy, which are recommendations about the management of a particular problem, may be more suitable. To minimize controversy and to encourage rapid acceptance of guidelines, it is important that the recommendations are based firmly on evidence drawn from reliable data and capable of leading to precise measurements of implementation and benefits.

The problem of implementating guidelines in the management of head injuries is complicated by the fact that neurosurgeons see only a minority of the immense number of people sustaining a head injury. In the United Kingdom, in a population of 55 million there are 1 million hospital attenders with a head injury. Only 18% of attenders are admitted and of these only the more severe cases are referred to neurosurgery, accounting for only about 4–8% of admissions. The problem is not only to optimize quality of care by implementating guidelines for management of obviously severe cases, but also to try to pick out the small proportion in a huge population who are at risk of delayed deterioration due to secondary complications and who easily can be successfully treated, if detected in time. The perspective in the management of head-injured patients is not just the tip of the iceberg, formed by the severe cases, but the entire mass usually invisible without deeper scrutiny.

Aspects of care, in which a standardized approach might be beneficial, are:

- Prehospital care
- Initial assessment/triage
- Resuscitation/transportation
- Radiological investigation
- Hospital observation or home observation
- Neurosurgical consultation
- Neurointensive care
- Surgical intervention
- Rehabilitation

In each of these areas, practice varies and different specialities are involved, not necessarily coherently linked to each other. Lack of clearly defined responsibility of management is a major obstacle to quality improvement. Nevertheless, in recent years neurosurgeons in Europe, Australia, and the United States have published (Study Group of Head Injury in Italian Society for Neurosurgery, 1996; Maas, Dearden, & Teasdale, 1997; Guidelines for Treatment of Head injury in Adults, Opinions of a Group of Neurosurgeons, 1958; Guidelines for the Management of Severe Head Injury, 1995; The Management of Acute Neurotrauma in Rural and Remote Locations, 1990) guidelines to assist doctors and health care professionals in making decisions about the appropriate level of care under specific clinical circumstances. International guidelines might seem to be a desirable goal, but throughout the world there is great variation in the arrangements and facilities available to treat head injuries. Even in developed countries, injured victims often are seen by junior medical staff and at a time that senior doctors are not available in hospital. Patients with multiple trauma often require a high-quality multidisciplinary approach, and consequently there is every chance for erroneous decisions.

Guidelines Formulation

In developing guidelines, the first step is to consider from which sources useful data can be obtained. After the data are assembled, reviewed, and validated, it is then possible for experts to come together to obtain some kind of consensus or agreement about which guidelines may be feasible or appropiate in a certain country, region, or state. Local involvement is important to counteract resistance to the development and implementation of guidelines. Implementation should be followed by auditing the uptake of the guidelines and their effect, both on the entire process of management and on patient outcome.

In 1984, guidelines for initial management for head injury in adults were published in the United Kingdom. They focused on early detection of traumatic intracranial hematoma based in firm data about risk factors. They dealt with indications for skull X ray, admission to hospital, and neurosurgical consultation (Briggs, 1984). This work was further elaborated on and published as a flow diagram describing a plan of management for patients with head injury (Teasdale, Murray, & Anderson, 1990). This approach has been adopted nationally in the United Kingdom. As stated before, auditing guidelines are an important measure in quality improvement. Does the implementation of guidelines change outcome? This question was answered positively in 1995, when data on patients with an extradural traumatic intracranial hematoma in Western Scotland showed a decline from a 28% rate of dead and vegetative state before guidelines to 8% in 1995, after national guidelines were in use.

In 1995, in the United States the results were published of the efforts of a committee of neurosurgeons formed in 1993 to analyze the evidence in published literature on the management of severe head injury. The committee was formed in collaboration between the Joint Section on Neurotrauma and Critical Care of the American Association of Neurosurgical Surgeons and the Congress of Neurological Surgeons. The work was organized and supported by the Brain Trauma Foundation.

One of the major goals of the guideline process was to evaluate the quality of existing literature in the field of traumatic head injury and to establish, if possible, valid recommendations based entirely on published peer-reviewed data. Fourteen topics were selected because they were considered to be fundamental in the management of severe head injury. Each topic was subjected to careful analyses of relevant scientific papers with special emphasis on clinical outcome. Literature searches were performed back to 1966, based on information as Medline. The publications selected were reviewed and the quality of evidence arranged into three classes, according to its quality and reliability:

- Class I evidence: Prospected randomized control trials, the gold standard of clinical practice.
- Class II evidence: Prospectivily collected data or retrospective analyses based on clearly reliable data on well-defined populations. This class included prospective trials that did not meet the strict criteria for class I, as well as nonrandomized studies, observational studies, cohort studies, and so forth.
- Class III evidence: Retrospective studies—clinical series, registries, case reviews, and expert opinions.

The strength of recommendations that emerged from the consideration of the data was also classified:

- Standards: These are based on class I evidence reflecting a high degree of clinical certainty and representing accepted principles of management.
- Guidelines: These are appropriate when data suggest moderate clinical certainty and represent a particular strategy or range of management strategies. These data are concerned provide class II evidence.
- Options: Patient management strategies in which there is unclear clinical certainty.

These recommendations are based on class III evidence.

Through the document, very precise statements link the data to the recommendations for management. In total, 2941 papers were reviewed and classified; 342 articles were used in the text but surprisingly yielded only three standards. In addition, 10 guidelines and 16 options were formulated. These guidelines do not represent a "cookbook" for practice, but are a synopsis of selected literature in the management of severe head injury. This approach clearly can facilitate the development of evidence-based protocols but also can stimulate further research and evolution of improved guidelines.

In 1996, the study group on head injury of the Italian Society for Neurosurgery published guidelines for management of adults with a minor head injury (Study Group of Head Injury in Italian Society for Neurosurgery, 1996). The aim was to provide comprehensive data and criteria to identify patients with minor head injury at risk of developing an acute intracranial hematoma. These guidelines are now accepted in Italy and have gained interest also in Spain and Portugal. This reflects increasing collaboration between neurosurgeons in various countries in Europe. In June 1997, neurosurgeons of the Scandinavian countries (49th Annual Meeting of the Scandinavian Neurosurgical Society, 1997) decided to establish a Scandinavian standardized model for head-injury management; consequently, the first meeting in Scandinavia was held early in 1998.

The European Brain Injury Consortium (EBIC) published their guidelines for management of head injury in adults in 1997 (Maas, Dearden, & Teasdale, 1997). The recommendations in this paper are of a pragmatic nature, arising from consensus and expert opinion, but also based on the efforts that led to the North American guidelines described above. The recommendations in the guidelines begin at the site of the accident and follow the management chain to the intensive care unit. Special attention is drawn to the consistency of treatment in the conduct of clinical trials in head injury.

A group of European neurosurgeons, brought together with support from an industrial sponsor (Bayer), also published their opinions on guidelines for treatment of head injury in adults in 1997. This work was intended to serve as a basis for discussion about national or local protocols and distinguished three levels of certainty to help young neurosurgeons to define neurosurgical requirements and to enhance the care of the head-injured patients including those with multiple injuries. The authors attempted to find common "denominators" on a European scale, even though the suggestions may not be appropriate for all countries or regions in Europe.

Conclusion

Although much clearly has been achieved in advancing quality inprovement in the acute phase of head injury management, the process is just beginning and more needs to be done. There is a need for more research, more published knowledge, refinement of guidelines, and analyses of their dissimination and implementation.

Audit of the use of guidelines and evaluation of their impact on outcome is an educational process. People who are going to use guidelines must have a feeling of ownership. Guidelines used in one country may not be applicable in another. There are major differences in the epidemiology of trauma, in geography, prehospital care systems, as well as hospital facilities. These factors must be taken into account in adapting guidelines produced from fundamental considerations to the environment in which they are going to be used. Standards should be applicable internationally, but guidelines can be developed on national bases and can lead to options evolved for local use.

The care of head injuries involves communication about individual patients, as well as between a great variety of specialities. It involves cooperation and coordination. In each of these three steps, guidelines can help and support quality improvement.

The development of validated guidelines and their use to improve the care and outcome of patients present a challenge to neurosurgeons and other specialities involved in trauma care, whether in acute phase or in later phases.

References

Baker, S. P., O'Neil, B., Hadden, W., & Leng, W. B. (1987). The Injury Severity Score: A method of describing patients with multiple injuries and evaluation of emergency cases. *Journal of Trauma, 14,* 187–196.

Boyd, C. R., Tolson, M. A., & Copes, W. S. (1987). Evaluating trauma care: The TRISS method. *Journal of Trauma, 27,* 370–378.

Briggs, M. (1984). Guidelines for initial management after head injury in adults: Suggestions from a group of neurosurgeons. *British Medical Journal, 288,* 983–985.

Champoun, H. R., Copes, W. S., & Sacco, W. J. (1990). The Major Trauma Outcome study: Establishing national norms for trauma care. *Journal of Trauma, 30,* 1356–1365.

Committee on Trauma. (1993a). *Advanced trauma life support programme for physicians.* Chicago: American College of Surgeons.

Committee on Trauma. (1993b). *Resources for optimal care of the injured patient.* Chicago: American College of Surgeons.

Guidelines for the Management of Severe Head Injury. (1995). New York: Brain Trauma Foundation.

Guidelines for Treatment of Head Injury in Adults, Opinions of a Group of Neurosurgeons. (1958). *Zentral B L Neurochirurgia, 58,* 72–74.

Maas, A. I. R., Dearden, M., & Teasdale, G. M. (1997). EBIC-Guidelines for Management of Severe Head Injury in Adults. *Acta Neurochirurgia (Wien), 139,* 286–294.

The Management of Acute Neurotrauma in Rural and Remote Locations. (1990). *A set of guidelines for the care of head and spinal injuries.* Brisbane: The Royal Australian College of Surgeons.

The Study Group of Head Injury in Italian Society for Neurosurgery. (1996). Guidelines for minor head injured patients' management in adult age. *Journal of Neurosurgery Science, 40,* 11–15.

Teasdale, G. M., Murray, G., & Anderson, E. (1990). Risks of traumatic intracranial hematoma in children and adults: Implication for managing head injuries. *British Medical Journal, 300,* 363–367.

The 49th Annual Meeting of the Scandinavian Neurosurgical Society. Aarhus, Denmark, June 1997.

2

Brain Injury and Theories of Recovery

DONALD G. STEIN

Function: 1. The action of performing. 2. Activity; the action of performance; the mode of action by which (something) fulfils its purpose. (*Oxford Universal Dictionary*) 3. An organism's complex adaptive activity, directed toward the performance of some physiological or psychological task. (Luria, 1966, p. 22)

Background and Introduction

Clinical neurologists have long known that some recovery of function after damage to the brain and spinal cord is possible, but the specific mechanisms mediating the process are still not completely understood. Part of the difficulty in defining the mechanisms of functional recovery stems from the fact that there may be multiple pathways leading to recovery. This is because brain and spinal cord injuries at the cellular and morphological level are not the result of a single causative event. Rather, they derive from an initial and relatively rapid biochemical cascade that then produces secondary cellular events leading to further destruction of nerve tissue. Many of the destructive events such as the breakdown of the blood–brain barrier, the excessive release of glutamate and other excitatory amino acids, dramatic changes in the levels of neurotransmitters such as gamma-aminobutyric acid (GABA) and norepinephrine, the production of oxygen free radicals, the release of arachidonic acid, lipid membrane peroxidation, and so forth are at the heart of much of the current research being conducted in university laboratories and pharmaceutical companies.

Following the initial, metabolic cytotoxic events, there are structural changes in neurons due to necrotic degeneration as well as genetically activated, or programmed, cell death known

This chapter originally appeared in: Goldstein, L. B. (Ed.) (1998) *Restorative neurology: Advances in pharmacotherapy for recovery after stroke*, Armonk, N.Y.: Futura Publishing. Reprinted with permission.

DONALD G. STEIN • Brain Research Laboratory, Department of Neurology, Emory University School of Medicine, Atlanta, Georgia 30322.

International Handbook of Neuropsychological Rehabilitation, edited by Christensen and Uzzell.
Kluwer Academic/ Plenum Publishers, New York, 2000.

as *apoptosis*. In turn, the neuronal loss and degeneration of dendrites and terminals, as well as alterations in neuron–glial relationships over time also can produce significant changes in the structure of remaining intact neurons, as these cells respond to the loss of their inputs. Thus, in response to injury, nerve cells alter their metabolic activities and structure in the cell body and at the level of their dendrites and terminal boutons. All these early as well as late changes in cellular activity can produce long-term alterations in cerebral organization and behavior, which in turn will determine the course and extent of the functional recovery.

For the most part, contemporary research on functional recovery after damage to the central nervous system (CNS) has focused on the molecular, genetic, and neurochemical mechanisms that are altered by trauma or disease. The primary goal of this effort is the discovery of new therapeutic agents that can expedite restoration of neural function at the cellular level. Because so much of this work is driven by practical and economic concerns, relatively little recent, scholarly effort has been directed to clarifying the theories of functional recovery, some of which have been around since the beginnings of the 20th century.* In this chapter, I have chosen a few of the concepts that have been most frequently used to explain how behavioral recovery and restitution of function after severe brain damage might occur.

In order to discuss some of these theories that have been used to explain how recovery occurs, there needs to be some understanding of what is meant by "recovery." In the field of neurorehabilitation, "recovery of function" is generally taken to mean that the cognitive, sensory, and motor impairments that follow brain injury are reduced or eliminated without necessarily specifying how such deficits are reduced or eliminated. In some cases, recovery is taken to imply that the postinjury behavior is the same as that seen prior to the injury; that is, in the face of severe damage to a specific brain region, behavior is spared and there is no loss of function. This type of "explanation" is a phenomenological definition of recovery because there is no causal set of physiological mechanism(s) proposed to account for the behavioral changes. As an extreme example, functional recovery is said to occur over time because there is "spontaneous reorganization." In this sense, the recovery is simply a description of a patient's behavior rather than an explanation of the processes involved. It is also a circular explanation with very little descriptive value because the spontaneous reorganization is inferred from the behavior. In other words, there is improved behavior because of spontaneous reorganization and spontaneous reorganization because there is improved behavior.

Another problem that can occur with a strictly phenomenological approach is that the extent to which deficits are reduced in order to claim recovery is not always clearly specified. What is expected of the patient may vary considerably, depending on who holds the expectations and who sets the criteria for determining what is and what is not recovery. For example, unless a patient were tested prior to a brain injury, how would it be possible to determine the extent to which postinjury behavior recovered to "normal" levels (see Almli & Finger, 1988, for more discussion of this issue)? A trauma surgeon could define recovery when the patient emerges from surgery alive, recognizes a relative, and can be removed from intensive care. Social workers and nursing staff might think recovery has occurred when the patient no longer needs hand-feeding or other personal attentions. The insurance company representative might define the recovery as complete when there is no longer any further benefit from rehabilitation training or speech therapy (or in the context of today's managed care programs, after a 6 week course of therapy), while the patient's lawyer might be satisfied only with a definition of recovery based on his or her client's ability to return to gainful and satisfying employment.

---

*For a more comprehensive and detailed discussion on theories of recovery, there are several books available; e.g., Finger and Stein (1982), Finger *et al.* (1988), and Rose and Johnson (1992).

None of the above definitions of "recovery" may take into consideration the patient's own perceptions of how he or she feels or self-perception after stroke or injury. Indeed, it is not uncommon for patients with moderate to minimal brain damage to be accused of malingering when they report that they cannot function as well on their jobs or in daily life as they did before their injuries. In some instances, they may be treated with the wrong medications, which can make their symptoms even worse (Goldstein, 1988, 1992; Schallert, Jones, Shapiro, Crippens, & Fulton, 1992).

Since it has been estimated that only about 15% of patients with serious head injury are capable of returning to their previous jobs, which of these definitions of recovery is most appropriate? Note that none of the above definitions would require the inclusion of a physiological or metabolic substrate to be useful. Indeed, some clinicians and researchers in the field of neurotrauma have suggested that once there is significant loss of neural tissue, no true recovery of function is possible. They might argue that focusing on the achievement of ends (goals) rather than the means by which such goals are accomplished and the lack of test sensitivity to subtle deficits can make it appear as if some functional recovery has occurred (see Finger & Stein, 1982; von Steinbüchel, von Cramon, & Pöppel, 1989; Stein, Brailowsky, & Will, 1995, for a more thorough discussion of this issue).

In a similar context, the term *neural plasticity* is often used to refer to changes in nervous system activity associated with repair processes, although usually at a more molecular level of analysis. Like the term *functional recovery*, neural plasticity can have different meanings that are sometimes difficult to fathom outside of the specific experimental parameters in which they are applied. For example, among other things, neural plasticity can refer to postinjury changes in the number (and types) of neurotransmitter receptors along membrane surface of a neuron. The same term can refer to increases (or decreases) in posttraumatic dendritic or terminal end-foot branching as well as to regeneration of axons in the peripheral nervous system. Plasticity has also been used to describe the alterations in receptive field characteristics of individual or groups or neurons after injury or rehabilitation training. Once again, the extent to which the plasticity occurs or even its relationship to behavioral recovery is not always specified. Indeed, in many molecular biological laboratories, changes in gene expression and regulation, in their own right, have been characterized as examples of neural plasticity without any reference whatsoever to the behaviors that might be affected by these alterations. This is a dangerous practice because injury-induced increases in gene regulation of a specific protein or neurotransmitter, or even the rerouting (sprouting or synaptogenesis) of terminal boutons into a deafferented CNS area may not always be beneficial to the organism, and in some cases may be detrimental, that is, lead to seizures, spasticity, or maladaptive behaviors (see Stein *et al.*, 1995, for examples). This is why behavioral assessment of putative treatments for CNS injuries must follow molecular and morphological studies. Even though there may be significant alterations in physiological parameters, the behavioral work is required to determine if the treatments are beneficial, detrimental, or without effect.

The lack of precision in defining what is meant by behavioral or morphological recovery and related terms like plasticity make it difficult to evaluate which of the various theories of recovery currently in vogue are most appropriate or most valid (see Almli & Finger, 1992, for more discussion). At the current state of our knowledge, we may have to accept that not everyone in the field of neurorehabilitation requires a molecular level of explanation, and therefore, different theories may be used to explain different components of the recovery process. Thus, the therapist who is primarily concerned with returning a patient to a more normal life may have a theory that intensive, physical therapy in a group situation, combined with strong family support and high levels of motivation may be fundamental to obtain recovery of cognitive and motor performance.

I doubt that many molecular biologists working with the expression of genes involved in neurotransmitter regulation would accept this theory of recovery, unless they were the patients in the therapeutic situation. Thus, some concepts of recovery of function may have face validity at one level of explanation (e.g., recovery of verbal behavior) and be of no help at another (e.g., explaining how the control of gene expression could lead to the prevention of apoptosis and/or the rescue of dying or injured neurons by increased synthesis of neurotrophic factors).

Fortunately, most clinical and molecular investigators can avoid the issue of developing a common and universal definition of functional recovery by creating operational definitions that meet their needs in a given experimental situation. In many animal investigations, recovery of function is defined in terms of a brain-damaged animal's ability to reattain the same criterion score that it was able to accomplish preoperatively. When treatment modalities are used, then the measurement of behavioral recovery is taken as the treatment group's ability to perform the task more rapidly (i.e., to achieve criterion) than untreated subjects with the same type of injury. Both injury groups are then usually compared to intact controls who are used to provide baseline or normative data. The same types of analyses can be applied in clinical drug studies; but when more subjective measures are used such as caregivers' or family members' reports of progress in activities of daily life, the problem of defining recovery becomes more subjective and more complex. For example, I think it would be difficult to assign specific physiological mechanisms to restoration of the ability to go shopping in a supermarket, while failing to be able to write a check or balance a checkbook. Although a critical discussion of these questions is warranted if a comprehensive theory of recovery is to be developed, such an effort is beyond the scope of this chapter.

Compensation, Restitution, and Substitution of Function

If we return to the Oxford Universal Dictionary definition of function, it is "the action of performing." To some, true recovery of function after serious brain injury is not possible because logic would dictate that once the neurons mediating a specific function are lost, the only way that any recovery could occur would be through a series of behavioral tricks permitting some degree of compensation, regardless of how sophisticated or how simple those tricks might be. Recently, Kolb (1995), a distinguished neuroscientist, described his own personal recovery from a migraine-induced ischemic stroke. He noted that when he awoke one morning, he was unable to see anything in the left half of his visual space. Although part of his visual world began to reappear within a few hours, Kolb seemed to have lost pattern vision in about one quarter of his foveal representation and he also had reduced acuity in the upper left quadrant of his visual field. He had difficulty reading and in recognizing people's faces because they were missing the left side. Eight years after his stroke, Kolb could report that he had substantially recovered his reading and facial recognition abilities. In describing his recovery, Kolb suggested that much of what he gained is similar to what a cat does when it has to walk using only three of its legs:

> I am able to read not because I see in the left upper fovea again but because I do not try to use this region to read with. Rather, I have learned to fixate so that parts of words that once fell in the upper left fovea now fall in the lower fields. I am told by people that I do this by tilting my head to one side, although I am not conscious of doing this. I should note that I did not specifically set out to learn this strategy but I apparently developed (it) "spontaneously." (Kolb, 1995, Chapter 3, p. 4)

Kolb's example and description of compensation is an excellent one and is used by many people to show that while the general behavior (of reading and facial recognition) we call reading has recovered, the original behavior, that is, the preinjury, specific and precise visual search strategy has not returned; rather, a new strategy has emerged (or has been substituted) to replace that which was lost by the injury. In this view, the fact that compensation occurs can be taken to mean that any possibility of true recovery of function is irretrievably lost. Indeed, LeVere (1988) has previously argued that the act of compensation or substitution of function could prevent recovery. He states that: "Compensatory strategies seem inappropriate and, in fact, could reasonably be considered the antithesis of realizing the full potential of the brain-injured individual" (p. 22). To some extent this notion has received experimental verification. For example, Taub, Pidikiti, DeLuca, and Crago (1996) demonstrated that recovery of function after peripheral nerve section in monkeys could be blocked by allowing the animals to use their unaffected limb. If the intact limb was restrained and the animals were forced to use their injured limbs to retrieve food and drink, some recovery did occur, although it may not have completely approximated preinjury levels of performance. Preliminary research with human stroke patients has revealed similar results; requiring them to use the affected limb by restraining use of the normal produced better quality of movement as well as "mastery of a large range of daily activities that they had not previously carried out with the affected arm" (Taub *et al.*, 1996, p. 142).

Is there any physiological evidence to indicate what processes might be involved in compensatory activities? In other words, following brain damage, is compensation just a question of using "tricks" (which would obviously depend on the functional capacity of remaining intact tissue) or is there some kind of neuronal reorganization that might mediate improved performance? The idea that brain-damaged organisms can show some adaptive capacity by using a different behavioral strategy does not necessarily imply that the injury is not producing widespread alterations in cerebral activity, both cortically and subcortically. For example, Payne and Cornwell (1994) reported that there are "significant anatomical and behavioral changes caused by restricted lesions of the primary visual cortex occurring in early life" which may account for the sparing of pattern discrimination, depth perception, and visual orienting in cats and monkeys.

In an important study, Rauschecker (1995) examined the effects of early visual deprivation in kittens and demonstrated a type of compensatory activity that might account for the behavioral recovery seen in these animals and those with traumatic brain injuries. It appears that visually deprived cats have a significantly improved auditory localization ability. In these animals, electrophysiological recording studies showed that the anterior ectosylvian visual area "was completely taken over by auditory and somatosensory inputs" (pp. 36–43). Moreover, there was a substantial hypertrophy of the cortical areas representing the facial vibrissae, which could play a critical role in developing compensatory maneuvers leading to adaptive behaviors:

> When blind cats are tested in a spatial-maze task, they are not impaired in learning and solving the task, even if it is changed from trial to trial. On closer inspection, it becomes obvious that the blind cats make extensive use of their facial vibrissae in forming a spatial image [or "cognitive map"] of their environment. (Rauscheker, 1995, p. 39)

This is a solid example of sensory substitution (see Bach-y-Rita, 1972, 1990, for the development of original ideas and concepts in this area) producing compensation and recovery; that is, the accomplishment of a specific goal (spatial navigation, orientation, and obtaining positive reinforcement) without consideration of the means by which the specific goals are achieved. In his discussion, Rauschecker raises an interesting philosophical question. If a blind individual has a reorganized brain in which the visual system becomes activated by auditory or tactile stimuli, is the percept determined by the input stimulation or is it formed by the brain region that receives the reorganized afferents?

In humans, recent positron emission tomography (PET) studies of cerebral blood flow after CNS injury and during the performance of cognitive tasks have shown that there are substantial changes in cortical metabolism taking place in areas both ipsi- and contralateral to the damaged site (Weiller, Chollet, Friston, Wise, & Frackowiak, 1992). For example, Weiller and co-workers studied regional cerebral blood flow (rCBF) and motor recovery in adult patients who had suffered from striatocapsular infarctions. The rCBF measurements were taken at rest in the stroke patients and for comparison in normal subjects. At rest, the patients had significantly lower blood flow in a number of brain structures including the basal ganglia, thalamus, sensorimotor cortex, the insula, the brain stem, the prefrontal cortices, and the ipsilateral cerebellum. The authors suggested that the alterations in rCBF showed the distribution of the dysfunction caused by the stroke. After recovery of the use of the affected hand, rCBF was increased in the contralateral cingulate gyrus area and in the premotor areas as well as in the caudate nucleus on the injured side of the brain; the patients also demonstrated higher rCBF bilaterally than did normal subjects.

From my perspective, it was interesting to note that as the use of the affected hand occurred, the pattern of rCBF activation during movement of the unaffected hand was also different from normal subjects. In other words, the unilateral injury to the brain created a new pattern of cerebral blood flow and metabolism that under normal circumstances might not have been implicated in the coordination of the unaffected hand's movement. These changes in rCBF, then, represent a complex reorganization of function produced by the infarct. The authors suggest that these "remote functional effects" could be the result of a "functional disinhibition" of the contralateral premotor cortex, which is, of course, not seen under normal conditions.

Significant individual variation may also play a role in determining which new structures or pathways may become implicated in the compensatory processes that are associated with the behavioral recovery (Weiller, Ramsay, Wise, Friston, & Frackowiak, 1993; Chollet & Weiller, 1994). Even with respect to language localization to the frontal cortex there appears to be considerable individual variation (Ojemann, 1992). Ojemann, a neurosurgeon, examined 88 patients who required left hemisphere surgery for the control of epilepsy. He first determined hemispheric dominance with the intracarotid amobarbital perfusion test. Prior to surgery, electrical stimulation mapping while the patients were conscious was conducted to determine localization of language function. The results of the stimulation indicated that all 88 patients had at least one site in the cerebral cortex that caused significant errors in naming when stimulated. In some patients, however, there were no areas deemed essential for naming anywhere in the frontal cortex. Ojemann concluded that there are some patients with left dominance for language in which Broca's area or any other lateral frontal sites are not required for language.

In observations similar to those reported by Jenkins and Merzenich (1992) and Chollet and Weiller (1994), Ojemann also noted that there are marked individual differences in the boundaries and extent of the language area. For the neurosurgeon who is performing surgical resections, these are important problems; but for us, Ojemann's findings can be taken to suggest that individual differences in CNS organization may be due to cognitive and environmental influences that shape and modulate cortical structure and function(s). Yet, the problem that remains is, if individual variation is so important and if it is just a question of substituting a new behavioral maneuver for one that is lost, then why do we often see specific and rather stereotyped responses emerge in response to brain damage? Are the range of "tricks" and compensatory maneuvers determined only by changes occurring at the physiological–morphological level or do psychosocial factors also play a role?

Evidence from studies based on recording of the activation or inhibition of individual or ensembles of neurons can also be taken to suggest that in adult subjects compensation and substitution of function may be dependent on injury- and/or experience-induced reorganization of neuronal activity. For example, Merzenich and colleagues in San Francisco have conducted an extensive series of experiments to map the cortical topography of neurons representing the skin surface of the hands and digits in owl monkeys. This is done by recording the electrical activity in individual neurons in area 3(b) of the somatosensory cortex during tactile stimulation of the hand or digits. Once the topographical mapping in normal subjects is completed, it is then possible to study the effects of training and peripheral or central nervous system injuries on the reorganization of these cortical map(s). Of the many interesting events described in these experiments, several are relevant to the points I wish to make here. First, the investigators showed that there is considerable variation (individual differences) in the functional inputs of the cortical maps, such that an almost infinite number of alterations in functional representations of sensory input can be created. These differences in the size and shape of the cortical maps is probably due to the differential use of the hand by the animals as well as their individual learning experiences throughout their development.

Second, as the animals learned specific tactile and motor tasks, the cortical representations, as measured by unit recordings, changed as a function of experience and training (see Jenkins & Merzenich, 1992, for a more detailed review of this work). In some cases, training increased the cortical territories representing the skin surfaces by as much as 500%. These data are important from my perspective because they reveal that cortical activity and probably cortical morphology reorganize as a result of training and experience. The training is what leads to the use of new strategies and new maneuvers. Does brain injury also produce a similar type of functional reorganization? The answer would appear to be a "yes," and brain injury followed by neurorehabilitation may provide for additional reorganization. Jenkins and Merzenich created small cortical lesions in area 3 hand representation region of digit 3 in owl monkeys and found that when representational mapping was done over time (sometimes taking as much as 3 months), there was extensive reorganization. The recordings revealed that representation of digit 3 reemerged, although the receptive fields for this finger were much larger than in intact animals. Also, the representation of all of the digits was reversed from the normal order: "That is, normally as one moves from lateral to medial in cortex, the normal representational sequence is from radial to ulnar (e.g., thumb to little finger) whereas we observed the reversed sequence from digit 5 to digit 4 to digit 3" (Jenkins & Merzenich, 1992, pp. 29–30).

We can suppose that shifts in cortical representation and in cortical activity are likely to occur in all CNS areas affected by a lesion or stroke and these changes may underlie either the functional recovery or contribute to the permanent behavioral deficits that are observed (e.g., see Chollet *et al.,* 1991; Weiller *et al.,* 1992;). Recently, Nudo and Milliken (1996) used intracortical, microstimulation to develop detailed functional maps of the hand representation area in adult squirrel monkeys before and after ischemic infarcts were created. Initially, Nudo and Milliken found that there was no spontaneous reorganization (compensation); that is, movements previously represented in the infarcted zone did not spontaneously reappear in the cortical region(s) surrounding the infarct. In fact, it seemed that the cortical representations of the hand movements that were recorded from the intact, neuronal tissue adjacent to the lesion were actually reduced compared to the territory occupied in intact animals.

In a second study, Nudo, Wise, SiFuentes, and Milliken (1996) combined the same recording and lesion techniques with extensive, preoperative and postoperative skilled motor training procedures for the affected hand (retrieving small food pellets) in order to determine whether both representational activity in the cortex as well as behavioral compensation–recovery could be induced. The infarct initially caused a severe deficit in the monkey's ability to retrieve food pellets from small wells; however, with rehabilitation training, the animal's performance improved over time to normal levels:

> Comparison of the cortical maps of movement representation before and after infarct revealed substantial rearrangement of the representations surrounding the lesion. Spared hand representations appeared to invade adjacent regions (that were) *formerly occupied by representations of the elbow and shoulder. This invasion occurred over distances of up to 3 millimeters* [italics mine]. (Nudo *et al.*, 1996, pp. 1792–1793)

In one animal, expansion resulted in a hand representation that was larger than the entire representation before the infarct, including the infarct zone.

It would appear from these data that postinjury physical training helps to prevent degradation of representation in the cortical fields underlying skilled finger movements. Further, it seems that the training helps to increase the size of the field in the intact, adjacent tissue directing it to "take over the damaged function." Recently, Kasten and Sabel (1995) examined the effects of rigorous training on restoration of visual function in 14 human patients who had suffered various types of traumatic injuries to the posterior cortex. All these patients had homonymous hemianopias. The patients received intensive training on tasks designed to respond to small light stimuli, to track moving stimuli, discriminate geometric shapes, and enhance color perception in the damaged visual field. Although two patients showed no improvement following this regimen, the remainder did evidence varying degrees of visual recovery within the hemianopic field beginning within 30 hours of training.

The Nudo, Kasten and Sabel, and Jenkins and Merzenich experiments leads me to agree with the latter in suggesting that for adult subjects the extent of recovery (or the severity of the functional deficit) is related to the distribution of inputs and outputs to a given cerebral area. In an area with highly restricted or highly specific connections (such as the visual cortex), less recovery would be expected than if a particular, partially damaged area had a distribution of inputs and efferents. However, there also is increasing evidence that some form of rehabilitation training and postinjury therapy may be necessary to "unlock" the recovery processes and help to shape adaptive, postinjury behavior. Unmasking, compensation, and the activity of spared neurons in the zone of injury may all contribute to the recovery process, if the right environmental and contextual conditions are present.

In concluding this section on "compensation" as one theory of recovery, I have to stress that while such compensatory changes may be more or less local, we cannot exclude the possibility that a more widespread interplay of excitatory and inhibitory processes also may be taking place in regions quite distant from the locus of the injury. Jenkins and Merzenich (1992) state the complex issues and the intriguing problems that researchers in this field must face if they intend to manipulate compensatory recovery surgically or pharmacologically:

> Functional reorganization in cortical areas not directly damaged by brain injury can also be expected. Brain damage will result in alteration of a lesion specific set of functional areas that constitute input sources to many other non-damaged cortical areas. New, fragmented distributions of input sources to other cortical fields should create novel representational constructs, *some of which must be unique to brain inured patients* [italics mine]. Another important implication of our findings is that even if a cortical lesion was anatomically identical in its locus and extent in any two individuals, the resultant representational and functional defects would be idiosyncratic, as would the course of subsequent recovery. Cortical representations [*and I would add, their reorganization*] are an emergent property of a dynamic self-organizing system, and are not attributable to a fixed "hard wired" system. The representational constructs

> that emerge in such a system reflect the cumulated stored histories of the patterns of neural inputs and the behavioral contexts in which the networks have evolved over the lifetime of a given individual. The constructs of no two individuals will be identical.
>
> Behavioral substitutions can also be expected to occur after brain injury. A new behavior can be substituted for a behavior that is lost or defective as a result of damage to requisite brain structures. And in these instances, distorted brain representations and substituted behaviors reciprocally feed each other. *The brain damage distorts behaviors, which in turn further drive brain regions to consolidate the distorted representations subserving novel emergent compensatory behavior* [italics mine]. Finally, in another class of substitution, a new cortical area can be the primary source of a behavior, while before injury it only contributed secondarily. (pp. 33–34)

Redundancy and Multiple Representation May Underlie Recovery

For at least several decades it has been generally accepted that complex functions (such as language, cognition, perception, memory, sensory information processing, and fine motor movements) implicate the involvement of CNS areas that are widely distributed throughout the cortex, diencephalon, and brain stem. For example, in their highly regarded book, Damasio and Damasio (1989) write that perceptuomotor interactions leading to cognitive processing

> is achieved by the retroactivation of fragmentary records as a result of feedback activity from convergence zones. According to this model, there is no single site for integrating sensory and motor processes and, there is no localizable, single store for the meaning of a given stimulus within a cortical region. Meaning is arrived at by widespread multiregional activation of fragmentary records pertinent to a stimulus within a large array of sensory and motor structures. (pp. 63–64)

This view stands in contrast to the popular idea of complex functions residing in specific, neuronal centers, or at the more reductionistic level, of "pontifical" or command cells being the final decision-making structure in making a visual response, for example.

Stimulation and recording of receptive field characteristics following training or injury (e.g., Jenkins & Merzenich cited above) or a PET scan and other noninvasive imaging techniques have helped to corroborate the idea of relatively diffuse, parallel, and serial systems acting to create psychological functions. This is one reason why Damasio and Damasio (1989) could report that one of their patients with complete bilateral destruction of the hippocampus (including the entorhinal cortex, hippocampus, and amygdala), the basal forebrain (bilaterally), the anterolateral and anteroinferior temporal cortex, and the bilateral orbitofrontal cortex had intact perception in all of his sensory modalities except olfactory: "The descriptions he produces of complex visual or auditory entities and events are indistinguishable from his examiners" (p. 68).

It is difficult to believe that the Damasio's patient is not profoundly impaired in his activities of daily life; nonetheless, the example they provided does begin to focus on the question of how, in the face of so much brain injury, can this individual function as effectively as he does on these neuropsychological tests? Part of the answer must lie in the fact that, despite the apparent genetic, anatomical, and physiological specializations of cerebral tissue, there is considerable redundancy with respect to CNS structure(s) mediating or controlling function(s). This can be taken to mean that there are multiple representations of complex behavioral and psychological functions distributed over a wide array of structures, even though we may not know the mechanisms by which the integration into meaningful behavior (perception, cognition, etc.) takes place.

In contemporary parlance we talk about serial and parallel circuits mediating complex cerebral functions, but the idea of distributed function or multiple representation is not new. At the beginning of the century, for example, Morton Prince (1910), the president of the American

Neurological Association, wrote that "cerebral function is the expression of a mechanism involving the cooperation of widely separated anatomical areas" (p. 348), and that focal lesions could create specific symptoms but could not destroy a whole function. Two decades later, Kurt Goldstein (1939) took a similar position in stating that: "the destruction of one part of the brain never leaves unchanged the activity of the rest of the organism, especially the rest of the brain" (p. 258). Injury may be the stimulus needed to "unmask" the parallel and/or redundant systems so that the behavior can unfold.

A modern example of this type of redundancy comes from the work of Finger and Simonds (1976). These investigators demonstrated that adult rats with bilateral somatosensory cortices removed in several stages, were still able to make tactile discriminations, if they were provided with appropriate training on the task. For the animals to relearn the task after brain damage in the same number of trials that it took to learn as an intact subject, or better, to show no deficit at all after such massive surgery can be taken to indicate that some redundancy or multiple representation of function may exist in the adult CNS.

Working in the visual system, K. L. Chow (1968) destroyed up to 85% of the optic tracts in cats causing massive degeneration of the lateral geniculate nucleus (LGN). In the face of this injury, the cats still retained a preoperatively learned brightness and pattern discrimination. With more injury (about 90% of the tracts and LGN destroyed), the cats could not retain what they had previously learned, but over an extended testing period were able to master the discrimination tasks.

Recently, Sautter and Sabel (1993) studied the effects of mild, moderate, or severe optic nerve crush on recovery of brightness discrimination in adult rats. After mild crush, about 28% of retinal ganglion cells could be labeled by retrograde transport of horseradish peroxidase injected into the superior colliculus; this dropped to about only 8% in rats with severe injury. By 2–3 weeks after the surgery, complete restoration of brightness discrimination could be seen in animals despite the fact that only about 11% of retinal ganglion cells survived the nerve crush operation. Do these findings suggest a kind of redundancy or parallel processing of information necessary to perform the tasks? Sautter and Sabel speculate that return of function may be mediated by compensatory processes taking place at other levels in the CNS that could be due to reorganization of sensory maps. In the light of all the recent evidence discussed here, this may be a real possibility.

Those of us who have had the patience to do extensive behavioral testing in bilaterally brain-damaged laboratory rats know that with enough time and despite massive injuries to almost any part of the cerebral mantle the animals will attain criterion on the tasks employed. Likewise, it has been suggested that, in the case of Parkinson's patients, about 95% of the fibers projecting to the striatum from the substantia nigra have to degenerate before the symptoms begin to emerge. If indeed this is the case, this would be another example of "within system" redundancy, or *equipotentiality* (functional equivalence), to use a term coined by Karl Lashley in the 1930s (Lashley, 1929, 1933). Lashley was convinced that within a given cortical association area all parts are equivalent for the mediation of the function. He based his hypothesis on a large number of lesion studies that demonstrated that visual habits and motor and maze learning would survive all but total removal of the system or could be relearned in about the same number of trials as it took before the surgery.*

*Some writers have taken issue with Lashley's (and others) ideas on equipotentiality and mass action. See, for example, Kolb & Whishaw (1988) and Norrsell (1988). Although somewhat dated and lacking in more molecular biological approaches, Finger *et al.* is still the only single source of materials discussing the theoretical issues surrounding research on recovery from brain damage.

The idea that there is multiple representation and redundancy of function involving a number of different structures in the CNS is compelling and may help to explain how recovery can occur in the face of massive injury to a specific brain region. However, if other structures "take over" the function of a destroyed or damaged area, how then do they mediate their own functions at the same time? Similar to equipotentiality, *vicariation theory* states that following trauma, the tissue surrounding the damaged area has an ability to take over the function of the damaged area. This vicarious substitution can theoretically be implemented in one of three ways: (1) function is transposed to similar tissue on the contralateral portion of the brain; (2) function is transposed onto other uninjured areas of the ipsilateral cortex; and (3) function is controlled via other structures at different levels of anatomical organization. Is there a price to be paid for this type of vicariation? In other words, if area A mediating function A is destroyed, is function A now shifted to area B, which now must mediate function A as well as B?

If such vicariation does occur, is there a price to be paid for this type of "crowding?" Brenda Milner (1974), a Canadian neuropsychologist, pioneered this type of investigation in the 1970s. Using the Wada technique mentioned earlier, she reported that in patients tested without damage or pathology in the left hemisphere, speech was localized in 96% of patients who were right handed. About 70% of left-handed patients had speech localized to the left hemisphere. In patients who had suffered brain damage during infancy, a different picture seemed to emerge. Here, about 80% of right-handed patients had localized speech in the left hemisphere and 12% had speech localized to the right hemisphere. In the left-handed patients with brain damage, speech localization in the left hemisphere dropped to about half.

Do these findings indicate a shift of function or an unmasking of function that was previously suppressed by the dominant hemisphere? Milner noted that the patients with early brain damage had low verbal and nonverbal IQs, a phenomenon that was not seen in adults with frontal lesions. These patients had clear and specific behavioral deficits but no general lowering of IQ. People who have examined this question have found that there is a diminution of general cognitive abilities after early brain lesions, despite the fact that there may be considerable compensation on specific types of tasks (for more details and discussion, see, for example, Woods, 1980; LeVere, Gray-Silva, & LeVere, 1988).

Diaschisis, Neural Shock, and the Unmasking of "Latent" Pathways in Recovery: The Remote Effects of Brain Injury

Diaschisis and Neural Shock

Although concepts such as compensation, multiple representation, equipotentiality, and vicariation may have some face validity after the fact of recovery, they do not provide for any specific physiological or morphological mechanisms that could be manipulated to determine how the recovery might actually take place. Just over 20 years ago, P. D. Wall (1975) took strong issue with many of the concepts I have described here. He stated that: "The usual process of submerging ignorance by nomenclature has been used as though to name is to explain. Shock, diaschisis and such words have no meaning or usefulness in pointing to an explanation" (p. 35). Despite Wall's complaint, it seems that one of the most persistent and now apparently testable (quasi?)physiological hypotheses can be attributed to the Russian neurologist, Constantin von Monakow (1853–1930). Von Monakow's concept of *diaschisis*, which I will review briefly, had an impact on generations of neurologists and neuroscientists right up to the present time.* The idea of diaschisis, in some respects, can be seen as a form of neural "shock" that is initiated by trauma or injury to the brain (Finger & Stein, 1982; Feeney & Baron, 1986). The shock, or transient inhibition (diaschisis), can spread to remote sites or in the fiber pathways leading from the injury to other brain areas. According to Riese (1977), the behavioral deficits produced by an injury are due to the sudden withdrawal of excitation of sites at a distance from the damage. This withdrawal of excitation would lead to an inactivation in related brain areas, which in turn would produce the symptoms associated with the injury. As the diaschisis regresses over time, activity would return to the suppressed areas with a concomitant return of function.

In more contemporary language, we can think of the phenomenon of diaschisis as being the result of varying degrees of neuronal deafferentation due to the initial injury. This deafferentation could be fairly rapid, local, and monosynaptic or it could be more gradual and more extensive because of retrograde or anterograde transneuronal degeneration. These types of neuronal changes occurring hand in hand with injury-induced depression of cellular metabolism, reduced blood circulation, and the dynamics of reperfusion can produce dramatic and widespread changes in CNS activity and function(s) at a distance from the injury.

Most recently, Feeney (1996) wrote that "remote functional depression" could be caused by sublethal levels of excitatory amino acid activation of receptors on neurons distant from a CNS injury. For example, Feeney cited the work of Globus *et al.* (1990) who used microdialysis to detect abnormally high levels of glutamate and aspartate in CNS areas distant from the site of a cerebral infarct or contusion. Areas indirectly affected by the injuries showed reduced cerebral blood flow and energy depletion (Feeney, 1996). He noted that the neurons in these affected regions were able to survive (although presumably at a lower level of function) because of an abundance of the inhibitory neurotransmitters GABA and glycine. One now classic study shows how additional brain surgery may be used to eliminate a source of diaschisis. Sprague (1966) created extensive unilateral lesions of the visual cortex in cats in order to produce a persistent and severe contralateral visual hemianopia in these animals. The results were as expected, except that in a subsequent surgical procedure Sprague damaged the superior colliculus contralateral to the cortical lesion and by so doing was able to reverse the hemianopia. Sprague suggested that the superior colliculus lesion removed the inhibitory influence of the opposite superior colliculus, an imbalance that was now detrimental to restoration of function in the cats with visual cortex lesions. Removing the inhibitory influences resolved the hemianopia. Could this be considered as a example of recovery from a form of diaschisis?

Von Monakow's concept of diaschisis continues to be employed in a number of studies using modern imaging technology such as PET, electroencephalography (EEG), computed tomography (CT), magnetic resonance imaging (MRI), and single photon emission computed tomography (SPECT) evaluations to perform quantitative analysis of measures such as rCBF, electrical activity, and cerebral metabolism.† One of the first investigators to provide direct examination of the concept was Warren Kempinsky (1958), who used electrophysiological recording techniques to measure spontaneous and evoked visual potentials in cats with unilateral lesions of the cortex caused by middle cerebral artery occlusion (MCAo). Kempinsky observed that electrical activity was temporarily depressed in the intact hemisphere following the initial injury. If the corpus callosum was sectioned several weeks prior to the MCAo, there were no changes in evoked potentials in the intact hemisphere and electrocorticograms recorded on the

*See, for example, writings of Prince (1910), Goldstein (1939), Riese (1958), Teuber (1974), Feeney & Baron (1986), Glassman & Smith (1988), and Meyer, Obara, & Muramatsu (1993).

†See Toole and Good (1996), for a recent overview of new developments in this area.

intact side were only mildly and briefly affected in approximately half of the animals studied. Kempinsky suggested that the distal changes he observed could not have been due to the direct disruption of blood flow in the affected areas because the depression of neural activity was seen in cortical regions with blood vessels that were not directly associated with the zone of injury. He concluded that the effects seen in the hemisphere contralateral to the injury were due to "the suspension of activity" caused by the interruption of nerve fibers coming from the zone of injury and crossing via the corpus callosum into the intact hemisphere. This diaschisis, then, presumably was caused by the removal of excitation provided by the callosal inputs.

In the 1980s, Meyer (1982) reexamined and confirmed Kempinsky's findings in baboons. Meyer created cerebral infarctions and observed depression of local cerebral blood flow in the contralateral hemisphere that was significantly reduced by prior section of the corpus callosum. More recently, Heiss *et al.* (1983) used PET scanning to show that patients suffering from strokes that interrupted thalamocortical projections without directly damaging the thalamus itself had decreased thalamic perfusion and depressed metabolism. Treatment with amphetamine, however, helped to eliminate depression in thalamic neurons and restored thalamic blood flow and metabolism to more normal levels.

The above findings notwithstanding, there have been questions raised as to whether diaschisis is truly a functional phenomenon that correlates with severity of the initial injury or consequent recovery, if it occurs. This problem was recently addressed by Infeld, Davis, Lichtenstein, Mitchell, and Hopper (1995), who examined crossed cerebellar diaschisis and brain recovery after stroke. Within 72 hours after onset of the stroke, these workers used SPECT to examine 47 patients with crossed cerebellar diaschisis (CCD) caused by acute middle cerebral artery territory cortical infarctions. Among other measures, they examined the relationship of CCD to infarct hypoperfusion and clinical severity. The latter was evaluated using a modified Canadian Neurological Scale and Barthel Index. Thirty-one of the patients were evaluated again at 3 months after stroke onset. For comparison, cerebellar blood flow asymmetry was measured in 22 healthy, age-matched subjects.

The results of their analyses showed that CCD after MCAo occlusion does correlate with infarct hypoperfusion volume as well as with the extent of the neurological deficits. However, after neurological recovery had occurred, the CCD persisted and was attributed to the destruction of cerebropontile connections causing the depression and continued vasoconstriction and "functional deactivation": "Severity of CCD remained unchanged both over the first 72 hours and between acute and outcome stages" (Infield *et al.*, 1995, p. 95). These findings can be taken to suggest that (1) diaschisis may not just have temporary effects, but may persist over very extended periods of time, and (2), chronic depression of some forms of neural and vasogenic activity can persist over time without direct functional consequences on standard tests of neurological outcome.

Finally, diaschisis is being seen in a somewhat different light by Andrews (1991), who suggests that the phenomenon may not just be taken to include remote *decreases* in cerebral blood flow or inhibition of neural activity. Instead, Andrews suggests that, in addition to these manifestations of diaschisis, remote *disinhibition* leading to neural hyperreactivity may also be triggered by certain types of injury. This hyperactivity in both hemispheres may be due to damaged neural structure and denervation supersensitivity. Andrews states that

> Although the notion of disinhibition or facilitation is contrary to the original view of Von Monakow that the remote effect of cerebral injury is inhibitory, there is evidence that diaschisis can be facilitative rather than inhibitive. Regarding intrahemispheric diaschisis, prefrontal injury recently has been shown to result in increased amplitude of both the somatosensory and auditory primary cortical evoked potentials. (1991, p. 947)

Can Andrews' hypothesis be taken to suggest that induced neuronal hypoactivity after CNS trauma could be neuroprotective? If this is the case, it might explain why some neurotrauma clinicians use barbiturate-induced coma as a putative therapy for head trauma patients.

Given all the different models and theories about what diaschisis is or is not, it seems that the full story on this hypothetical construct still remains to be told. Is it simply a shortcut term that describes a variety of injury-induced changes in the nervous system that occur shortly after the damage? As I noted, there are many short- and long-term proximal and distal changes in the brain after injury. Which events can be attributed specifically to diaschisis and which to other mechanisms such as degeneration, apoptosis, alterations in neuron–glia relationships, or attack on cell membranes by injury-liberated free radicals and other toxic substances still remains to be determined. One has to be careful in applying the concept to all injury-related events lest it lose explanatory value; that is, where almost every detrimental change in CNS function is seen as an example of diaschisis. Nonetheless, it is interesting to see how a concept developed almost a century ago took so long to attract serious, scientific interest and experimental and clinical confirmation. It is also interesting to note that von Monakow's concept had to wait almost 100 years for the development of cutting edge technology before it could be scientifically validated.

Unmasking and Latent Pathways

The brief review of some of the literature on diaschisis provides a good start for the discussion of another mechanism that has been suggested as a possible basis for functional recovery after brain injury. One of the key components of the principle of diaschisis that researchers have now found more compelling is the idea that the symptoms (or syndrome) associated with different types of brain damage may be the result of large-scale alterations in neuronal and metabolic activities taking place in areas quite remote from the site of the injury itself. As noted above, many of these changes are thought to take place rapidly, too rapidly to be attributed to changes in morphology or metabolism resulting from degeneration or necrosis per se. I also commented on recent work (Andrews, 1991) suggesting that diaschisis could exert excitatory as well as inhibitory influences on sites distal to the injury zone. In this context, we also can consider that some of the beneficial (as well as potentially detrimental) remote effects of focal brain injury might be due to the unmasking of functional activity in previously existing pathways whose activity is suppressed, diminished, or ineffective in intact organisms.

One of the first investigators to explore (and name) this phenomenon was Patrick Wall. In an early study, Wall and Egger (1971) damaged the gracile nucleus in adult rats and then made single-cell recordings in the ventral posterior lateral nucleus (*vpln*) of the thalamus. This is the subcortical area receiving somatosensory information on its way to the somatosensory cortex. Wall and Egger found that the thalamic cells that once responded to stimulation of the hindlimb fell silent after gracile nucleus damage; however, stimulation of the forelimb, which previously did not excite cells in the *vpln,* now did so. In fact, by 7 days postinjury the area of *vpln* responding to stimulation of the forelimb expanded to occupy about two thirds of the area that had previously responded to stimulation of the leg. This activation did not begin to occur until about 3 days after the gracilis lesion, so the authors initially explained their results in terms of being mediated by collateral sprouting (see next section of this chapter for discussion of this topic). In another study, Merrill and Wall (1972) severed dorsal root ganglia whose receptive fields were first recorded in lamina IV of the spinal cord and which responded to stimulation of the hindleg. After transection of the dorsal roots, the corresponding cells in lamina IV fell silent, but then within a few hours became excited by stimulation of the abdomen, a condition that was never seen in the intact cat.

In subsequent experiments, Merrill and Wall (1978) decided to use cryoblocking to see whether they could obtain reversible unmasking of these latent and somewhat anomalous pathways. Accordingly, they blocked the entire dorsal columns of the spinal cord at the Lumbar Level. They found that most of the cells that had their receptive fields on the cat's lower leg became unresponsive to tactile stimulation, but response returned to normal once the effects of the cold had worn off. However, there were a number of cells in the cord that, during the cold block, "switched" their receptive fields to the abdomen and upper leg and then disappeared when the exposed area of the cord was rewarmed. The rapid (virtually immediate) reorganization and the reappearance of normal responsiveness observed in these experiments precluded the possibility that regeneration of new terminals or collateral sprouting could account for the findings.

Could similar "unmasking" of latent pathways be observed in various brain regions as well as the spinal cord? Could the unmasking of previously ineffective synapses account for some degree of functional recovery after CNS injury? Brandenberg and Mann (1989) examined this question by studying unilateral sensory nerve crush followed by unit recording in the somatosensory cortex of both hemispheres. Over time and as recovery to tactile stimulation proceeded, the receptive fields in the somatosensory cortex increased in size compared to intact animals. In addition, the appearance of cortical cells that responded to *bilateral* sensory stimulation increased dramatically. Such bilateral representation does not exist in normal controls. These authors attributed their results to unmasking of previously existing pathways that were suppressed by normal sensory input.

In the visual system, an early paper by Berman and Sterling (1976) could be taken to suggest that retinocollicular input to the visual cortex is normally suppressed by descending corticocollicular afferents. These investigators deprived cats of monocular vision at birth. Under these circumstances, the superior colliculus responded almost exclusively to visual stimulation of the nondeprived eye. When the cortex ipsilateral to the normal eye was removed, the contralateral, initially deprived eye now controlled excitation of the colliculus. This switch in dominance occurred within 15 minutes to 1 hour after lesion of the visual cortex and represents a complex interplay of excitatory and inhibitory mechanisms suggestive of both diaschisis and the unmasking of latent pathways that are suppressed in normal subjects.

In another more recent study, Chino *et al.* (1992) first made laser lesions of one eye in mature cats causing the formation of a small scotoma, which was mapped by recording in the visual cortex. After these recordings were completed, the investigators removed the intact, contralateral eye. Almost immediately, the scotoma caused by the lesion of the contralateral eye disappeared. Another group of animals were allowed to survive for about 2 months after the monocular, retinal lesion and then had the intact eye removed. The scotoma caused by the initial laser surgery did not disappear until after the removal of the intact eye, indicating that for the duration of time studied, inputs from the intact eye actively *suppressed* restoration of function, which could occur only once the inhibition controlled by the intact eye was eliminated. This phenomenon, too, can be seen as a confirmation of the Sprague effect discussed earlier (i.e., the injury-induced inhibition of one system by another), while at the same time suggesting that active unmasking of neural pathways following injury to the CNS may be implicated in the recovery process.

Although the research on unmasking is providing new insights into the potential for and mechanisms of reorganization of neural function in adult brain-damaged subjects after CNS injury, there is some evidence to suggest that the phenomenon may have maladaptive consequences. For example, Ramachandran, Stewart, and Rogers-Ramachandran (1992) examined patients who had undergone upper limb amputation. In one patient, stimuli applied to the face caused highly precise, referred sensations in individual digits (which, of course, were no longer there). In another patient, somatotopic representations of the phantom limb were found on the face and chest, indicating the appearance of abnormal maps in regions quite distal from the stump itself. In a recent confirmation of these results, Yang *et al.* (1994) found that deafferentation of the upper limb in adult rhesus monkeys led to a substantial reorganization of cortical somatosensory receptive fields, resulting in a significant enlargement of cortical areas responsive to stimulation of the face. The investigators then used magnetic source imaging technology to map somatosensory receptive fields in normal human controls and in two patients who had had their upper arm amputated. In the injured hemisphere, the investigators observed a significant expansion of facial representations into the digit and hard areas—a finding similar to that seen in monkeys.

It is difficult to imagine, from these examples, how such neural reorganization in response to injury could be considered as "adaptive." Sensory awareness of where a limb is in space is essential for visually guided and tactile reaching and grasping behavior. In the absence of the limb, stimulation of the face leading to a highly organized sensation of digits or limbs that are no longer there can hardly be considered to be an example of adaptive plasticity that would enable an organism to cope more effectively with its environment. The changes that do occur could be attributed to injury-induced anomalous growth of axon collaterals, if the reorganization takes place over a long period of time, if it is homotypic, and if it is more or less topographic or "equipotential." However, we have already seen that massive reorganization can take place very rapidly (i.e., within hours to days after the deafferentation or cortical injury) and is subject to wide individual variation and environmental influences such as training and prior experiences (Merzenich *et al.*, 1987; Jenkins, Merzenich, & Recanzone, 1990; Jenkins & Merzenich, 1992).

The role of neurons that survive after a CNS lesion also needs to be more carefully examined with respect to the role that they might play in mediating adaptive or maladaptive response to injury. Along with the unmasking or topographic reorganization, spared neurons might be expected to contribute to the overall pattern of activity generated by these injury-induced changes to normal morphology and circuitry of the brain. For example, Cowey and Stoerig (1989) examined four adult monkeys with long-standing partial ablations of the visual cortex. Using retrograde labeling techniques, they were able to show that some neurons within the lateral geniculate body survive retrograde degeneration caused by cortical lesions because they project their terminals to regions outside of the striate cortex. Cowey and Stoerig suggest that these spared neurons may be implicated in the residual vision involving stimulus detection, localization in space, and discrimination. It is possible that, in addition to any masking and/or sprouting, these types of fibers may play a role, for better or worse, in the reorganization of cognitive maps seen in the studies discussed here.

Sprouting and Synaptogenesis in Recovery of Function

In terms of the numbers of papers dealing with plasticity in the central nervous system, I would venture a guess that more has been written about neuronal sprouting than any other subject in this area. Despite the wealth of effort and output, there still is remarkably little known about whether what has been called anomalous, collateral sprouting is responsible, wholly or in part, for functional and behavioral recovery from brain damage. This is not to say that there is no research at all, because I will be discussing some of the relevant material in this final section. There are literally hundreds of studies and reports each year on the genetics, molecular biology, morphology, and neurochemistry of anomalous growth in the brain and spinal cord. The problem is that there is hardly any behavioral follow-up to evaluate whether such alterations are beneficial, detrimental, or of no particular consequence to the functioning organism. This can be a dangerous situation because drugs or molecular biological procedures than can enhance sprouting and regeneration by altering the metabolic machinery of cells (neurons and glia) could lead to maladaptive behavior(s) that render the organism worse. If it is done at all, overly simplistic testing "to get it out of the way" also reveals a negative bias toward behavioral and psychological research as somehow being less worthy or less important than physiological studies.

The notion that some form of axonal growth can occur in the adult nervous system is about as old as the concept of diaschisis. As early as 1885, Exner speculated that regeneration could occur following peripheral nerve injury, but his ideas in this domain were basically ignored until the late 1940s and 1950s, when a number of investigators began to examine the possibility of this type of plasticity in spinal cord preparations more thoroughly (see Cotman & Nadler, 1978; Finger & Stein, 1982, for selected overviews of this work). Although there are now a number of different forms of morphological plasticity (see, for example, Steward, 1989; Steward and Rubel, 1993, for excellent and comprehensive reviews), lesion-induced axonal sprouting and the formation of new synapses (reactive synaptogenesis) is not ordinarily taken to mean the regeneration of previously existing connections. In general, axonal sprouting and reactive synaptogenesis indicate that either surviving neurons in an injured brain region extend collateral branches into vacated synaptic spaces or that axonal fibers of passage that are not part of the same system form new branches of their terminals and make new synapses where there are previously vacated sites. In some cases, there may be competition for vacated synaptic spaces in which heterotypic terminals are more "successful" in forming new synapses than homotypic, surviving axons.

With respect to morphological plasticity in the brain itself, perhaps the study with the most initial impact was generated by Geoffrey Raisman (1969). Raisman was one of the first to use light electron microscopy to examine sprouting after partial denervation of the septal nuclei in adult rats, and his work generally established the experimental paradigm for subsequent studies examining sprouting in the CNS. Raisman chose to focus on this particular structure because it receives two distinctly different sets of afferent fibers. One set of afferents arise in the hippocampus and travel to the septum via the fimbria–fornix. The other fiber system originates in the hypothalamus and terminates in the septum via the medial forebrain bundle. Axons coming from the hippocampus terminate on the dendrites of the septal neurons, whereas those coming from the hypothalamus tend to concentrate on the septal cell bodies.

After determining the normal pattern of septal innervation, Raisman made selective lesions in either the hippocampal or the hypothalamic pathways in different groups of animals and then allowed for long-term survival. After an interval of 3–6 months, Raisman damaged the remaining pathway(s) to study the degeneration patterns caused by the second lesion. He found that if the hippocampal fibers were damaged in the first operation, fibers from the hypothalamus grew new axonal terminals that made contacts on the dendritic sites that were evacuated by the degenerating hippocampal fibers.

If the hypothalamic fiber tracts were damaged first, then the hippocampal–fimbrial fibers sprouted new terminals into the septal areas vacated by the dying hypothalamic cells. Although this was not neuronal regeneration per se, the "sprouting" was a clear example of morphological reorganization in the nervous system of adult brain-damaged mammals. Raisman noted that this was an example of heterotypic reorganization, because the two fiber systems came from completely different CNS regions and in their normal state the cells produced different neurotransmitters. Here, after brain injury, new connections were established that did not exist in the normal brain. Raisman (1969) wrote that: "on *a priori* grounds, it would be predictable that this heterotypic re-innervation would impose, in addition to the original loss of afferent information, further functional confusion by establishing connexions which do not normally exist" (p. 45).

Raisman's initial concerns would imply that behavioral recovery in the presence of such sprouting might actually be impaired rather than enhanced by this type of plasticity. In fact, in early development, anomalous sprouting into deafferented zones has been shown in a number of instances to be maladaptive (see Meyer & Sperry, 1974; Schneider & Jhaveri, 1974, for earlier examples of this phenomenon).

More recent work by Sur, Garraghty, and Roe, 1988, and by Rauschecker, 1995 (cited above), provide further evidence to show that aberrant projections can have complex and perhaps detrimental consequences. Sur and colleagues studied the outcome of unilateral ablations of the superior colliculus and visual cortical areas 17 and 18 in neonatal ferrets to determine what type of rerouting of retinal afferents would occur in these preparations when they were examined as adults. In addition, the inferior colliculus was damaged so that retinal afferents would have a vacated "target" that they could innervate. Anatomical tracing studies in these animals revealed that, in the absence of superior colliculus and visual cortex, fibers from the retina would grow into a shrunken and degenerated lateral geniculate body of the thalamus, but they also grew into the medial geniculate body and other auditory thalamic nuclei. The retinal projections occupied up to one third of the medial geniculate volume, while fibers originating in the medial geniculate projected to the auditory cortex. Subsequent electrophysiological recordings were used to show that the retinal projections could "impart visual functions (that is visual driving and discernable receptive field properties) to cells in nonvisual thalamus" (Sur *et al.*, 1988, p. 1439). The authors then suggested that, at least in early development, modality-specific inputs might determine the function of the thalamus or cortex receiving them, a possibility that was also discussed by Rauschecker (1995) and reviewed earlier in this chapter. Since no cognitive or discriminative behavior was examined in the ferrets, I do not know whether or not their visual or auditory functions were intact, improved, or seriously impaired.

The many developmental studies on reorganization after early lesions are interesting but beyond the purview of this chapter; here, it is more relevant to ask whether such sprouting can occur after injury in adult subjects and whether or not it has any beneficial or detrimental consequences. Thanks to the work of Carl Cotman and Oswald Steward and their students and colleagues since the 1970s, we know that the injury-induced sprouting in the hippocampal formation and its related structures is a reliable phenomenon that occurs in adult subjects and can have beneficial effects on behavioral recovery of function.

One of the key behavioral experiments in this area was performed by Loesche and Steward (1977). These investigators looked at spatial alternation behavior in adult rats following unilateral, entorhinal cortex (EC) damage created to deprive the hippocampus of its primary afferent input. Behavioral performance on this task was disrupted by the lesion but gradually returned to preoperative, normal levels by about 10–12 days after the injury. What is important here is that Loesche and Steward were able to show that the time it took to observe functional recovery corresponded rather precisely to the time that it took for EC fibers to cross over from the contralateral, intact homologue and reinnervate the vacated synaptic sites in the ipsilateral hippocampus (how such innervation coming from the contralateral side of the body might be implicated in mediating the animal's ability to localize itself in three-dimensional space is not completely clear).

To make sure that the contralateral projections were involved in the recovery, Loesche and Steward cut the fimbria–fornix to eliminate the sprouting and the spatial alternation deficit was reinstated. Subsequent research showed that excitatory postsynaptic potentials in the previously denervated hippocampus could be generated by microstimulation of the contralateral EC. It is worthwhile to note that task difficulty may play a role in determining whether collateral sprouting is necessary to mediate functional recovery.

Some years ago, Ramirez and Stein (1984) replicated the work of Loesche and Steward and found similar correspondence between the time of recovery and the appearance of sprouting; however, when the rats were tested within 2 days after the injury with a very brief intertrial interval, the animals with unilateral EC lesions were able to perform the task as well as intact controls long before fibers from the contralateral intact EC could have reinnervated the deafferented hippocampus.

On a supposedly more difficult task, Glasier, Janis, and Stein (1996) created unilateral EC lesions in adult rats and then tested the animals in the Morris water maze and on a series of increasingly complex maze problems in the Hebb–Williams maze. The animals in this experiment showed persistent deficits for up to 6 months after injury; that is, over a time period in which maximum sprouting, by all accounts, should have occurred. There are a number of speculations about how and when such lesion-induced sprouting can play a role in functional recovery, but more systematic behavioral studies need to be done to demonstrate direct causality. Nonetheless, there is even some evidence to show that synaptic reorganization similar to that seen in rodents also occurs in humans. Grady, Jane, and Steward (1989) examined the brains of one male (56 years old) and one female patient (61 years old) who had clinical evidence of uncal herniation at the time of autopsy. Their histopathology was compared to that of brain tissue taken from patients who did not have neurological disorders at the time of death. In both cases, the patients showed a depletion of stellate neurons in the EC compared to normals as well as what appeared to be terminal proliferation, which could be attributed to sprouting and which was not seen in normal brain tissue. The authors speculated that such reactive synaptogenesis might account for the significant behavioral recovery that is seen in human patients following brain injury.

In a recent critical review of hippocampal function, Ramirez (1997) discussed many of the possibilities concerning how plasticity in hippocampal circuitry could contribute to recovery of function; for example, sprouting of remaining intact fibers might "amplify signals" needed to activate neurons implicated in the circuitry controlling the behavior. Ramirez also postulates that sprouted inhibitory circuitry and "enhancement of glutamatergic and/or GABAergic transmission" might also be necessary under some conditions for recovery to occur. Ramirez speculates that GABAergic sprouting contributes to recovery by inhibiting inhibitory interneurons that innervate granule cells of the hippocampus. He suggests that this disinhibition (analogous to removal of diaschisis?) could increase baseline levels of excitability in the hippocampal granule cells, and thereby lead to an enhancement of their information processing capacity.

Regardless of which neurotransmitters might be involved, there is also some evidence to suggest that behavioral experience may play a critical role in determining the extent and functional significance of lesion-induced synaptogenesis. Recently, Schallert and Jones (1993) created unilateral injury to the forelimb representation area of the sensorimotor cortex in adult rats. This injury produced a substantial and transient expansion of the size of the homologous, contralateral cortex, which they attributed to enhanced dendritic arborization (a form of reactive synaptogenesis). This dendritic arborization was greatest 18 days after the lesion and it did not return to control levels (as measured in intact rats) even after 120 days postoperatively.

Schallert and Jones noted that the dendritic overgrowth appeared to correspond in time to the animal's use of its intact forelimb to provide support for standing and movement; there was "overdependence" on the intact forelimb for these behaviors. Eventually, the forelimb asymmetry decreased the time frame that corresponded to the decreases in dendritic branching that were noted over time (the dendritic "pruning" effect).

By creating special restraint jackets for the rats, Schallert and Jones were able to restrict the use of the affected or normal limbs. What they found was that restricting the use of the intact limb prevented the dendritic overgrowth that was seen in the intact sensorimotor cortex in nonrestricted animals; no similar effects on dendritic morphology were seen in nonoperated controls.

These findings can be taken to indicate that lesion-induced neuronal plasticity can be directly affected by environmental and experiential factors, which would include training. In a way, these results are similar to those of Jenkins and Merzenich (1992), which were discussed earlier in this chapter, showing that training and experience can shape morphology and function in the damaged brain. Although the mechanisms underlying these events are not completely understood, it does highlight again the importance of doing careful behavior studies to determine what if anything is the outcome of the phenomena we have called "neuronal plasticity." In addition, with respect to sprouting and synaptogenesis, it is important that investigators conducting experiments at the molecular and morphological levels not overlook the fact that the handling and environments of their experimental preparations may be playing a role in affecting the parameters they wish to study.

Finally, there has to be some concern about whether plasticity is beneficial or pathological, as I have noted above. In a review, Cotman, Cummings, and Pike (1993) also make this point in reviewing the role of trophic factors in CNS plasticity. They point out that patients with Alzheimer's disease (AD) also show various types of compensatory sprouting in the hippocampus (see also Grady *et al.,* 1989, cited above), which possibly could play a role in maintaining cognitive functions before there is complete deterioration as the disease progresses. In AD patients, the authors also noted enhanced synaptogenesis, which apparently was stimulated by and contributed to the formation of senile plaques. Cotman *et al.* (1993) observed that as the sprouting progressed in these patients, it appeared to be attracted into the areas containing senile plaques rather than to innervate functionally active brain regions. If such compensatory sprouting is directed toward senile plaques, neuronal and behavioral dysfunction might be augmented rather than decreased. Thus, for example, providing neurotrophic factors or other growth-promoting substances to AD patients could actually make them worse, according to Cotman *et al.* This is yet another reason why detailed behavioral assessments are so important in clinical studies on functional recovery; the increases in morphological and neurochemical parameters sought at the laboratory bench may not be sufficient to warrant too much enthusiasm over neuroprotection until we know how the whole functioning organism will respond in the long run.

Conclusions

The field of restorative neurology as its own discipline within the broader domain of neuroscience has made enormous progress in finally recognizing that functional recovery after brain and spinal cord injuries is both possible and probable. Resistance to the idea of any form of adaptive neuronal plasticity following brain injury in adults is no longer the problem it was in terms of obtaining credibility and funding for research in this critical area of inquiry. As this chapter describes, there are a number of interesting concepts describing and attempting to explain how recovery of function might occur. As with many areas of science, there is considerable disagreement over which might be the most appropriate approach to studying and manipulating injury-induced CNS plasticity.

Despite all the work and thinking done thus far, we still do not have a "magic bullet" treatment that will cure any of the degenerative diseases of the CNS, nor do we have an effective, universally accepted clinical treatment for brain and spinal cord trauma (indeed, it is interesting to note that research on behavioral and functional recovery from brain damage is one of the least-funded areas of research sponsored by the National Institutes of Health and no funding in this area is provided by the National Science Foundation). Fortunately, the field now has moved away from the simplistic idea that a single mechanism such as sprouting, for example, is going to provide "the answer" to how recovery of function occurs.

Although some writers (including this one) have previously taken more of an absolutist position on defining recovery, that is, recovery *must* equal a return to exactly the same behavior as existed prior to brain damage (see Almli & Finger, 1988), it now seems more likely that much of what is attributed to "recovery of function" is really compensation or substitution of function initiated by brain injury. In other words, while it may be possible to mimic "normal" behavior, the neural processes mediating that behavior may be very different from those mediating behavior in the intact organism. Here, we can think back to the self-report of Kolb (1995) described earlier on the resolution of his ischemic stroke that impaired his visual capacity. It is even possible to think that "efficiency" or compensation of function could be enhanced over those of the intact organism by reorganizational processes that are triggered by CNS injury. One example that comes to mind is that monkeys with lesions of the lateral frontal, parietal cortex, or amygdala can learn visual discrimination, tactile discrimination, and delayed reaction tasks faster than normal controls, although they are impaired on other cognitive tasks compared to normals (Irle, 1990). This phenomenon itself is an important area of study, because we need to know what types of manipulations or rehabilitation strategies should be applied to enhance compensatory mechanisms, be they at the neuronal or behavioral levels of analysis. It is important to be aware of the fact that drugs used to enhance or modify a physiological substrate or to control one aspect of a disorder (e.g., postinjury seizure control) could be disruptive to mechanisms underlying functional recovery (Schallert *et al.,* 1992; Cotman, Gómez-Pinilla, & Kahle, 1994). Thus, it is entirely possible that application of the wrong rehabilitation technique (including pharmacotherapy) could lead to serious maladaptive consequences, as discussed above. If the goal of restorative neurology and neuroscience is to provide effective and long-lasting benefits to the victims of brain and spinal cord trauma, it is becoming clear that much more interdisciplinary research (including behavioral) will need to be done before we can fully understand and control the cascade of destructive and potentially beneficial phenomena that follow damage to the brain.

ACKNOWLEDGMENTS I would like to thank my graduate students Jeffrey Smith and Kimberly Grossman for helping me research and find many of the documents cited in this chapter and for their critical reading of the manuscript. Dr. Zoltan Fulop, my valued colleague, also was of great help in preparing the final version of this manuscript.

References

Almli, C. R., & Finger, S. (1988). Toward a definition of recovery. In S. Finger, T. E. LeVere, C. R. Almli, & D. G. Stein (Eds.), *Brain injury and recovery: Theoretical and controversial issues* (pp. 1–14). New York: Academic Press.

Almli, C. R., & Finger, S. (1992). Brain injury and recovery of function: Theories and mechanisms of functional reorganization. *Journal of Head Trauma Rehabilitation, 7,* 70–77.

Andrews, R. J. (1991). Transhemispheric diaschisis. *Stroke, 22,* 943–949.

Bach-y-Rita, P. (1972). *Brain mechanisms in sensory substitution.* New York: Academic Press.

Bach-y-Rita, P. (1990). Brain plasticity as a basis for recovery of function in humans. *Neuropsychologia, 28,* 547–554.

Berman, N., & Sterling, P. (1976). Cortical suppression of the retino-collicular pathway in the monocularly deprived cat. *Journal of physiology, 255,* 263–273.

Brandenberg, G. A., & Mann, M. D. (1989). Sensory nerve crush and regeneration and the receptive fields and response properties of neurons in the primary somatosensory cerebral cortex of cats. *Experimental Neurology, 103,* 256–266.

Chino, Y. M., Kaas, J. H., Smith, E. L. d., Langston, A. L., & Cheng, H. (1992). Rapid reorganization of cortical maps in adult cats following restricted deafferentation in retina. *Vision Research, 32,* 789–796.

Chollet, F., & Weiller, C. (1994). Imaging recovery of function following brain injury. *Current Opinion in Neurobiology, 4,* 226–230.

Chollet, F., DiPiero, V., Wise, R. J. S., Brooks, D. J., Dolan, R. J., & Frackowiak, R. S. J. (1991). The functional anatomy of motor recovery after stroke in humans: A study with positron emission tomography. *Annals of Neurology, 29,* 63–71.

Chow, K. L. (1968). Visual discriminations after extensive ablation of optic tract and visual cortex in rats. *Brain Research, 9,* 363–366.

Cotman, C. W., & Nadler, J. V. (1978). Reactive synaptogenesis in the hippocampus. In C. W. Cotman (Ed.), *Neuronal plasticity* (pp. 227–271). New York: Raven Press.

Cotman, C. W., Cummings, B. J., & Pike, C. J. (1993). Molecular cascades in adaptive versus pathological plasticity. In A. Gorio (Ed.), *Neuroregeneration* (pp. 217–240). New York: Raven Press.

Cotman, C. W., Gómez-Pinilla, F., & Kahle, J. S. (1994). Neural plasticity and regeneration. In G. J. Siegal *et al.* (Eds.), *Basic neurochemistry: Molecular, cellular and medical aspects* (5th ed., pp. 607–626). New York: Raven Press.

Cowey, A., & Stoerig, P. (1989). Projection patterns of surviving neurons in the dorsal lateral geniculate nucleus following discrete lesions of striate cortex: implications for residual vision. *Experimental Brain Research, 75,* 631–638.

Damasio, H., & Damasio, A. R. (1989). *Lesion analysis in neuropsychology.* New York: Oxford University Press.

Exner, S. (1885). Notiz zu derfrage von der fasvertheilung mehrerer nerven in einem muskel. *Pflüger's Archiv fur die gesante Physiologie, 36,* 572–576.

Feeney, D. (1996). Pattern of brain damage in a traumatic brain injury model: Noradrenergic pharmacotherapy promotes recovery of function. In J. Toole & D. C. Good (Eds), *Imaging in neurologic rehabilitation* (pp. 91–124). New York: Demos Vermande.

Feeney, D., & Baron J-C. (1986). Diaschisis. *Stroke, 15,* 817–830.

Finger, S., & Simons, D. (1976). Effects of serial lesions of somatosensory cortex and further neodecortication on retention of a rough-smooth discrimination in rats. *Experimental Brain Research, 25, 1*83–197.

Finger, S., & Stein, D. G. (1982). *Brain damage and recovery: Research and clinical applications.* New York: Academic Press.

Finger, S., LeVere, T. E., Almli, C. R., & Stein, D. G. (Eds.). (1988). *Brain injury and recovery: Theoretical and controversial issues.* New York: Plenum Press.

Glasier, M. M., Janis, L. S., & Stein, D. G. (1993). Persistent deficits in Hebb–Williams Maze performance are shown by rats with unilateral entorhinal cortex lesion. *Abstracts of International Behavioral Neuroscience Conference,* Washington, D.C.

Glassman, R. B., & Smith, A. (1988). Neural space capacity and the concept of diaschisis. In S. Finger *et al.* (Eds.), *Brain injury and recovery: Theoretical and controversial issues* (Chapter 4). New York: Plenum Press.

Globus, M. Y., Busto, R., Martinez, E., Valdes, I., & Dietrich, W. D. (1990). Ischemia induces release of glutamate in regions spared from histopathological damage in the rat. *Stroke, 21, 1*143–1146.

Goldstein, K. (1939). *The organism.* New York: The American Book Company.

Goldstein, L. B., & Davis, J. L. (1988). Physician prescribing patterns following hospital admission for ischemic cerebrovascular disease. *Neurology, 38, 1*806–1809.

Grady, M. S., Jane, J. A., & Steward, O. (1989). Synaptic reorganization in the human central nervous system following injury. *Journal of Neurosurgery, 71,* 534–537.

Heiss, W. D., Ilsen, H. W., Wagner, R., Pawlik, G., Wienhard, K., & Eriksson, L. (1983). Decreased glucose metabolism in functionally inactivated brain regions in ischemic stroke and its alteration by activating drugs. In J. S. Meyer, H. Lechner, M. Reivich, & E. O. Ott (Eds.), *Cerebral vascular disease,(4),* (pp. 162–168). Amsterdam: International Congress Series, Excerpta Medica.

Infeld, B., Davis, S. M., Lichtenstein, M., Mitchell, P. J., & Hopper, J. L. (1995). Crossed cerebellar diaschisis and brain recovery after stroke. *Stroke, 26,* 90–95.

Irle, E. (1990). An analysis of the correlation of lesion size, localization and behavioral effects in 283 published studies of cortical and subcortical lesions in old-world monkeys. *Brain Research Review, 15,* 181–213.

Jenkins, W. M., & Merzenich, M. M. (1992). Cortical representational plasticity: Some implications for the bases of recovery from brain damage. In N. von Steinbüchel, D. Y. von Cramon, & E. Pöppel (Eds.), *Neuropsychological rehabilitation* (pp. 20–35). Berlin: Springer-Verlag, Berlin.

Jenkins, W. M., Merzenich, M. M., & Recanzone, G. (1990). Neocortical representational dynamics in adult primates: Implications for neuropsychology. *Neuropsychologia, 28,* 573–584.

Kasten, E., & Sabel, B. (1995). Visual field enlargement after computer training in brain-damaged patients with homonymous deficits: An open pilot trial. *Restorative Neurology and Neuroscience, 8,* 113–127.

Kempinsky, W. H. (1958). Experimental study of distal effects of acute focal injury. *Archives of Neurology and Psychiatry, 79,* 376–389.

Kolb, B. (1995). *Brain plasticity and behavior.* Mahwah, NJ: Lawrence Erlbaum.

Kolb, B., & Whishaw, W. (1988). Mass action and equipoteniality reconsidered. In S. Finger *et al.* (Eds.), *Brain injury and recovery: Theoretical and controversial issues* (pp. 103–114). New York: Plenum Press.

Lashley, K. S. (1929). *Brain mechanisms and intelligence.* Chicago: University of Chicago Press.

Lashley, K. S. (1933). Integrative functions of the cerebral cortex. *Physiology Review, 13,* 1–42.

LeVere, T. E. (1988). Neural system imbalances and the consequences of large brain injuries. In S. Finger *et al.* (Eds.), *Brain injury and recovery: Theoretical and controversial issues* (pp. 15–41). New York: Plenum Press.

LeVere, N. D., Gray-Silva, S., & LeVere, T. E. (1988). Infant brain injury: The benefit of relocation and the cost of crowding. In S. Finger *et al.* (Eds.), *Brain injury and recovery: Theoretical and controversial issues* (pp. 133–150). New York: Plenum Press.

Loesche, J., & Steward, O. (1977). Behavioral correlates of denervation and reinnervation of the hippocampal formation of the rat: Recovery of alternation performance following unilateral cortex lesions. *Brain Research Bulletin, 2,* 31–39.

Luria, A. R. (1966). *Higher cortical functions in man* (2nd ed.). New York: Basic Books.

Merrill, E. G., & Wall, P. D. (1972). Factors forming the edge of a receptive field. The presence of relatively ineffective afferents. *Journal of physiology, 226,* 825–846.

Merrill, E. G., & Wall, P. D. (1978). Plasticity of connection in the adult nervous system. In C. W. Cotman (Ed.), *Neuronal plasticity* (pp. 97–111). New York: Raven Press.

Merzenich, M. M., Nelson, R. J., Kaas, J. H., Stryker, M. P., Jenkins, W. M., Zook, J. M., Cynader, M. S., & Schoppmann A. (1987). Variability in hand surface representations in areas 3b and 1 in adult owl and squirrel monkeys. *Journal of Comparative Neurology, 258,* 281–297.

Meyer, J. S. (1982). Changes in local CBF and lambda values following regional cerebral infarction in the baboon. *Advances in Bioscience, 43,* 153–165.

Meyer, J. S., Obara, K., & Muramatsu, K. (1993). Diaschisis. *Neurology Research, 15,* 362–366.

Meyer, R. L., & Sperry, R. L. (1974). Explanatory models for neuroplasticity in retinotectal connections. In D. G. Stein, J. J. Rosen, & N. Butters (Eds.), *Plasticity and recovery of function in the central nervous system* (pp. 45–64). New York: Academic Press.

Milner, B. (1974). Sparing of language functions after early unilateral brain damage. *Neuroscience Research Bulletin, 12,* 213–217.

Norrsell, U. (1988). Arguments against redundant brain structures. In S. Finger *et al.* (Eds.), *Brain injury and recovery: Theoretical and controversial issues* (pp. 151–164). New York: Plenum Press.

Nudo, R. J., & Milliken, G. W. (1996). Reorganization of movement representations in primary motor cortex following focal ischemic infarcts in adult squirrel monkeys. *Journal of Neurophysiology, 75,* 2144–2149.

Nudo, R. J., Wise, B. M., SiFuentes, F., & Milliken, G. W. (1996). Neural substrates for the effects of rehabilitative training on motor recovery after ischemic infarct. *Science, 272,* 1791–1794.

Ojemann, G. (1992). Localization of language in frontal cortex. *Adv. Neurol., 57,* 6–36.

Payne, B. R., & Cornwell, P. (1994). System-wide repercussions of damage to the immature visual cortex. *Trends in Neuroscience, 17,* 126–130.

Prince, M. (1910). Cerebral localization from the point of view of function and symptoms. *Journal of Nervous and Mental Disorders, 37,* 337–354.

Raisman, G. (1969). Neuronal plasticity in the septal nuclei of the adult rat. *Brain Research, 14,* 25–48.

Ramachandran, V. S., Stewart, M., & Rogers-Ramachandran, D. C. (1992). Perceptual correlates of massive cortical reorganization. *Science, 258,* 1159–1160.

Ramirez, J. J. (1997). The functional significance of lesion-induced plasticity of the hippocampal formation. *Advances in Neurology, 73,* 61–82.

Ramirez, J. J., & Stein, D. G. (1984). Sparing and recovery of spatial alternation performance after entorhinal cortex lesions in rats. *Behavior and Brain Research, 13,* 55–61.
Rauschecker, J. P. (1995). Compensatory plasticity and sensory substitution in the cerebral cortex. *Trends in Neuroscience, 18,* 36–43.
Riese, W. (1958). The principle of diaschisis. *International Record of Medicine, 171,* 73–82.
Riese, W. (1977). *Selected papers on the history of aphasia.* In R. Hoops & Y. Lebrun (Eds.), *Neurolinguistics, 7,* (pp. 123–142). Amsterdam: Swets & Zeitlinger.
Rose, F. D., & Johnson, D. A. (1992). *Recovery from brain damage: Reflections and directions.* New York: Plenum Press.
Sautter, J., & Sabel, B. A. (1993). Recovery of brightness discrimination in adult rats despite progressive loss of retrogradely labeled retinal ganglion cells after controlled optic nerve crush. *European Journal of Neuroscience, 5,* 680–690.
Schallert, T., & Jones, T. A. (1993). Exhuberant neuronal growth after brain damage in adult rats: The essential role of behavioral experience. *Journal of Neural Transplantation & Plasticity, 4,* 193–197.
Schallert, T., Jones, T., Shapiro, L., Crippens, D., & Fulton, R. (1992). Pharmacologic and anatomic considerations in recovery of function. In S. Hanson & D. M. Tucker (Eds.), *Neuropsychological assessment: Physical medicine and rehabilitation: State of the art reviews* (Vol. 6, pp. 375–393). Philadelphia: Hanley and Belfus.
Schneider, G. E., & Jhaveri, S. R. (1974). Neuroanatomical correlates of spared or altered function after brain lesions in newborn hamster. In D. G. Stein, J. J. Rosen, & N. Butters (Eds.), *Plasticity and recovery of function in the central nervous system* (pp. 65–110). New York: Academic Press.
Sprague, J. M. (1966). Interaction of cortex and superior colliculus in mediation of visually guided behavior in the cat. *Science, 153,* 1544–1547.
Stein, D. G., Brailowsky, S., & Will, B. (1995). *Brain repair.* New York: Oxford University Press.
Steward, O. (1989). Reorganization of neuronal connections following CNS trauma: Principles and experimental paradigms. *Journal of Neurotrauma, 6,* 99–145.
Steward, O., & Rubel E. W. (1993). The fate of denervated neurons: Transneuronal degeneration, dendritic atrophy and dendritic remodeling. In A. Gorio (Ed.), *Neuroregeneration* (pp. 37–60). New York: Raven Press.
Sur, M., Garraghty, P. E., & Roe, A. W. (1988). Experimentally induced visual projections into auditory thalamus and cortex. *Science, 242,* 1437–1441.
Taub, E., Pidikiti, R. D., DeLuca, S. C., & Crago, J. E. (1996). Effects of motor restriction of an unimpaired upper extremity and training on improving functional tasks and altering brain behaviors. In J. Toole & D. C. Good (Eds.), *Imaging in neurologic rehabilitation* (pp. 133–154). New York: Demos Vermande.
Teuber, H.-L. (1974). Recovery of functions after lesions in the central nervous system. *Neuroscience Research Progress Bulletin, 12,* 197–209.
Toole, J., & Good, D. C. (1996). *Imaging in neurologic rehabilitation.* New York: Demos Vermande.
Von Steinbüchel, N., von Cramon D. Y., & Pöppel, E. (Eds.). (1992). *Neuropsychological rehabilitation.* Berlin: Springer-Verlag.
Wall, P. D. (1975). Signs of plasticity and reconnection in spinal cord damage. In *Outcome of Severe Damage to the Central Nervous System* (pp. 35–63). Ciba Foundation Symposium #34 Amsterdam: Elsevier.
Wall, P. D., & Egger, M. D. (1971). Formation of new connections in adult rat brains after partial deafferentation. *Nature, 232,* 542–545.
Weiller, C., Chollet, F., Friston, K. J., Wise, R. J. S., & Frackowiak, R. S. J. (1992). Functional reorganization of the brain in recovery from straitocapusular infarction in man. *Annals of Neurology, 31,* 463–472.
Weiller, C., Ramsay, S. C., Wise, R. J., Friston, K. J., & Frackowiak, R. S. (1993). Individual patterns of functional reorganization in the human cerebral cortex after capsular infarction. *Annals of Neurology, 33,* 181–189.
Woods, B. T. (1980). The restricted effects of right hemisphere lesions after age one: Wechsler test data. *Neuropsychologia, 18,* 65–70.
Yang, T. T., Galler, C. C., Ramachardran, V. S., Cobb, S., Schwartz, B. J., & Bloom, F. E. (1994). Noninvasive detection of cerebral plasticity in adult human somatosensory cortex. *Neuroreport, 5,* 701–704.

3

Neuroimaging Evidence of Diaschisis and Reorganization in Stroke Recovery

GEORG DEUTSCH AND JAMES M. MOUNTZ

Background: Recovery After Stroke

In general, two competing but not necessarily mutually exclusive models can explain the mechanisms underlying the often observed recovery of neurological and cognitive function (e.g., limb movement, speech production, language comprehension, perceptual skills) after stroke. One is that recovery essentially reflects resolution of a temporary cessation of function in brain tissue not directly destroyed by the stroke but nevertheless affected via deafferentation and a consequent "diaschisis." The second is that recovery involves spared brain taking on functions previously performed by damaged brain tissue, for example, the cortical representation of the hand or other damaged sensory–motor regions extends into adjacent tissue, or the uninvolved hemisphere takes on the cognitive capacities of the infarcted side. Thus, the first model emphasizes changes associated with temporarily affected brain, whereas the second accentuates reorganization in noninvolved brain ("plasticity").

Evidence for cerebral reorganization in the sense of uninvolved brain taking on new functions poststroke is mostly provided by studies of recovery from aphasia following left hemisphere injury. Evidence that the right hemisphere is responsible for improved language function comes from data such as Kinsbourne's (1971) demonstration of speech arrest in recovered aphasics during right carotid barbiturate injection and from case studies of patients who, after recovering from left hemisphere stroke-induced aphasia, had subsequent right hemisphere strokes and became aphasic again. An earlier attempt to study this issue with electrophysiological recordings during language processing in recovered aphasics generated data supporting the view that restitution of language entails reorganization of brain function with

---

GEORG DEUTSCH AND JAMES M. MOUNTZ • Department of Radiology, University of Alabama at Birmingham, Birmingham, Alabama 35233.

International Handbook of Neuropsychological Rehabilitation, edited by Christensen and Uzzell.
Kluwer Academic/ Plenum Publishers, New York, 2000.

increased participation of the nondominant hemisphere (Papanicolaou, Moore, Deutsch, Levin, & Eisenberg, 1988). More recent imaging studies using positron emission tomography (PET) have provided evidence of increased activity in contralesional hemisphere, but also indicated there was individual variability and evidence for recruitment of areas outside the infarct in the damaged hemisphere during certain conditions. A single-case PET study of a recovered aphasic showed focal increased activity in a right hemisphere region exactly homologous to the left hemisphere lesion during a speech task (Buckner, Corbetta, Schatz, Raichle, & Petersen, 1996). Also using O-15 PET measures of regional cerebral blood flow (rCBF), Ohyama and colleagues (1996) showed both right hemisphere activation and activation of spared left hemisphere regions during spontaneous speech production in a group of patients recovering from aphasia.

Motor Recovery

Damage to the pyramidal system is almost always partial due to its bilateral organization. Only the most distal forelimb functions have an exclusively contralateral projection (Lawrence & Kuypers, 1968). Although the ipsilateral component is relatively small (~10%), there is substantial evidence that it can mediate functional recovery in pathological conditions. Patients with infantile hemiparesis who undergo subsequent hemispherectomy often show excellent proximal motor functions on the hemiparetic side: they can walk with a barely perceptible limp and can use their arm for many purposes, even when the hemispherectomy is performed at adult age (Muller, Kunesch, Binkofski, & Freund, 1991). Using O-15 H_2O PET, Ramsay, Wise, Friston, and Frackowiak (1993) showed recovery-related recruitment of areas in the damaged hemisphere after capsular infarction, but also indicated there was considerable individual variability and, as in the studies of recovery from aphasia, frequent evidence of increased activity in the contralesional hemisphere.

Cortical Plasticity

Recently there has been considerable interest and a number of investigations into the extent to which cortical representation of hand and other motor functions may "remap" into adjoining regions following infarction or other damage to primary sensory–motor regions (Freund, 1996; Nudo, Wise, SiFuentes, & Milliken, 1996; Seitz & Freund, 1997). Some animal studies (Nudo *et al.*, 1996) and magnetoencephalography (MEG) and PET studies in humans have indeed reported evidence for such activation patterns in subjects recovering the use of initially impaired motor skills.

In patients with lesions of the motor cortex, movements of the contralesional hand activate areas outside the former hand representation. In patients with tumors occupying the hand area of motor cortex, activation has been shown to occur completely outside the motor cortex (Seitz *et al.*, 1995). These results provide evidence that show large-scale reorganization can occur that is not confined to changes within the somatotopic body representation in sensory–motor cortex.

Motor Training

There is some debate concerning preventing, through intensive motor training, what appears to be additional motor dysfunction that occurs due to longer-term loss of cortical representation areas after the acute stage of stroke (Nudo *et al.*, 1996). The value and effects of longer-term intervention, even a year or more poststroke, in terms of intense training of affected limbs, is also in debate (Taub, 1995) and may ultimately be dependent on which mechanism of recovery—reorganization or resolution of diaschisis—is in fact operating in individual cases.

Diaschisis

Diaschisis and the role it plays in recovery of function has a long history, beginning with Von Monakow's (1969/1914) classic article. Many neurologists can attest to the fact that the improvement observed in function post-left middle cerebral activity (MCA) stroke, for example, progression from hand and leg weakness with aphasia to just hand weakness, appears linked to anatomy adjacent to the cerebral infarction. Von Monakow defined diaschisis as reduced regional functioning resulting from deafferentation or the interruption of normal input to a region not directly involved in the stroke. PET and single photon emission computed tomography (SPECT) studies have demonstrated remote effects in rCBF consequent to focal infarction (e.g., Feeney & Baron, 1986; Feldmann, Voth, Dressler, Henze, & Felgenhauer, 1990). Distinguishing between regional ischemia and depressed neurometabolic activity is aided by calculating regional oxygen extraction fraction (OEF) by comparing simultaneous measurements of rCBF and cerebral metabolic rate for oxygen ($CMRO_2$) (Herold *et al.*, 1988; Ackerman *et al.*, 1984). Although reports of "ischemic penumbra" (Astrup, Siesjo, & Symon, 1981) and "luxury perfusion" (Baron, 1985) persisted poststroke, some studies reported normal oxygen extraction in regions surrounding stroke, suggesting a greater role of diaschisis rather than ischemia in the reduced activity levels (Raynaud, Rancurel, Samson, & Baron, 1987). A PET study of six stroke patients with motor hemineglect reported significant diaschisis in frontal and parietal cortices ipsilateral to but outside of the infarction. Edema and ischemic penumbra were ruled out as likely explanations for most of the observed hypometabolism via oxygen extraction analysis (Fiorelli, Blin, Bakchine, Laplane, & Baron, 1991).

Metabolic rates of the diaschisis region as measured by local glucose consumption is also decreased. Using a unilateral carotid and middle cerebral artery occlusion model in cats, Ginsberg, Reivich, Giandomenico, and Greenberg (1977) demonstrated mildly suppressed 14 C-2-deoxyglucose utilization in the contralateral hemisphere. Thus, diaschisis can involve areas outside the lesion in the affected hemisphere as well as areas in the other hemisphere (e.g., "cross hemispheric" or "cross callosal" diaschisis). It also should be kept in mind that not all poststroke neurometabolic reductions may be due to diaschisis; selective neuronal loss may be involved, especially in cases of long-standing hemodynamic vascular territory constraint (Mountz, San Pedro, Mason, Deutsch, & Hetherington, 1997).

Identifying Diaschisis with Neuroimaging

Methods to Separate Vascular and Metabolic Dysfunction

Blood Flow and Oxygen Methods

Regional cerebral blood flow (rCBF) is a sensitive indicator of cerebral status outside the infarction poststroke, including identification of diaschisis. However, there are some confounds inherent in interpreting both "normal" and "reduced" resting state rCBF (Yudd, Van Heertum, & Masdeu, 1991). Decreased resting rCBF may occur as a result of impaired vascular supply (ischemia) or it may reflect reduced neurometabolic activity, such as that resulting from neuronal loss, diaschisis, or other parenchymal dysfunction. It is often difficult to know whether reduced rCBF outside of infarcted tissue reflects ischemia, that is, true vascular constraints, or whether it is simply a secondary manifestation of reduced neurometabolic activity due, for example, to neuronal loss or disconnection effects such as diaschisis.

There are several methods for discriminating between an rCBF reduction that represents a primary vascular constraint and that which is a secondary manifestation of reduced neurometabolic activity. One is oxygen extraction analysis during PET scans, in which it is determined whether a greater than usual percentage of O_2 is being extracted from regions that appear to have reduced rCBF. If the oxygen extraction is abnormally high, then the rCBF reduction does in fact represent a vascular constraint to an area with normal metabolism; an ischemic condition exists. If, on the other hand, oxygen extraction is normal, then the rCBF reduction indicates a reduced metabolic rate in the region and is simply reflecting the close coupling between flow and metabolism. Another method is vascular reactivity or "stress" testing, which can be performed with standard clinical brain SPECT as well as with PET.

It is generally agreed that cerebrovascular reactivity to increases in CO_2 represents an index of vascular reserve, that is, the limit of increases in rCBF is governed by the condition of the vasculature. Cerebrovascular reactivity to CO_2 has been shown to be reduced in patients at risk for stroke (Levine *et al.*, 1989) and to correlate well with changes in oxygen extraction fraction and rCBF–cerebral blood volume ratios (Herold *et al.*, 1988; Kanno *et al.*, 1988). Diamox (acetazolamide) also produces a strong vasodilatory challenge via carbonic anhydrase inhibition and a resultant increase in blood gas CO_2 (Matsuda *et al.*, 1991). There is a high degree of equivalence between studies of CV reactivity in vascular disease patients using either 5% CO_2 or a 1 gram Diamox intravenous injection.

We have demonstrated that regions of reduced metabolic activity show an unusual degree of increase in rCBF during CO_2 or Diamox stress (Mountz, Deutsch, & Khan, 1993; Mountz, Deutsch, Kuzniecky, Rosenfeld 1994c; Deutsch, Mountz, Liu, & San Pedro, 1996b). The increase is larger relative to that in tissue with normal metabolic rate, probably because of a nonlinearity in vessel response: constricted vessels react more to CO_2 than dilated blood vessels (in the absence of vascular constraints). This has been reported previously as "the law of initial values" (Rogers, Meyer, Mortel, Mahurin, & Thornby, 1985) and as normalization of the rCBF pattern in Alzheimer's disease during CO_2 stress (Bonte *et al.*, 1989; Deutsch, Halsey, & Harrell, 1991). Thus, cerebrovascular reactivity testing typically exaggerates an rCBF defect pattern that is a result of hemodynamic constraints but reduces the pattern abnormality in patients who have rCBF defects arising purely from metabolic or parenchymal reductions in cerebral activity.

Magnetic Resonance Spectroscopic Imaging

Identification of the reason for reduced activity in cerebral regions also can be accomplished by magnetic resonance spectroscopic imaging (MRSI) of certain cerebral metabolites. This is an evolving area of research, but there are now several hypotheses about the significance of several metabolites imaged by MRSI for distinguishing ischemia, diaschises, and neuronal loss.

For example, MRSI evidence for elevation of lactate in the stroke penumbra distant to the rim provides evidence of ischemia as a result of its production during the anaerobic glycolysis accompanying oxygen insufficiency. Proton MRSI also can image the distribution of *N*-acetyl aspartate, creatine, choline, glutamate, and glutamine, although the exact role of each of these in indicating aspects of neuronal function is somewhat controversial. Later, we will discuss the role of some of these metabolites in identifying cerebral injury as we present MRSI patient data.

SPECT Methods

Acquisition Parameters. State-of-the-art brain SPECT involves the use of rotating Anger gamma camera systems with at least two heads. We currently use a Picker triple-head prism 3000-XP (Picker International Inc., Cleveland, OH). In this system, each head rotates 120° at 3° increments at 45 seconds per stop to acquire projection images over the entire 360°. The basic principle of modern gamma scintillation cameras, developed in the 1950s, is still used today (Anger *et al.*, 1967). Briefly, photon emissions from the Tc-99m-labeled hexamethyl-propyleneamine oxime (HMPAO) blood flow tracer, which is incorporated into the brain, penetrate the face of the scintillation detector heads and pass through a collimator system. This system consists of a honeycomb of thin lead columns that only allow gamma rays emitted perpendicular to the detector to strike a sodium iodine crystal and produce a small amount of light (scintillation), which is detected by an array of photomultiplier tubes. The light signal intensity is amplified through electronic circuitry to yield the *X* and *Y* position of where the photon struck the crystal. The precision to which the photomultiplier tubes can determine the *X* and *Y* position yields the intrinsic resolution of the detector head. Typical intrinsic detector head resolution on contemporary Anger gamma cameras is approximately 2–3 mm full width at half maximum (FWHM), although several other factors determine the actual extrinsic resolution of a scanning procedure.

Procedure: Subjects receive an intravenous injection of approximately 20 mCi Tc-99m HMPAO in an environment where ambient light and noise are reduced as much as possible. SPECT image acquisition is performed by the Picker Prism triple-head gamma camera set to make 40 equal angular stops for each head at 45 sec/stop. This typically yields ~16 million counts over 360° per total brain SPECT acquisition. The camera is equipped with low-energy, high-resolution collimators. Camera extrinsic resolution for a 25-cm field of view using a 128 × 128 matrix in air is approximately 7 mm FWHM for an average brain acquisition rotation radius of 12.5 cm. Data are stored and processed on an ADAC Pegasys workstation/analysis system in a 128 × 128 digital matrix. Typical reconstruction parameters for the Picker Prism 3000-XP employ a Butterworth filter with frequency cutoff of 0.28, order of 8. The pixel size in the computer image matrix is ~2 mm on edge. Images are displayed in the transverse, coronal, and sagittal planes using 4 mm for in-plane thickness and retaining the 2 mm resolution in plane for optimizing region of interest (ROI) delineation (described below). Images are displayed in a standard fashion, preferably parallel to and sequentially above the canthomeatal (CM) line, which is an imaginary line connecting the auditory meatus and lateral canthus of the eye.

Annular cortical ROIs are defined on SPECT using a semiautomated ROI method yielding the values of maximum and average pixel in 15° or 30° sectors circumferentially around the brain, progressing clockwise from the 12 o'clock position. The outer border is defined by counts per pixel values at 50% of the mean total brain counts per pixel. The inner border is defined at an equal angular distance of 10 to 20 pixels (1.96 to 3.92 cm) from the outer border. The value for the ROI is the average the top 90% of counts per pixel within that ROI. In practice, data values are obtained for slices from approximately CM + 2cm to CM + 9cm, since the lower and higher slices are not easily amenable to this semiautomated ROI technique (Deutsch, Mountz, Katholi, Liu, & Harrell, 1997a; Mountz, 1991).

A reference system device (described below) is used during all SPECT as well as all MRI scans to aid in localization of anatomic structure on functional images. The reference system device allows identification of image level in millimeters above the CM line for consistent selection of a desired brain level and direct comparison with structures seen on MRI as shown in Fig. 1. This figure shows the levels for three representative rCBF brain SPECT scan sections, parallel to and above the CM line, routinely analyzed by automated semiquantitative software developed at University of Alabama at Birmingham (UAB).

Coalignment of SPECT and Structural MR images. Most brain rCBF SPECT scan data require analysis in conjunction with an anatomic image. In order to maximize the complementary observations of structure and function simultaneously, several methods are available to orient the final SPECT scan brain images in space so that they can be coregistered with an anatomic image such as an MRI scan. At our institution we routinely place a reference device on the patient prior to MRI and SPECT procedures to accomplish this. The current reference system is held on the head by a glasseslike framework anchored in the external auditory meatus and positioned adjacent to the CM line (Mountz, Wilson, Wolff, Deutsch, & Harris, 1994a). The reference system geometry is configured as two isosceles triangles. The two isosceles triangles are reproducibly positioned on the head by orientation adjacent to the CM line. Thin intravenous (IV) tubing coursing the edges of the triangles provides a linear array of external fiduciary reference points visible on all scan planes after injection with the appropriate contrast agent. This permits accurate and reproducible oblique reconstruction of all SPECT data, such that the transverse sections are oriented parallel to the CM line.

By analyzing the relative positions of the array of fiduciary dots produced on scan cross sections, the spatial orientation of sets of transverse brain images are correlated between modalities. The dot position analysis is performed by a least-squares fit algorithm developed at UAB and which now operates on several computing platforms (Harrison Medical, Helena, AL). The method permits rapid point translation or whole three-dimensional image set coreg-

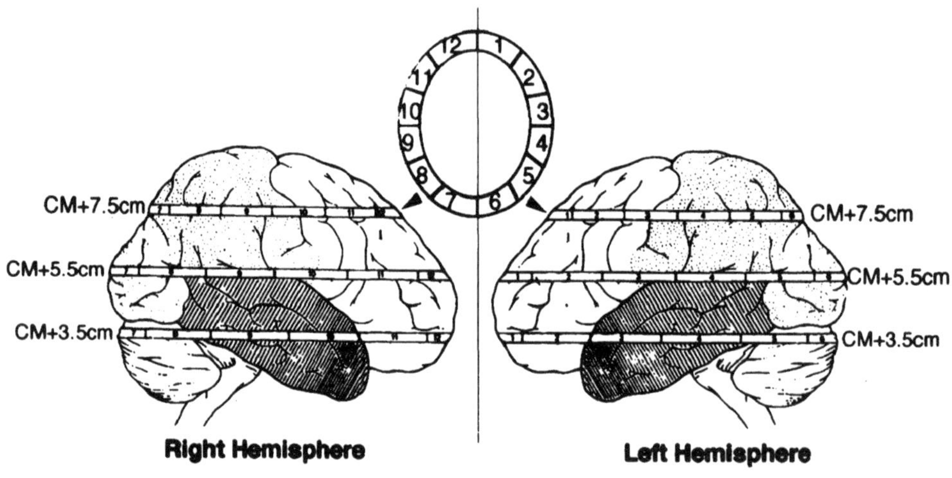

FIGURE 1. Lateral view diagrams of the left and right cerebral hemispheres, showing the positions of the sections typically sampled in the automated region-of-interest (ROI) analysis. The three levels are positioned at 3.5, 5.5, and 7.5 cm above the canthomeatal (CM) line. The oval illustrates the position of each ROI as used in our circumferential plots of cortical rCBF, progressing from the anterior left hemisphere (region 1) clockwise to the anterior right hemisphere (region 12).

istration between SPECT image data sets and MRI image data sets (Mountz, Zhang, Hong-Gang, & Inampudi, 1994b).

Diamox Stress SPECT. Two rCBF SPECT acquisitions are performed to obtain both a resting baseline and vasodilatory response scan. This can be done in one session using a low dose–high dose method, or each scan can be conducted on a separate day. In the split dose (low dose–high dose) method, a 7 mCi Tc-99m HMPAO dose is first injected at rest and scanned. One gram Diamox (acetazolamide) is then administered intravenously, allowing approximately 15 minutes for it to take effect, followed by a 28 mCi Tc-99m HMPAO injection and a second scan.

In order to obtain the highest resolution images for both rest and stress scans, it is preferable to conduct each study with a normal (high) HMPAO dose. This requires that the patient be brought back on separate days for each scan, allowing radioactive decay and clearance of a normal initial dose rather than depending on masking an initial low dose with a subsequent higher dose.

Note that most typical Diamox tests are intended to accentuate rCBF deficits in cases involving marginal flow or ischemia. We also use Diamox to help verify the presence of diaschisis, where rCBF actually improves with Diamox, as we shall show in the case examples presented later.

Quantifying Diaschisis and Stroke Defect Volumes. As we have discussed, in patients who have had a stroke, the flow deficit size on a SPECT image is often much larger than the abnormality visualized on CT or MRI. We use a quantitative method to calculate the extent of the rCBF deficit compared to the anatomical stroke volume. This method to measure SPECT defect size in unilateral stroke patients involves comparing rCBF in the involved versus the uninvolved hemisphere and is explained in detail in previous reports (Mountz, 1989; Mountz *et al.*, 1990). The method allows calculating the volume of impaired rCBF on SPECT in cubic centimeters that would correspond to an equivalent volume with total loss of flow. On each SPECT slice that shows any rCBF abnormality on the stroke side, an ROI is drawn around the entire area of reduced rCBF. The ROI is then mirrored onto the same area of the unaffected hemisphere and the fraction of the counts lost in the stroke side compared to the uninvolved side is calculated. This is done for all slices showing any rCBF reduction on the stroke side. Summing the data from all affected slices yields a hypothetical volume of zero perfusion tracer uptake: the volume of brain that would have no blood flow if all fractional reductions were combined. This index provides an objective method to quantify SPECT defect size relative to the MRI scan defect size in comparable units of measure. MRI defect size is defined by the sum of all areas of low signal (infarcted tissue) visualized on serial T1 weighted MRI sections. Any difference in size must be attributed to a decrease in function of viable brain tissue.

Results: Identifying Diaschisis with SPECT

The physiological basis for the initial neurological and cognitive impairment associated with stroke is due to the combined effect of absent tissue (infarction) and reduced neurometabolic activity outside of the infarction (both local and distant). Since the amount of neural tissue with diaschisis identifies the amount of affected brain that has the potential for recovery, it is hypothesized that quantification of the diaschisis volume is highly correlated with stroke recovery.

We discussed several methods for identification of diaschisis. In the patient examples presented here we do so by determining the volume of brain with reduced rCBF but with good cerebrovascular reactivity using resting state rCBF SPECT compared with stress rCBF SPECT measurements. When available we also examine metabolite abnormalities in the regions with presumed diaschisis by ^{1}H MRSI.

Case 1

The application of our SPECT semiquantitative method in stroke is demonstrated in the case of a 76-year-old male who was studied by brain MRI and Tc-99m HMPAO SPECT 4 weeks and approximately $1^1/_2$ years after a left anterior MCA territory infarction (color Plate I). The patient was recovering from the resulting right hemiplegia and aphasia at the time of the initial evaluation. Two initial and two follow-up Tc-99m HMPAO brain SPECT scans were performed (during each evaluation the scans were performed using the back-to-back low dose–high dose protocol). The initial evaluation involved a rest scan using 7 mCi Tc-99m HMPAO immediately followed by 1 gram Diamox IV, and after a 15-minute wait, 28 mCi 99mTc-HMPAO was injected and the second SPECT scan was obtained. The patient underwent follow-up SPECT in an identical manner $1^1/_2$ years poststroke (as shown in color Plate I). The 4-week poststroke 4.1 T MRI scan shows a region of low signal intensity corresponding to a left anterior middle cerebral artery territory infarction. The left side of color Plate I displays a transverse 7-mm 512 × 512 MR image from the patient at CM + 7cm above the CM line.

All four brain SPECT scans were analyzed using the SPECT defect volume formula described above. On the 4-week SPECT scan the effective volume of zero perfusion on the resting SPECT scan was calculated to be 68.1 cc, while the volume on the Diamox challenge scan was calculated to be 14.3 cc. The reduction in SPECT volume is expected in diaschisis (reverse Diamox effect), while an increase is expected in ischemia. This is compared to an MRI volume of 13.7 cc. The Diamox challenge study showed that there was no vascular reserve limitations in the stroke penumbra, indicating the rCBF reduction in the penumbra was consequent to lowered neurometabolic activity, most probably reflecting diaschisis. The issue addressed in follow-up evaluation was, did the SPECT volume excess at rest (i.e., 68.1 cc –14.3 cc = 53.8 cc) decrease over time?

At 18-month follow-up the effective volume of zero perfusion on the rest SPECT scan was calculated to be 16.8 cc, while the volume on the Diamox challenge scan was 14.5 cc. The significant reduction in rest volume indicates neurometabolic recovery of brain function over the follow-up period. One should especially note how the resting state SPECT at 18 months has a similar appearance to the Diamox stress test SPECT scan at 4 weeks. (Also note how the initial Diamox finding contrasts with the more traditional effect of Diamox on cerebral blood flow in cases of ischemia, where rCBF asymmetries are exaggerated, rather than diminished.)

The patient's scores on the Neurobehavioral Cognitive Status Examination (NCSE) administered at the Spain Rehabilitation Center showed a dramatic improvement over the same time period. The patient initially demonstrated moderate to severe impairments in most of the 10 domains tested (orientation, attention, comprehension, repetition, naming, construction, memory, calculation, similarity, judgment). At 18 months poststroke, his performance was within the average range for all but three of these (attention, repetition, similarity). Since it is a basic screening instrument, the NCSE may miss more subtle cognitive deficits. Nonetheless, the patient clearly experienced a very substantial recovery, which is what would have been expected given the substantial area of initial diaschisis (i.e., brain tissue affected but capable of recovery) measured by the neuroimaging procedures.

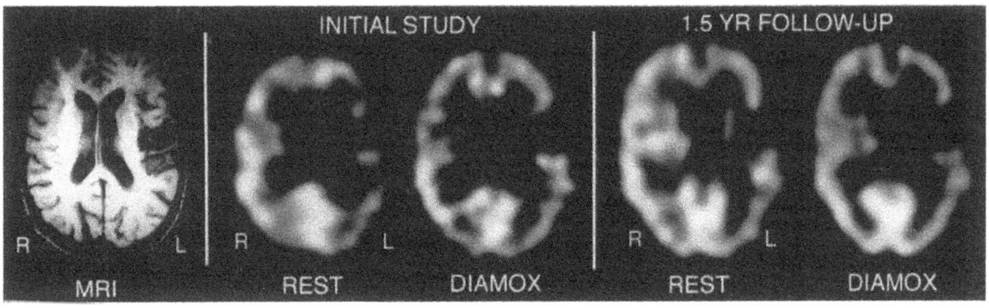

PLATE I. Stroke patient with left hemisphere diaschisis that resolves at follow-up.

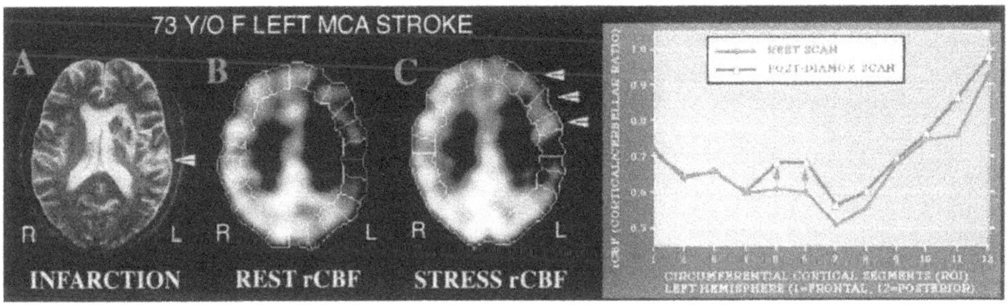

PLATE II. Verification and quantification of diaschisis in left MCA stroke.

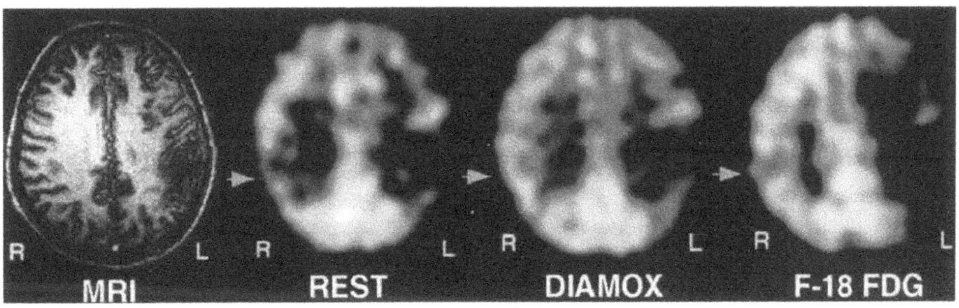

PLATE III. Cross hemispheric diaschisis verified by stress test and FDG scan.

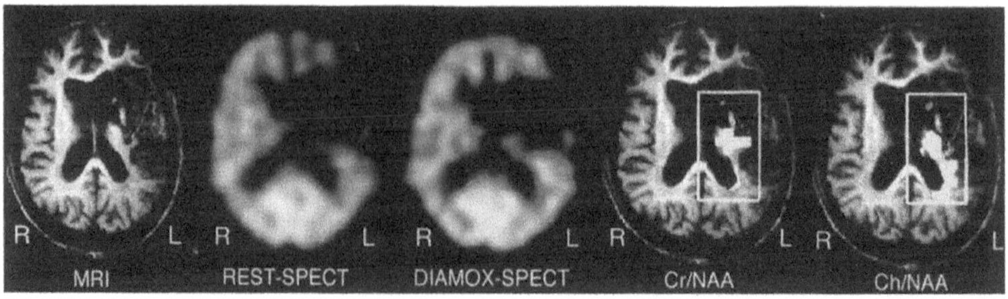

PLATE IV. MRSI identifies metabolite abnormalities in white matter underlying diaschisis.

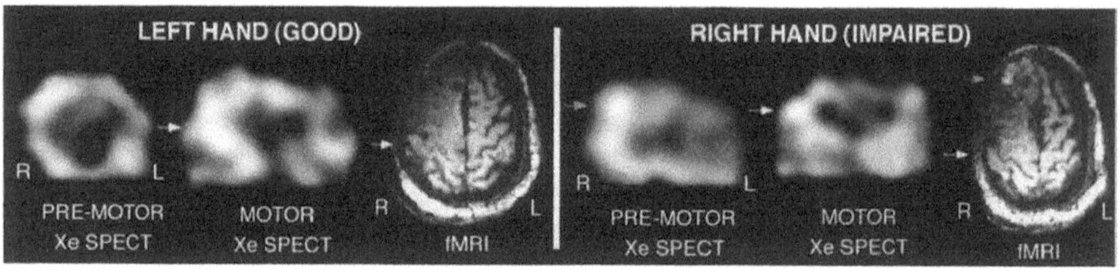

PLATE V. Xe SPECT and fMRI show ipsilateral activity during recovered hand movement.

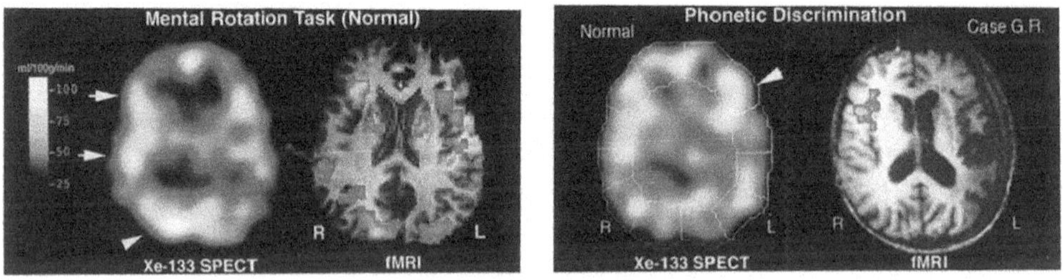

PLATE VI. (a) SPECT and fMRI of subject during spatial task. (b) Speech task evaluated by SPECT in normal control and by fMRI in a patient.

Case 2

Color Plate II shows a patient with a left internal capsule and anterior left cortical lesion producing diaschisis in adjacent regions (more evident on higher transverse slices). We use this case as an additional illustration of our method for quantification of the rCBF defect size associated with a lesion, in the course of evaluating the reduced activity outside an infarct. The SPECT images show the circumferential ROI analysis used and the graph plots the rCBF values in each ROI, starting at the left frontal ROI (1 o'clock position) and proceeding around the brain in clockwise fashion.

The patient is a 73-year-old female with a left MCA territory infarction 6 weeks post-stroke. She has a right hemiparesis (right upper extremity 6/10, right lower extremity 4/10) and severe expressive aphasia (1/10). The MRI anatomic scan (A) shows a moderately large infarction in the left MCA territory with a defect volume of 14 cc. The rest rCBF scan (B) shows a diaschisis penumbra extending from the 1 o'clock to the 3 o'clock position (SPECT defect volume of 21 cc). On Diamox stress (C) there is a reduction in the rCBF defect volume size (17 cc), particularly involving the anterior portion of the hemisphere (arrowheads). The graph of left hemisphere rCBF shows the region of diaschisis (green arrows at regions 5 and 6). The patient's neuropsychological tests showed deficits in left frontal lobe cognition.

Case 3 (Cross-Hemispheric Diaschisis)

Color Plate III illustrates a patient with a posterior left temporal–parietal infarction with evidence for cross-callosal (cross-hemispheric) diaschisis, as well as some ipsilateral peri-infarct diaschisis. Diamox stress increases rCBF in this region, indicating that the reduction is not due to vascular constraints. Additional confirmation is provided by an F-18 fluorodeoxyglucose (FDG) PET study (performed on our ADAC coincidence detection imaging camera) that shows reduced glucose utilization in the same region. We see cross-hemispheric diaschisis effects in patients with such posterior lesions, but much less frequently in patients with more anterior lesions.

Combined ^{1}H Spectroscopy and SPECT Data in Stroke

Before presenting combined SPECT and MRSI data in stroke, we will briefly describe the MRSI techniques used.

Proton (^{1}H) Spectroscopy Methods

All ^{1}H spectroscopic images have been acquired using the 4.1T whole body imaging spectrometer developed by UAB and Philips Medical Systems with a double-tuned quadrature headcoil designed specifically for high-field use (Vaughan, Hetherington, Otu, Pan, & Pohost, 1994). The pulse sequence used is based on a slice-selective excitation pulse and a spin echo. Water suppression is performed using a binomial selective refocusing pulse and balanced gradient crushers. Two dimensions of phase encoding are performed with sinusoidal gradients in the plane of the slice (Hetherington *et al.*, 1994).

A single-slice scout image is acquired in 1.5 minutes with resolution of 256 mm × 256 mm and is acquired to provide point to point reference for the spectroscopic imaging (SI) data. For the spectroscopic image, the repitition time (TR) was 2 sec, echo time (TE) 50 msec, 1-cm slice thickness, 32 × 32 phase encode steps over a 240 × 240mm field of view (FOV) resulting in

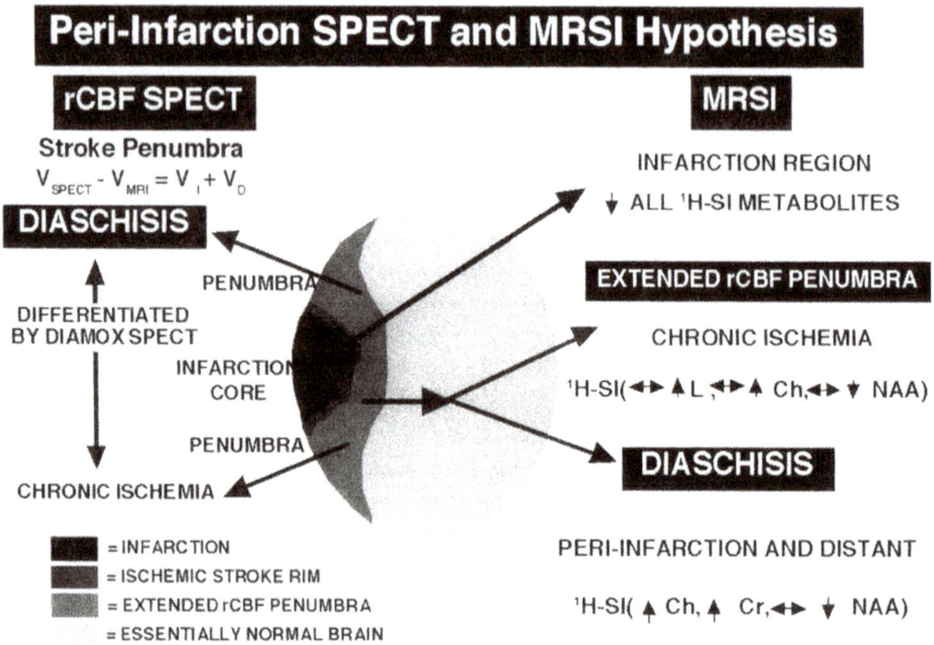

FIGURE 2. Diagram illustrating the most likely relationships between poststroke cerebral areas and metabolite levels measured by ^{1}H MRSI.

0.75 mm × 0.75 mm in plane resolution and 0.50 cc voxel resolution. The entire duration of the study including calibrations and SI acquisition is approximately 70–90 minutes.

All voxels within the ROI were analyzed using NMRI and the line width, resonance area, and chemical shift were determined. From this data the creatine–*N*-acetyl aspartate (Cr–NAA), choline–*N*-acetyl aspartate (Ch–NAA), and lactate–*N*-acetyl aspartate (Lac–NAA) ratios were determined for all pixels. A database of metabolite ratios from 20 healthy volunteers for gray and white matter volumes for structures within the parietal, occipital, frontal, and temporal lobes was used for comparison. To visualize those regions in patients that show significant differences from normal data, all voxels within the selected ROI were compared with the normal data using a highlighted color scale to demonstrate those ratios that were greater than two standard deviations for normal white matter and gray matter.

Hypotheses Regarding Metabolites

As we mentioned, this is a complex, still-evolving area, but there are now several hypotheses about the significance of several metabolites imaged by MRSI for distinguishing ischemia, diaschisis, and selective neuronal loss. A relatively established hypothesis is that elevated lactate provides evidence of ischemia as a result of its production during the anaerobic glycolysis accompanying oxygen deprivation. The exact role of NAA, Cr, and Ch in indicating aspects of neuronal function is more controversial. We have used the following working hypotheses in MRSI studies of recovering stroke patients.

In regions of "pure" diaschisis in the cortex, steady-state ^{1}H MRSI regional measurements of NAA, Cr, Ch, and Lac are all expected to be normal, since the reduced metabolism is presumed to be due solely to deafferentation of normal stimulatory input to the region and not to any real rCBF or metabolite constraints. However, if selective neuronal loss is contributing to the low rCBF, NAA will be reduced. NAA appears to be a "neuronal marker" and is expected to be low in regions with neuronal loss (as well as in the "chronic" ischemic conditions). Choline, as an indicator of increased membrane breakdown, may be increased in areas of neuronal loss (as well as in the ischemic conditions described above) but should be normal in "pure" cortical diaschisis. Creatine is an intracellular compound that serves as a marker for cell integrity. Creatine is reduced where cells are dead but can be elevated in gliosis (Fig. 2 illustrates the most likely relationships between poststroke cerebral areas and metabolite levels measured by ^{1}H MRSI).

SPECT and MRSI Data on Patients with Varying Cerebrovascular Compromise

Additional support for the role of diaschisis, as well as potentially improved cerebral status information, is provided by combined SPECT and MRSI studies. As we shall see, MRSI shows quite different findings in cortical gray matter versus that in white matter in cerebral regions showing rCBF reduction and diaschisis on SPECT scans.

Case 4

Figure 3a,b are data from a patient who suffered a right MCA territory stroke with resulting left hemiparesis. The SPECT data showed no significant diaschisis volume or ischemic residual. The calculated right MCA territory defect from the anatomic scan was 57.9 cc. The rest and Diamox SPECT (Fig. 3a) show almost no change and have essentially equal volumes of hypothetical zero perfusion (67.4 cc and 63.3 cc, respectively).

MRSI showed abnormal metabolite levels, including elevated Lac in the stroke rim. Figure 3b shows thresholded images of abnormal metabolite levels superimposed on structural MR scout images. All pixels within the white rectangle were analyzed. The highlighted pixels

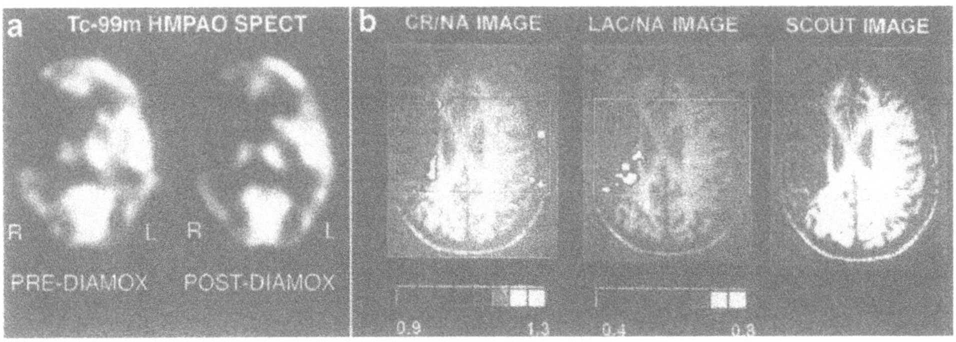

FIGURE 3. SPECT and MRSI data from a patient who suffered a right MCA territory stroke. (a) The rest and Diamox SPECT show almost no change and have essentially equal volumes of hypothetical zero perfusion (67.4 cc, and 63.3 cc). This is very close to the calculated anatomical defect of 57.9 cc, indicating no significant diaschisis volume or ischemic residual. (b) Thresholded images of abnormal metabolite levels superimposed on structural MR scout images. All pixels within the white rectangle were analyzed. The highlighted pixels in the Cr–NA image represent pixels that had a Cr–NA ratio more than 0.9 (two standard deviations higher than that observed in parietal gray matter in healthy controls). Since lactate (LAC) is not normally detected in the 0.5-cc voxels of healthy controls, the observation of lactate in quantities comparable to NA (more than 40% of the resonance area) is highly significant. The scale beneath each image displays the correspondence between the highlighted color and the measured metabolic ratio.

in the Cr–NAA image represent pixels which had a Cr–NAA ratio more than 0.9 (four standard deviations higher than that observed in parietal white matter and two standard deviations higher than that observed in parietal gray matter in healthy controls. Since Lac is not normally detected in the 0.5-cc voxels of healthy controls, the observation of Lac in quantities comparable to NAA (more than 40% of the resonance area) is highly significant.

Case 5

Figure 4a,b shows data from another patient presenting with right-sided neurological deficits. The rCBF SPECT scan showed an area of diminished perfusion in the left posterior parietal region that dramatically improved during a Diamox stress test, suggesting cortical diaschisis (Fig. 4a). The patient suffered a white matter stroke inferior to the MRI section (Fig. 4b) selected for spectroscopic analysis. A stacked plot of the ^{1}H spectra (posterior to anterior cortex along the vertical line shown in Fig. 4b) in the zone of diaschisis found on SPECT shows normal Lac, with normal Ch and Cr to NAA ratios (Fig. 4c). The normal metabolite levels in the same cortical region showing rCBF reduction and good Diamox reactivity supports our hypothesis concerning rCBF and MRSI changes in areas of "pure" diaschisis.

Case 6

A patient example is presented to illustrate the expected findings in selective neuronal loss, in this case, probably due to long-standing chronic ischemia. The patient had transient neurological deficits predominantly involving the left extremities. The Diamox SPECT (Fig. 5a) shows only slight reduction in relative rCBF to the right midtemporal region compared to the baseline study. The MRI scan (Fig. 5b) shows diffuse nonspecific signal changes in this region. The ^{1}H spectra (Fig. 5c) obtained at the seven regions illustrated demonstrates marked changes in Ch and Cr to NAA ratios, which suggest an abnormality not due to diaschisis. The Ch, Cr, and NAA levels are most abnormal at cortical region 7, but similar trends of abnormal ratios are seen to a lesser extent at cortical region 1.

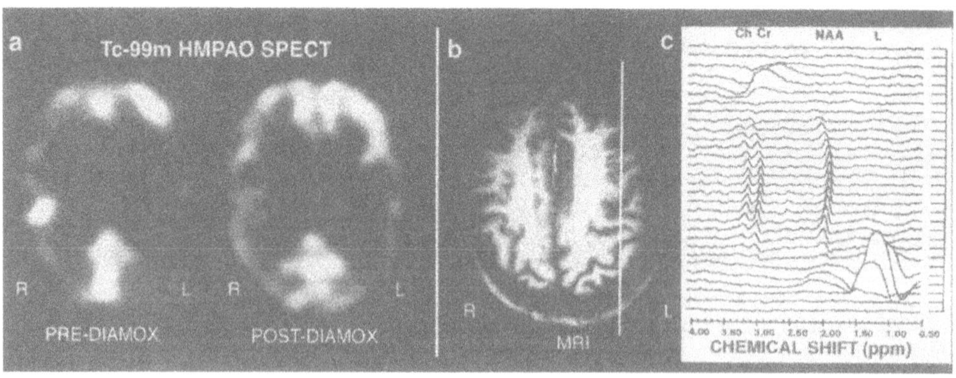

FIGURE 4. SPECT and MRSI data from a patient presenting with right-sided neurological deficits. The rCBF SPECT scan showed an area of diminished cortical perfusion in the left posterior parietal region that dramatically improved during a Diamox stress test, suggesting cortical diaschisis (a). The patient had a white matter stroke inferior to the SPECT section shown in (a) and (b) the MRI section selected for spectroscopic analysis. A stacked plot of the ^{1}H spectra (posterior to anterior cortex along the vertical line shown in b) in the zone of diaschisis found on SPECT shows normal lactate, (c) with normal Ch and Cr to NAA ratios.

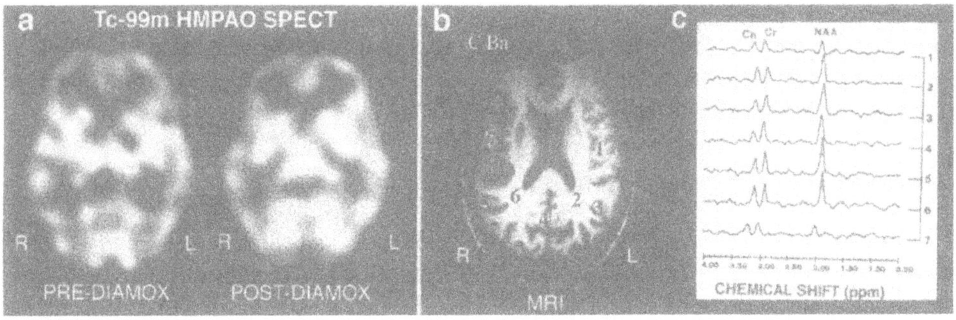

FIGURE 5. A patient illustrating SPECT and MRSI findings in selective neuronal loss, probably due to long-term chronic ischemia. (a) Diamox SPECT shows slight reduction in rCBF to the right mid-temporal region compared to the baseline study. (b) The MRI scan shows diffuse nonspecific signal changes in this region. (c) The ^{1}H spectra obtained at the seven regions marked on (b) demonstrate an abnormality in Ch, Cr, and NAA levels at cortical region 7, and to a lesser extent at cortical region 1.

Case 7

As we showed previously, in most patients there is a reduction in the size of the rCBF SPECT defect volume at Diamox stress compared to rest, indicating there is a diaschisis component of the penumbra. This result is illustrated in color Plate IV, the case of an 81-year-old male with a large left MCA stroke who was aphasic and hemiparetic from the stroke.

Color Plate IV shows the scout MRI and corresponding 6-week rest and Diamox rCBF brain SPECT scan sections (top row). The MRI demonstrates that the left MCA infarction spares some of the white matter of the left corona radiata. Perfusion to the left corona radiata is absent on the rest rCBF SPECT but present on the Diamox SPECT scan, indicating diaschisis. There is also peri-infarction diaschisis in the frontal lobe (12 o'clock to 1 o'clock) and in the left posterior temporal lobe (3 o'clock to 5 o'clock). The left internal carotid artery (ICA) carotid Doppler was normal. Surprisingly, the transcranial Doppler of the left MCA (anterior and posterior branches) was also normal.

There were abnormal Cr–NAA ratio levels and Ch–NAA ratio levels in the left corona radiata (white matter). This is indicated by the superimposed yellow highlighted pixels, which represent metabolite values within the area of measurement greater than 2 SD from normal.

On higher sections the rCBF SPECT scan showed normal perfusion in the leg region of the somatomotor cortex. The patient was evaluated at 3 months and has regained motor function to his lower extremity. All imaging results support the conclusion that the principal component of the penumbra in this patient is diaschisis. Furthermore, abnormal Ch in adjacent white matter suggests that the diaschisis is associated with membrane breakdown. Intracellular integrity loss is indicated by abnormal Cr. As hypothesized, when diaschisis (in the absence of chronic ischemia) is the principal component, the patient has a greater probability of regaining recovery from the stroke-induced neurological deficits.

Case 8 (Subcortical Lesion)

Distant, presumed diaschisis effects are also evident in subcortical infarcts. A 27-year-old female patient suffered hemiparesis and mild cognitive impairment from a stroke in the right putamen–right posterior limb of the internal capsule. The initial rest rCBF SPECT study showed reduction in right cortical blood flow above the lesion at a level where structural MRI showed normal anatomy. MRSI showed abnormal Ch–NAA, Cr–NAA, and Cr–Ch in the ipsilateral (right) centrum semiovale (white matter) underlying this cortical region. This may reflect axonal membrane catabolism in the subacute poststroke phase and may account for some of the disconnection effects leading to the cortical diaschisis.

Summary Comments Regarding MRSI Findings

In conclusion, MRSI shows quite different findings in cortical gray matter versus that in white matter in cerebral regions showing rCBF reduction and diaschisis on SPECT scans. Whereas the metabolites we have measured so far are in most cases normal in cortical regions of suspected diaschisis (as we originally hypothesized), they appear to be abnormal in adjacent or underlying white matter. This is perhaps not very surprising, considering that diaschisis is supposed to arise from "disconnection effects," and thus involve white matter integrity. At this time we cannot say whether the metabolite abnormalities seen in white matter adjacent to the infarct or in white matter tracts underlying regions of cortical diaschisis represent axonal damage or reflect repair and reorganizational processes. Overall, the MRSI data support the idea that the rCBF reductions in cortical gray matter observed on SPECT poststroke are usually due to diaschisis. In some cases, usually involving long-standing chronic ischemia, rCBF reductions may reflect more parenchymal damage and selective neuronal loss. Other metabolite imaging capabilities are becoming available, such as MRSI of glutamate and glutamine, tricarboxylic acid cycle (Krebs cycle) flux, and phosphorus-based SI of various stages in cell energetics. These will provide more comprehensive information on the status of specific cerebral regions poststroke.

Examining Activation Patterns during Motor and Cognitive Recovery

Task activation studies offer the primary method by which to assess the extent to which stroke recovery involves reorganization or relearning in unaffected brain. They also provide a method to further evaluate the status (functional viability–contribution to cognition) of areas judged to be diaschitic by the physiological measures.

Regional CBF activation by tasks is a measure of metabolic response to the sensory–motor and cognitive demands of the task, reflected indirectly by the very precise parenchymal control of the vasculature. In addition to validating simple sensory–motor tasks for the study of hand function recovery, we have worked to identify test conditions best suited for generating reliable asymmetries in hemispheric activation of cortical rCBF that can be applied to the study of recovery of function in stroke and trauma patients. Tasks that are hemisphere or region specific should be very useful in monitoring the compensation that takes place in regional activation during recovery from any cerebral injury.

Methods

Although HMPAO SPECT can be used for activation studies (sometimes very effectively due to its ability to "capture" or "lock in" the rCBF pattern at the time of tracer injection, allowing the actual scan to be performed afterward without stimulation accoutrements), it has several drawbacks. Multiple scans cannot be performed in one session due to the long tracer clearance and HMPAO distribution is not linear with absolute rCBF: it underrepresents higher rCBF values, resulting in poorer sensitivity to greatest rCBF changes. Studies of multiple task conditions are therefore best performed by methods employing dynamic tracer clearance methodology, such as O15 PET or Xe-133 clearance methods. Because PET is very expensive and not widely available clinically, we have employed new Xe-133 clearance SPECT methods for activation studies requiring repeatability and quantification. Though also not widely available, Xe SPECT capability will increase as more hospitals obtain the new generation of triple-head SPECT cameras that are now used for multiple clinical imaging purposes. Functional MRI (fMRI) is another method allowing the study of multiple activation task conditions, and although it is nonquantitative and suffers from several limitations in assessing brain-damaged patients, we show how it, too, can contribute to studying cerebral reorganization.

Xe SPECT Rationale

Xe-133 SPECT offers a cost-effective method to obtain quantitative, immediately repeatable (multiple condition) whole-brain scans that are very sensitive to sensory–motor and cognitive activation (the dynamic clearance method records all changes in flow rate and is not flow rate limited as in techniques using stably distributed tracers, such as HMPAO SPECT). The freely diffusable tracer technique is the original "gold standard" of rCBF measurement, providing sensitive and accurate estimation of all physiological flow rates. This is particularly useful in the evaluation of physiological stress, sensory–motor, and cognitive activation effects (Deutsch, Bourbon, Papanicolaou, & Eisenberg, 1988; Deutsch, Katholi, & Mountz, 1996a; Deutsch *et al.,* 1997b; Deutsch, Mountz, Liu, Sutor, & Roubin, 1997c). The rapid clearance of the tracer also allows conducting consecutive multiple studies in the same session. True quantitation of rCBF allows much better interpretation of activation studies compared with just redistribution or pattern change information. Whole-brain information, including transverse, transverse oblique, coronal, and sagittal reconstructed slices without gaps provide superior capability in evaluating true condition-induced changes without the potential confounds of motion- or orientation-induced changes in individual slice planes.

The only disadvantage of Xe SPECT at the current time is the lower spatial resolution (12.5 mm) compared to state of the art HMPAO SPECT (7–9 mm). This resolution is perfectly adequate, however, to evaluate the focal regional changes associated with most sensory–motor and cognitive tasks (Deutsch *et al.,* 1997b, 1998). Furthermore, we use HMPAO SPECT to provide collaborative, high-resolution information with respect to rCBF in small cortical regions and subcortical structures. The Xe SPECT technique will continue to be refined; a new fan beam collimator is being designed for 11-mm resolution and the anticipated introduction of Xe-127 should result in 9-mm resolution.

Xe-133 SPECT rCBF Imaging Method

We employ a Prism 3000-XP tomograph (Picker, Cleveland, OH), which yields three-dimensional images representing rCBF quantitatively in milliliters/minute per 100 grams. High-sensitivity collimators, a Xe-133 inhalation unit, and a CdTe lung probe are integrated with gantry electronics to perform complete scans every 10 sec for 7 min with a spatial resolution of 12–14 mm (FWHM) (Devous, Gong, Payne, Harris, 1993; Deutsch *et al.,* 1997b,c). Subjects undergo a brief (1–2 min) adaptation period with a nose clamp occluding the nostrils and a scubalike mouthpiece in place. Care is taken to ensure that there are no leaks around either the mouthpiece or nose clamp. Subjects inhale Xe-133 gas in an air mixture (20 m Ci/liter) during the first minute of the scan and then breathe room air for the remainder of the scan of Xe-133 washout. Xe-133 is delivered through a Diversified Diagnostics model 4000 xenon delivery unit. End tidal Pco_2, blood pressure, and respiratory rate are recorded during the measurement.

Projection images are acquired at 3° intervals into a 64 × 64 matrix. Each detector head acquires 40 projection images at a radius of 13 cm over a 120° circular orbit. Complete scans are acquired every 10 sec for 7 min. The input function is monitored with a scintillation probe placed over the lungs (right upper quandrant). The lung curve is stored time-locked with the projection data. Typically, only 4 min of data are used for analysis, starting with the first files during xenon inhalation that show brain activity. Transverse images of each of the next 24 10-sec scans are obtained by using the back-projection algorithm.

Two algorithms are used for calculating rCBF from SPECT data. The first is a slightly modified version of the original Kanno–Lassen algorithm, and the second is a new method called the deconvolution (DCV) algorithm (Devous *et al.,* 1993). Our standard ROI technique, as described for HMPAO SPECT above, is also used for Xe SPECT analysis.

fMRI Background

For some time it has been known that local increases in the concentration of deoxyhemoglobin in the blood can cause NMR signal reductions in tissues, and therefore these changes in the NMR signal can be used to infer changes in blood oxygenation. This effect is termed a BOLD (blood oxygenation level dependence) effect and is usually observed using a gradient-echo (T2*-weighted) MRI sequence (Ogawa, Lee, Kay, & Tank, 1990).

Since the first reports of functional imaging based on the BOLD effect (Kwong *et al.,* 1992; Ogawa *et al.,* 1993) abundant studies have demonstrated the utility of the BOLD-associated signal changes in identifying the location of activated cortical neurons. The fMRI techniques that have evolved are used in a wide range of applications, producing images of regional function in the brain with spatial resolution significantly greater than that of other functional imaging techniques (e.g., PET or SPECT). Because fMRI can be performed in many existing clinical systems, it has become increasingly more widely used. Even though some basic questions remain to be resolved regarding the relationship of these fMRI signals with cortical activation, fMRI is already taking its place with PET and SPECT as a useful technique for studying cortical function.

The principal mechanism for the local NMR signal change accompanying activation in T2*- and T2-sensitive functional images is thought to be an autoregulatory blood flow increase leading to a local decrease in deoxyhemoglobin concentration, leading in turn to a locally increased (typically by several percent) NMR signal. This signal increase typically begins within a few seconds of the onset of activation, reaches a peak within several seconds to 10 sec, and has been reported to persist for as long as 20 min (Bandettini *et al.,* 1995).

It should be noted that fractional signal increases due to activation are larger in high-field systems such as the UAB 4.1T system, and NMR sensitivity is higher as well, providing a double advantage to high-field functional MRI measurements. This advantage in principle can be realized as an increased sensitivity to small activation-associated changes or as an increased spatial resolution in the activation images obtained at high field. In functional imaging studies performed using our 4.1 T system, typical activation-related signal changes in activated regions not including larger veins are about 5–10%, while in 1.5 Tesla clinical MRI systems, typical signal changes are about 2–5%.

Combined Use of Xe SPECT and fMRI

Xe SPECT and fMRI can be used in a complementary manner. Xe SPECT can provide quantitative absolute rCBF maps that will allow identification of low-flow areas and diaschisis surrounding or adjoining the completed infarct through the combined use of resting and CO_2 stress scans. (Xe SPECT of CO_2 reactivity can establish the nature of such areas of reduced activity, just as in the HMPAO SPECT Diamox studies described earlier.) Xenon SPECT can also provide quantitative reactivity information to motor activity and cognitive tasks, which then can be further investigated through fMRI protocols allowing more control conditions as well as higher spatial and temporal resolution. fMRI by itself would be limited because baseline rCBF information (neither absolute flow or distribution) is not available, thus not allowing any understanding of the extent of activity reduction, diaschisis, and any distance effects of the stroke.

We will first present normal control and patient studies of motor recovery and then present data on recovery of more "cognitive" functions.

Results: Motor Tasks and Recovery

Normal Data

Two different tasks involving hand or finger movements were tested in five normal subjects during Xe SPECT scans. One was the sequential finger–thumb opposition task, used by many neuroimaging studies to activate motor cortex. The other was a task we have been developing to study both motor activation and an ideational cognitive component, a task involving stereognostic "recognition" of small complex shapes with the fingers of one hand. Both tasks showed robust focal activation of the motor cortex, so the sequential finger–thumb opposition task was chosen for our initial studies of motor recovery in stroke patients. Left-hand finger motion resulted in focal increases in right sensory–motor cortex averaging 107 ml/100 g per min, compared to 82 ml/100 g per min in homologous left hemisphere cortical regions. Figure 6 graphs the normal rCBF pattern changes for one brain section.

High Field fMRI Studies: Motor Tasks

The sequential finger–thumb opposition task used in our Xe SPECT studies has been well validated in fMRI studies by other investigators. We have also tested a simpler motor task using fMRI on 10 normal subjects designed for studying more impaired stroke patients: simple

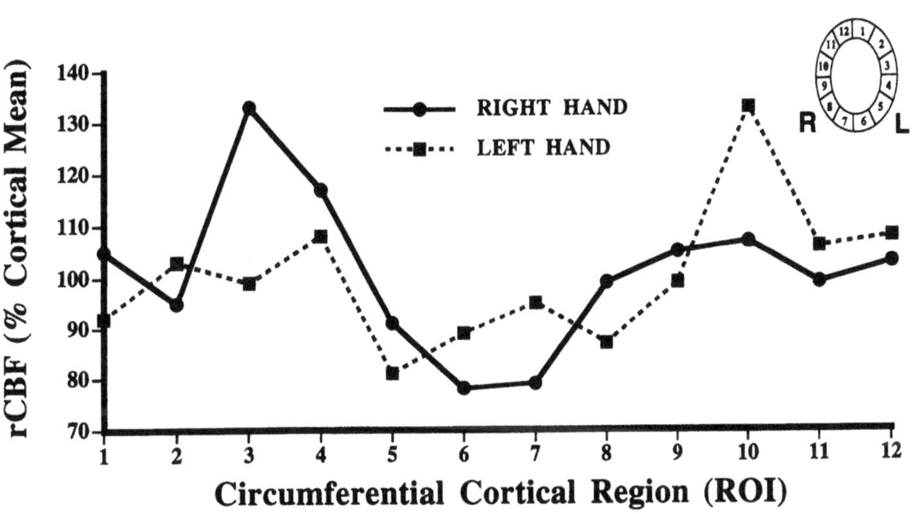

FIGURE 6. Finger Opposition Task. Level CM+6cm (N=5) Circumferential cortical profiles of rCBF pattern changes associated with a left-hand and a right-hand motor task in normal control subjects for one transverse brain section. MANOVA profile analysis showed a significant ($P < 0.001$) difference between the rCBF pattern at rest and both left and right tasks.

hand flexion and extension. In all subjects activation was observed contralateral to the hand motion of the task, validating the use of this very basic hand movement in fMRI studies of stroke recovery.

Case 9 (Motor Recovery)

Color Plate V illustrates Xe SPECT and fMRI activation studies in a patient recovering from a left internal capsule stroke. The patient's Fugl-Meyer test (Duncan, Propst, & Nelson, 1983) scores for wrist and hand had gone from 23/30 at 6 weeks to 30/30 at 6 months poststroke. Imaging was conducted while the patient performed the sequential finger–thumb opposition task with his recovering right hand and with his normal left hand. Xe SPECT images (coronal sections) are shown in the figure, from both the premotor region and the slightly more posterior motor cortex. The left-hand task increased rCBF slightly in right premotor cortex and substantially in the right motor cortex (as expected). Performing the task with the impaired but recovering right hand showed an increase in rCBF in the right frontal and premotor cortex, as well as some rCBF increases in the right motor cortex. The graph in Fig. 7 plots the patient's rCBF pattern compared with normal data.

fMRI (transverse images) showed a similar pattern of activation, with focal activation appearing in right prefrontal and motor regions during the right hand task. The left-hand task showed the expected activation of right motor cortex.

Case 10 and Other Cases

Another case has shown essentially the same effects during recovery of hand function. The left hand and fingers had partially recovered from a paresis due to a right internal capsule infarction. The patient's Fugl-Meyer test scores for wrist and hand had gone from 24/30 at weeks to 28/30 at 6 months poststroke. Xe SPECT scans showed the expected rCBF activa-

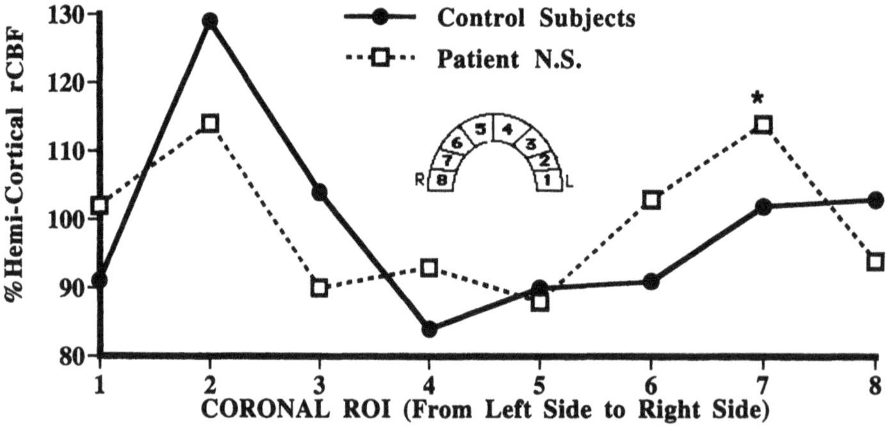

FIGURE 7. Left stroke patient using recovered right hand. Graph of rCBF pattern changes during a motor task involving a stroke patient's impaired right hand compared with normal data (Case 9). The data are plotted for a coronal section of the brain (illustrated in the inset) that passes through premotor cortex.

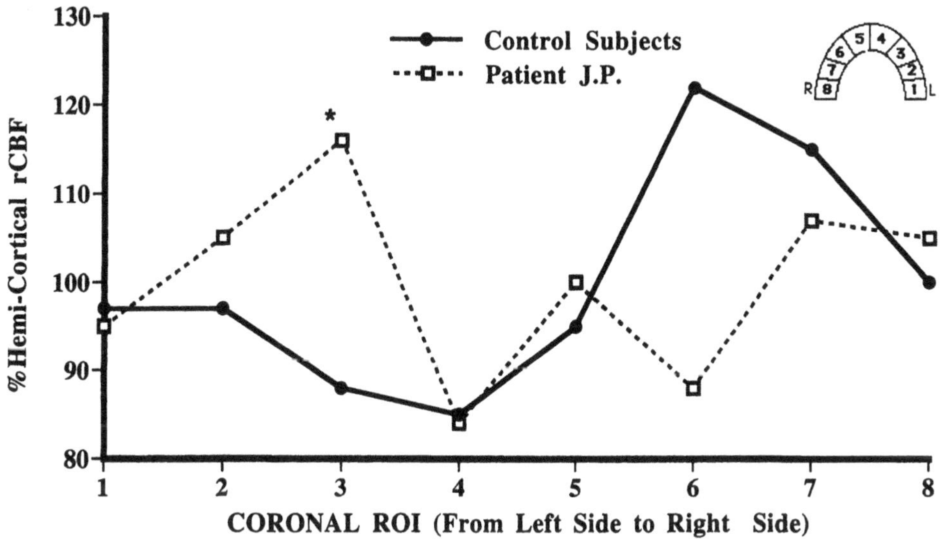

FIGURE 8. Right stroke patient using recovered left hand. Graph of rCBF pattern changes during a motor task involving a stroke patient's impaired left hand compared with normal data (Case 10). The data are plotted for a coronal section of the brain (illustrated in the inset) that passes through premotor cortex.

tion in left motor cortex during right-hand finger movements. Finger movements of the initially impaired left hand also show, anomalously, activation of left motor cortex and a very marked increase in the left thalamus. The graph in Fig. 8 plots the patient's rCBF pattern compared with normal data. Two other capsular infarct patients also showed increased activation in contralesional premotor regions. These findings are suggestive of ipsilateral recruitment for a motor function normally under contralateral control.

Baseline Activity Changes on SPECT and 18F-FDG

It is of particular interest that *resting state* SPECT and fluorodeoxyglucose (FDG) PET of each of the patients discussed above (case 9 and 10) showed increased premotor activity in the spared hemisphere 6 months poststroke. Resting state scans of case 9 showed an evolving area of hyperactivity in the right premotor cortex, apparently associated with the reduced activity in the left hemisphere. In addition, an 18F-FDG PET scan showed that the rCBF increase was indeed associated with increased glucose metabolism in the same region. This increased neurometabolic activity may reflect right hemisphere reorganizational changes homologous to the diaschisis in left cortical regions.

Case 10 showed very similar findings in her unaffected left hemisphere, also suggesting reorganizational changes homologous to the diaschisis in right cortical regions. A limited retrospective examination has yielded three other patients with multi-imaging modality evidence for unusual resting baseline changes in the initially unaffected hemisphere poststroke. This was not seen initially since it is only present on the 6 month to 1 year poststroke studies. In examining the resting state scans of all five patients and comparing the 1-year to the 6-week poststroke study, there was a mean increase of 10.6 + 5.7% (range, 4.2 to 18.6%) in rCBF in premotor cortex in the hemisphere opposite the lesion.

Motor Recovery Summary and Conclusions

Patients showed significantly increased activity in the premotor and motor regions of the unaffected hemisphere during movements of the impaired hand. One right hemisphere stroke patient showed a dramatic increase in thalamic activity in the left hemisphere during complex movements of her initially impaired left hand, as well as some increases in left motor cortex.

Additional fMRI studies, conducted in two of the patients, provided independent validation for reorganizational changes in the unaffected hemisphere consistent with the Xe SPECT activation data. Thus, recovery of motor function from unilateral stroke, especially involving lesions of the internal capsule, appears to involve increased activation of regions in the hemisphere contralateral to the lesion but not necessarily in primary motor cortex; premotor cortex, prefrontal cortex, and the thalamus often seem to be involved. This unusual activity may represent compensatory reorganization in spared brain areas homologous to those affected by the infarct.

Finally, resting state SPECT and FDG data also showed changes in contralateral premotor cortex over a 6-month period. Although the causal relationship of these changes to the recovery of motor deficits in these patients cannot be established, the data are provocative and worthy of continued investigation, especially in light of the coincident increased rCBF activation (both Xe SPECT and fMRI) shown in the same regions during movement of the recovered hand.

Results: Cognitive Tasks and Recovery

Normal Data

As mentioned earlier, we have worked to identify test conditions best suited for generating reliable asymmetries in hemispheric activation of cortical rCBF that can be applied to the study of recovery of function in stroke and trauma patients. Tasks that are hemisphere or region specific should be very useful in monitoring the compensation that takes place in regional activation during recovery from cerebral injury.

We identified a task—mental rotation—that robustly and reliably activates the right hemisphere (Deutsch *et al.,* 1988, 1997b). This task involves viewing slides of two arrays of cubes and deciding if they are the same but just oriented differently in space. We also have identified a verbal task—acoustic phonetic discrimination—that is easy enough for even most aphasic patients to attempt, yet generates reliable hemispheric and regional activation patterns. This task requires the subject to discriminate between speech sounds such as "br" and "pr" (Deutsch, Papanicolaou, Loring, & Eisenberg 1985a,b; Deutsch *et al.,* 1997b).

Both the visuospatial and verbal conditions result in "global" (bilateral) increases in flow within which can be distinguished hemisphere and region specific components. The region-specific asymmetries associated with each task are appropriate for the study of recovery from middle cerebral artery (MCA) strokes. The speech sound discrimination task involves Broca's area and the left temporal region, areas either directly or indirectly (via diaschisis) involved in most aphasic syndromes accompanying left MCA stroke. The rotation task elicits asymmetric region specific increases in right posterior temporal–parietal areas, regions also typically affected either directly or via diaschisis in right MCA strokes.

Xe SPECT Quantitative Task Effect Analyses

Color Plates VI a,b show Xe SPECT images of a normal control subject while performing the mental rotation task and speech sound (phonetic) discrimination task. Visual inspection shows prominent activation of posterior and right frontal–temporal regions at this level, canthomeatal (CM) + 5 cm, during the rotation task and prominent activation of left frontal operculum (at CM + 6 cm) (Broca's area) during the phonological task.

We have conducted analysis using multivariate techniques and also have attempted to generate normal 95% (±2 SD) "confidence limits" using group resting data that permit subsequent case-by-case analysis of individual patients in clinical settings. The rotation task, for example, results in increases at or exceeding the +2 SD level for normal resting rCBF at six locations, four involving the primary visual cortex and adjacent areas in each hemisphere (as would be expected from a visual task) but two others involving association cortex of the right hemisphere. The latter probably reflect more cognitive, asymmetrically distributed, cerebral operations associated with mental rotation

Much analysis of activation data in PET, SPECT, and fMRI modalities involves *relative* changes in rCBF distribution between conditions. This is due in part to technique limitations and/or technical difficulties and in part due to the prevailing assumption that pattern changes and not fluctuations in absolute rCBF represent the important data regarding brain activity–sensory/cognitive activity relationships. Since we are measuring absolute rCBF with xenon clearance SPECT, we have attempted to perform as much analysis as possible using "nonnormalized" quantitative rCBF before continuing with just pattern analysis. In addition to the changes evident in our standard circumferential profile analysis, the tasks showed significant changes in the left–right hemispheric symmetry observed at rest. The analysis in Fig. 9 shows the quantitative differences between rest and mental rotation: the rotation task showing a right greater than left increase in regions 2 and 3. Figure10 shows a similar hemispheric difference analysis for the phonetic task, in which significant left greater than right rCBF increases occur, especially in posterior left frontal regions corresponding to Broca's area.

We are increasing the number of verbal tasks in order to more appropriately monitor recovery from aphasia. The single phonetic task has been supplanted more recently by a computer-presented series of four hierarchical language tasks, including acoustic phonetic discrimination, rhyme judgment, lexical decision, and synonym judgment. Xe SPECT has shown increased rCBF in the left posterior temporal–parietal region (Brodmann areas 39, 40) during the synonym- or semantic-processing task in normal control subjects.

FMRI during Cognitive Tasks

Normal fMRI data has been acquired for the rotation and speech sound discrimination task, as well as some preliminary data on our newer hierarchical language series, intended to help assess recovery from aphasia. Visual stimuli were presented on a rear projection screen and viewed through a prism located above viewing ports built into the head coil. Auditory stimuli were presented through tubing connected to each ear with a custom-made earmold. A cross-correlation analysis compared the active and control states to determine activation. Significant activation was defined as a correlation coefficient of 0.35 or better between the waveform of intensity changes and task condition changes in at least five contiguous pixels. (This correlation is roughly equivalent to a *t*-test at the 99.5 % confidence level.) Pixels within the brain that passed the correlation test were then overlayed as colored patches on scout images, with percent signal increase designated by different colors [from 0.5% (red) to 10% (bright yellow)].

Color Plate VIa shows fMRI activation results in a normal control subject during the same mental rotation task for which Xe SPECT activation data is shown in the figure. The fMRI study shows a more bilateral activation pattern in this subject compared to the group SPECT data, but nevertheless involves right parietal and frontal association cortex to a greater

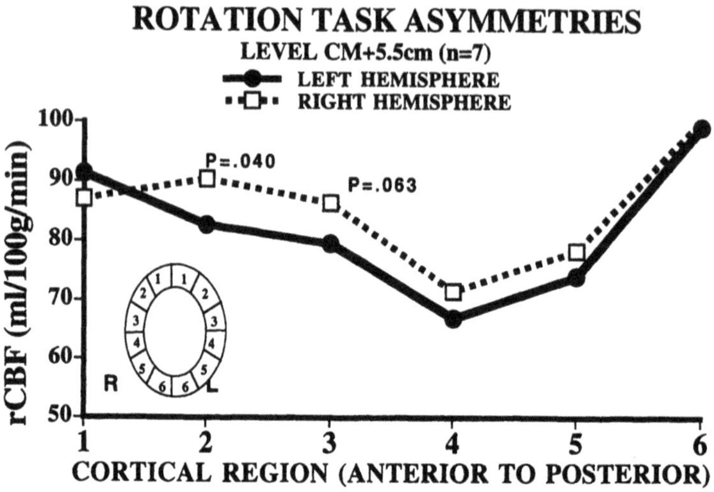

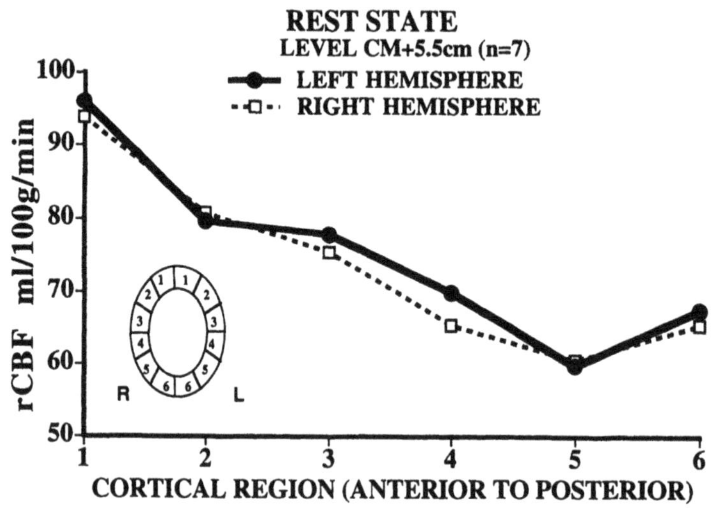

FIGURE 9. Graphs showing mean rCBF for six regions in each hemisphere for normal control subjects performing the mental rotation task. RCBF is highly coupled at rest. During the task, rCBF increases bilaterally but shows a right greater than left asymmetry. (An example Xe SPECT scan image of this task is shown in color Plate VIa.)

extent than the left. The activation is fairly extensive, reflecting the cerebral demands of the task and the fact that the control condition used in this study was "rest," to allow direct comparison with the previous SPECT data.

Analysis of the significant fMRI activation during synonym judgments compared to a speech sound control condition showed prominent changes in a high temporal region (Brodmann area 39) near the left angular gyrus. This result is consistent with our Xe SPECT data, neuropsychological data on language deficits, and models that postulate a high-level language-processing role for the posterior temporal lobe and its intersection with parietal and occipital regions.

Patient Data: Case Studies

Mean Hemispheric Changes in Stroke Recovery. Preliminary studies using the phonological task and rotation task during Xe-133 inhalation measurements of cortical rCBF have been conducted in 16 recovered stroke patients (1–3 years poststroke) to determine whether there is increased involvement of the spared hemisphere during tasks normally utilizing the damaged hemisphere. The group included 11 left hemisphere patients who had a good recovery from an initially documented aphasia and 5 right hemisphere patients who had shown a good recovery from an initial hemiplegia–hemiparesis and visual inattention with "neglect" and "denial" symptoms. Baseline rCBF studies showed reduced hemispheric mean flow levels

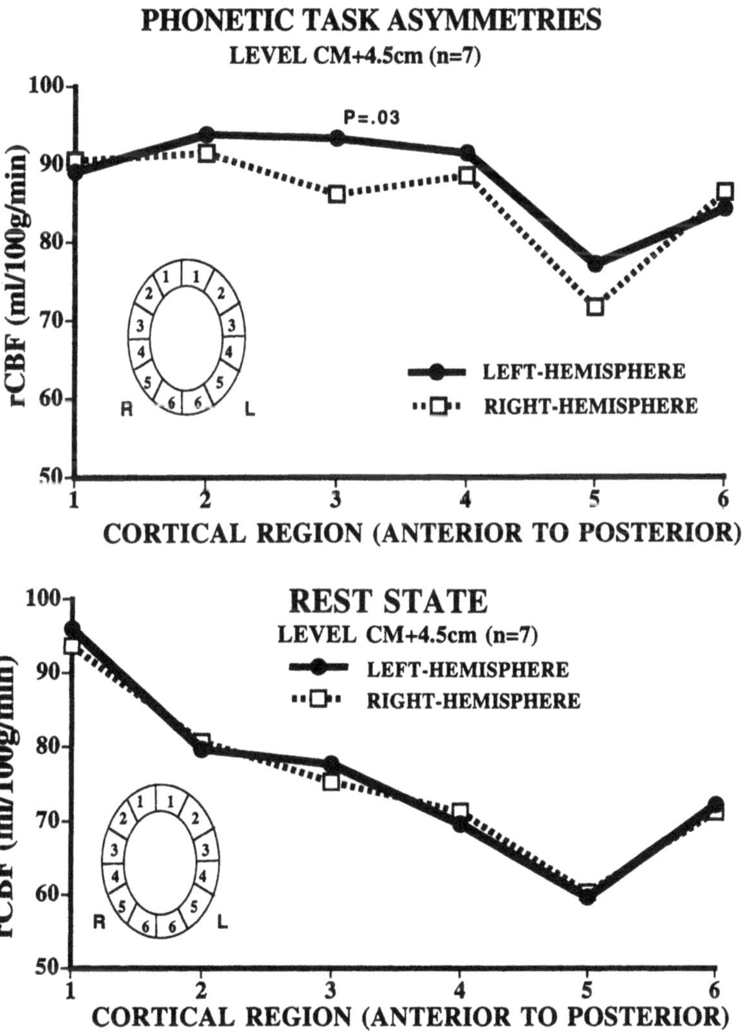

FIGURE 10. Graphs showing mean rCBF for six regions in each hemisphere for normal control subjects performing the phonetic discrimination task. RCBF is highly coupled at rest. During the task, rCBF increases bilaterally but shows a left greater than right asymmetry. (An example Xe SPECT scan image of this task is shown in color Plate VIb.)

consistent with side of lesion. Despite the large asymmetries in baseline flow, recovered stroke patients showed task-induced rCBF increases of similar magnitude to that seen in our normal subjects, in both the impaired and spared hemisphere. Figure 11 graphs the mean hemispheric flow changes. There was a trend, though not statistically significant for the group, of greater increased flow in the undamaged hemisphere in patients performing the task thought to normally involve the stroke side. In Figure 11, this is indicated by the rCBF increases associated with the hemisphere *not* specialized for a given task, which are most obvious for the left hemisphere during the spatial, mental rotation, task.

Recovery from Aphasia: Case 11. Figure 12 shows Xe SPECT and fMRI results in a patient performing several subtests of our hierarchical language series. The patient was 12 months poststroke, recovering from a fairly extensive left cortical infarction. His comprehension had recovered substantially, but speech production was still very limited. On testing on our language subtests, he performed auditory discrimination (nonword speech sounds) at 92% accuracy, rhyme judgment at 76% accuracy, and synonym judgment at 56% accuracy. Auditory stimuli were computer generated and presented through a hollow tube acoustic system fitted to custom-made silicone earmolds, allowing the patient to hear clearly despite the magnet noise. Task and control conditions alternated every minute for a total acquisition time of 8 min, resulting in 115 successive images of each slice.

Speech sound discrimination resulted in activation of the right superior frontal temporal region (Brodmann area 22, auditory association cortex) on Xe SPECT and fMRI. Figure 12 shows the fMRI results for one transverse slice, indicating activation in right superior frontal temporal cortex (area 22). Xe SPECT during this task condition also showed a right superior frontal temporal increase in rCBF. Figure 13 plots the patient's rCBF activation compared to controls.

Synonym judgment (compared to a nonword control condition) resulted in activation of right high posterior temporal–parietal regions (border of Brodmann areas 39 and 40) on Xe SPECT and fMRI. fMRI also showed activation of peri-infarct regions in the left hemisphere. On Xe SPECT,.mean rCBF at the two peri-infarct locations (arrows in Fig. 12) increased

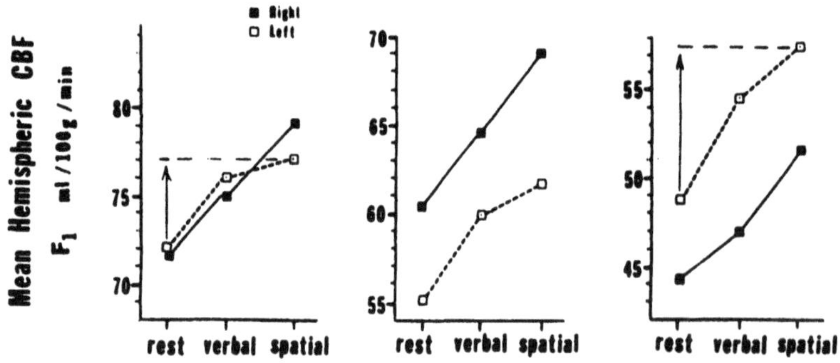

FIGURE 11. Mean hemispheric flow changes during a verbal (phonetic discrimination) and spatial (mental rotation) tasks in recovering stroke patients compared to normal controls. There was a trend for greater rCBF increases in the undamaged hemisphere in patients performing the task thought to normally involve the stroke side. This is indicated by the rCBF increases associated with the hemisphere *not* specialized for a given task, which is most obvious for the left hemisphere during the spatial task.

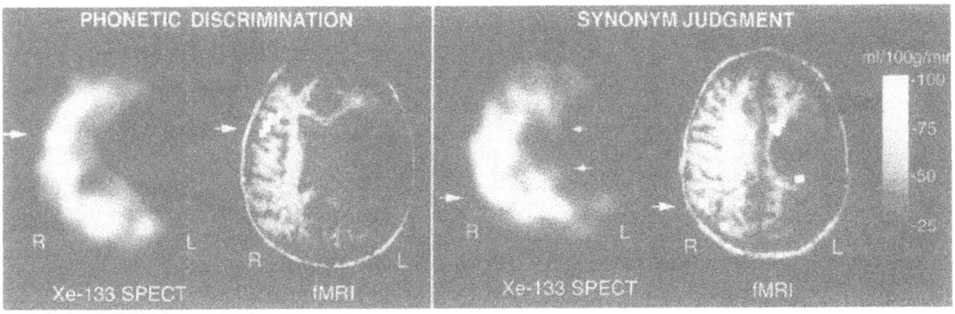

FIGURE 12. Recovered aphasic patient performing phonetic discrimination and semantic processing (synonym task). The patient underwent both Xe-133 SPECT and fMRI scans while performing these tasks.

from 34 to 48 ml/100 g per min, helping to confirm that the fMRI activation there was not an artifact.

Case 12. Color Plate VIb, which showed a SPECT scan of a normal subject performing the phonetic discrimination task, also shows fMRI results in a patient performing the same task (acoustic phonetic speech sound discrimination subtest of our hierarchical language series). The patient was 14 months poststroke, recovering from an extensive left cortical infarction. His comprehension had recovered substantially, but speech production was limited. He performed acoustic phonetic discrimination (nonword speech sounds) at 90% accuracy and rhyme judgment at 72% accuracy. Extensive activation is seen in areas 44, 45 in the spared right hemisphere during the speech sound discrimination task. This is the right hemisphere region homologous to Broca's area in the left. The rhyme task also activated areas 44, 45 in the right, but to a lesser extent.

Customizing Tasks for More Severe Impairments: Case 13. The patient's stroke involved the left internal capsule and cortical regions with severely impaired speech and language comprehension. Although, due to the nearly global aphasia, this patient could not perform our language subtests as initially designed, we modified the protocol to examine passive viewing of real words versus nonwords. The fMRI study compared word viewing to nonword viewing, and indeed indicated activity in several language–lexical-processing areas in this very aphasic subject, including left frontotemporal (Brodmann area 38) and higher left temporal–parietal (area 39), as well as several right hemisphere areas. The study was repeated and showed a very similar but less extensive activation pattern. This study represents an example of adjusting task demands to study implicit processing even in a globally aphasic patient, normally incapable of performing at any measurable level of competence on our standard series. Although not typical of the majority of our stroke studies, we believe this example provides evidence for how functional imaging can indeed examine cerebral operations in even severe stroke.

Language Recovery Summary and Conclusions

The two imaging modalities concur in providing evidence for some compensatory changes in the intact hemisphere during recovery from unilateral stroke, as well as task-related peri-infarct activation during certain conditions. In recovered aphasic patients, simple speech

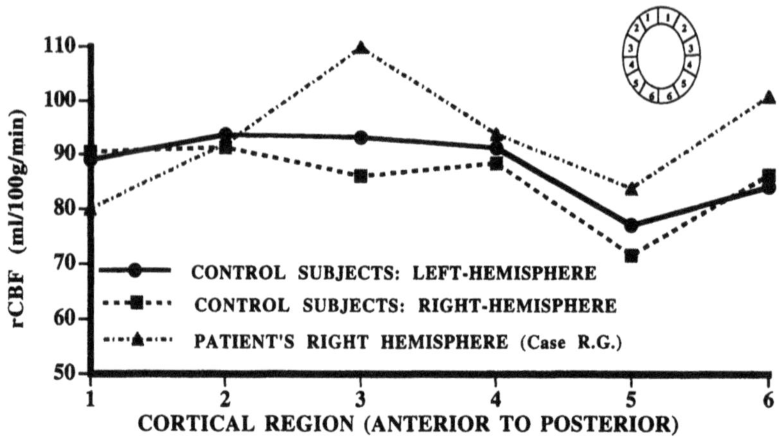

FIGURE 13. Phonetic task: Recovered left stroke patient. Level CM+4.5cm. Xe SPECT rCBF activation pattern during speech sound (phonetic) discrimination in stroke patient recovering from aphasia compared to normal control data. (The patient is case 11 whose images are shown in Fig. 12 above.) The patient showed activation of the right superior frontal temporal region homologous to left hemisphere region activated by controls.

sound discrimination can rely on the right hemisphere. Semantic judgment shows activation of a right hemisphere region homologous to that seen in the left hemisphere of normal subjects but also shows peri-infarct activation, possibly indicating greater demand on any intact left hemisphere mechanisms during the "higher level" task.

Implications

The Comprehensive, Multi-imaging Modality Approach to Stroke Recovery

Although the mechanisms of stroke recovery here discussed are not new (a number of investigations have suggested evidence for cortical plasticity in terms of electrophysiological and neuroimaging data suggesting "spread" of cortical sensory–motor representation), the combination of techniques discussed here offer a more comprehensive approach to evaluating plasticity and reorganization. We have provided a model and techniques that take into account local and distant baseline brain activity impairments and longitudinal changes in these impairments. Changes in activation patterns need to be viewed and interpreted in the context of any changes in underlying baseline activity, including (separating) permanent morphological damage, diaschisis, and selective neuronal loss or incomplete infarction.

This is accomplished through the use of rest–stress cerebrovascular reactivity scans and a method for quantifying resting rCBF impairment. We have demonstrated that this technique identifies areas of temporarily affected but viable brain, which is predictive of a certain degree of recovery of function. Furthermore, we introduce a highly sensitive and cost-effective quantitative rCBF technique using a truly diffusable tracer (whole-brain Xe SPECT) and combine it with high-field state of the art fMRI to provide truly sensitive measures of cerebral activity patterns during motor and cognitive tasks.

Significance of Functional Neuroimaging to Stroke Rehabilitation

Recovery is quite variable across stroke victims and this variability may be due, at least in part to differences in the extent to which a patient's initial disabilities are attributable to permanent damage versus potentially recoverable diaschisis. Continued refinement of the neuroimaging procedures described here should result in the ability to determine the extent to which an individual patient's disability is attributable to diaschisis. Neuroimaging of task activation provides somewhat more theoretical data on reorganizational processes and cerebral plasticity, but nevertheless should help ascertain which of the recovery mechanisms is most prominent within specific categories of stroke, leading to better intervention strategies.

Cerebrovascular disease, occurring in 500,000 people each year (Delisa, 1988) in the United States alone, represents a major health concern in this country. Due to the high incidence and the resulting chronic disabilities, stroke rehabilitation is recognized as a major concern of health care professionals (Ottenbacher & Jannell, 1993). Despite this recognition, the value of rehabilitation in stroke patients remains controversial (Anderson, 1990; Pedro-Cuesta, Widen-Holmquist, & Bach-y-Rita, 1992; Reding & McDowell, 1989; Dobkin, 1989). Presently, rehabilitation of stroke patients is composed of varying combinations of compensatory and facilitatory techniques. Compensatory training techniques emphasize attention to unaffected neuromuscular components to improve functional status. Facilitatory techniques attempt to promote or hasten the recovery of affected extremities to a normal movement pattern. Different facilitatory techniques exist (e.g., Brumstrom (Sawner & LaVigne, 1992), Bobath (Bobath, 1990), proprioceptive neuromuscular facilitation (Voss, Ionta, & Myers, 1985) that have varying emphases on the importance of assisting pathologically uninhibited spastic movement of muscle groups affected by a stroke in order to facilitate motor recovery. Despite the extensive variety of facilitation techniques used, studies have not been able to show a superiority of one technique over others in the rehabilitation of stroke patients (Kraft, Fitts, & Hammond, 1992; Dickstein, Hocherman, Pillar, & Shaham, 1986; Wagenaar, Meijer, & van Wieringen, 1990). Due to time constraints and concern for health care costs, rehabilitation of stroke patients appears to be shifting to a greater percentage use of compensatory techniques in an attempt to obtain a high enough functional level to allow the patient to return to the community earlier. However, it is unclear how the shift away from emphasis on facilitatory techniques is affecting long-term neurological and functional recovery. Part of the difficulty studies encounter in attempts to prove the value of stroke rehabilitation in general or the superiority of one therapeutic technique over another is due to the heterogeneity of stroke patients. Another area of difficulty is the lack of understanding of the processes of neurophysiological recovery from a stroke. The resolution of diaschisis is one theory of neurological recovery; reorganization in unaffected brain is another. These mechanisms are clearly not mutually exclusive; we have shown evidence for both in the data presented here.

Rationale for Rehabilitation Techniques and Patient Selection

It is possible that presence or absence of diaschisis has been a confounding variable in selection of treatment programs in studies that have compared facilitatory and compensatory techniques. Facilitatory techniques, applied either to affected limbs or cognitive operations, may be of greater benefit to patients with a significant diaschisis component. As an example, it is generally agreed that patients with global aphasia do not benefit from inpatient therapy techniques. However, patients with a large component of diaschisis in areas associated with language control may represent a subgroup with a greater prognosis for recovery that deserve facilitatory intervention.

Evidence that a functional deficit is rooted in permanent morphological damage and whose recovery appears to require cerebral reorganization would suggest the use of compensatory techniques, that is, an emphasis on alternate strategies to accomplish movement or cognitive operations affected by the stroke. Evidence for plasticity (reorganization of unaffected brain) can be confused with evidence for resolution of temporary damage, but the technologies described in this chapter provide the means to evaluate changes in baseline cerebral activity (resolution of diaschisis or other temporary damage) as well as evidence for true reorganization of intact brain. The extent to which each mechanism is primary can be identified in individual patients. Thus neuroimaging should provide a better understanding of the stroke recovery process and lead to rehabilitation strategies tailored to the individual patient's deficits.

Prognosis for Recovery

By being able to document diaschisis and show an association between neurological recovery and resolution of diaschisis, we hope to be able to advise patients and families earlier concerning chances for and extent of recovery. Neuroimaging activation studies also should eventually provide data on reorganizational plasticity potential in different forms of stroke. Improved ability to provide prognosis should assist patients and families in coping with the disabilities secondary to a stroke and assist in long-term planning for the disposition and needs of the patient. Accurate prediction of rehabilitation potential will become increasingly important when allocating scarce treatment resources.

ACKNOWLEDGMENTS Supported in part by grant R01 AG06432 to Dr. Deutsch and grant R01 HD32100 to Dr. Mountz from the National Institutes of Health.

References

Ackerman, R. H., Alpert, N. M., Correia, J. A., Finklestein, S., Davis, S. M., Kelley, R. E., Donnan, G. A., D'Alton, J. G., & Taveras, J. M. (1984). Positron imaging in ischemic stroke disease. *Annals of Neurology, 15*(Suppl.), S126–S130.

Anderson, T. P. (1990). Studies up to 1980 on stroke rehabilitation outcomes. *Stroke, 21*(Suppl. II), II-43–II-45.

Anger, H. O., Powell, M. R., van Dyke, D. C., Schaer, L. R., Fawwaz, R., & Yano, Y. (1967). Recent applications of the scintillation camera. *Strahlentherapie—Sonderbande, 65,* 70–93.

Astrup, J., Siesjo, B. K., & Symon, L. (1981). Thresholds in cerebral ischemia—The ischemic penumbra. *Stroke, 12,* 723–725.

Bandettini, P. A., Davis, T. L., Kwong, K. K., Fox, P. T., Jiang, A., Baker, J. R., Belliveau, J. W., Weisskoff, R. M., & Rosen, B. R. (1995). FMRI and PET demonstrate sustained blood oxygenation and flow enhancement during extended visual stimulation. *Abstracts of the Society for Magnetic Resonance Annual Meeting, 1995,* 453.

Baron, J. C. (1985). Positron tomography in cerebral ischemia: A review. *Neuroradiology, 27,* 509–516.

Bobath, B. (1990). *Adult hemiplegia evaluation and treatment* (3rd ed.). Heinemann Medical Books, Oxford. New York: Oxford University Press.

Bonte, F. J., Devous, M. D., Reisch, J. S., Ajmani, A. K., Weiner, M. F., Hom, J., & Tinter, R. (1989). The effect of acetazolamide on regional cerebral blood flow in patients with Alzheimer's disease or stroke as measured by SPECT. *Investigative Radiology, 24,* 99–103.

Buckner, R. L., Corbetta, M., Schatz, J., Raichle, M. E., & Petersen, S. E. (1996). Preserved speech abilities and compensation following prefrontal damage. *Proceedings of the National Academy of Sciences USA, 93,* 1249–1253.

Delisa, J. A. (Ed.). (1988). *Rehabilitation medicine principles and practice.* Philadelphia: Lippincott Raven.

Deutsch, G., Papanicolaou, A. C., Loring, D. W., & Eisenberg, H. M. (1985a). Left hemisphere blood flow during acoustic, phonetic and semantic target tasks. *Journal of Clinical and Experimental Neuropsychology, 7,* 632.

Deutsch, G., Papanicolaou, A. C., Loring, D. W., & Eisenberg, H. M. (1985b). CBF during tasks intended to differentially activate the cerebral hemispheres: New normative data and preliminary application in recovering stroke patients. *Journal of Cerebral Blood Flow and Metabolism, 7,* S306.

Deutsch, G., Bourbon, W. T., Papanicolaou, A. C., & Eisenberg, H. M. (1988). Visuospatial tasks compared via activation of regional cerebral blood flow. *Neuropsychologia, 26,* 445–452.

Deutsch, G., Halsey, J. H., Jr., & Harrell, L. E. (1991). Regional CO_2 reactivity of cortical blood flow in Alzheimer's disease. *Journal of Cerebral Blood Flow and Metabolism, 11*(Suppl. 2), S22.

Deutsch, G., Katholi, C. R., & Mountz, J. M. (1996a). The relationship of absolute rCBF activation response to age, gender and baseline flow. *NeuroImage, 3,* 575.

Deutsch, G., Mountz, J. M., Liu, H. G., & San Pedro, E. C. (1996b). Cerebrovascular stress tests in parenchymal versus vascular disease. *Journal of Nuclear Medicine, 37,* 88P.

Deutsch, G., Mountz, J. M., Katholi, C. R., Liu, H. G., & Harrell, L. E. (1997a). Regional stability of cerebral blood flow measured by repeated Tc-HMPAO SPECT: Implications for the study of state dependent change. *Journal of Nuclear Medicine, 38,* 6–13.

Deutsch, G., Mountz, J. M., Liu, H., Katholi, C. R., San Pedro, E., & Yester, M. (1997b). Mental rotation and phonological tasks investigated with a new xenon rCBF SPECT method. *NeuroImage, 5,* S-128.

Deutsch, G., Mountz, J. M., Liu, H. G., Sutor, R. J., & Roubin, G. S. (1997c). Xenon SPECT sensitivity to cerebrovascular status in baseline and diamox stress studies. *Journal of Cerebral Blood Flow and Metabolism, 17,* S-199.

Deutsch, G., Mountz, J. M., Twieg, D. B., Southwood, M. H., San Pedro, E. C., & Liu, H. G. (1998). Xenon SPECT, fMRI and FDG evidence for reorganization poststroke. *NeuroImage, 7, S-498*

Devous, M. D., Gong, W., Payne, J. K., & Harris, T. S. (1993). Comparison of technetium-99m-ECD to Xenon-133 SPECT in normal controls and in patients with mild to moderate regional cerebral blood flow abnormalities. *Journal of Nuclear Medicine, 34,* 754–761.

Dickstein, R., Hocherman, S., Pillar, T., & Shaham, R. (1986). Stroke rehabilitation three exercise therapy approaches. *Physical Therapy, 66,* 1233–1238.

Dobkin, B. H. (1989). Focused stroke rehabilitation programs do not improve outcome. *Archives of Neurology, 46,* 701–703.

Duncan, P. W., Probst, M., & Nelson, S. G. (1983). Reliability of the Fugl-Meyer assessment of sensorimotor recovery following cerobrovascular accident. *Physical Therapy, 63,* 1606–1610.

Feeney, D. M., & Baron, J. C. (1986). Diaschisis. *Stroke, 17,* 817–830.

Feldmann, M., Voth, E., Dressler, D., Henze, T., & Felgenhauer, K. (1990). 99mTc-Hexamethylpropylene amine oxime SPECT and X-ray CT in acute cerebral ischaemia. *Journal of Neurology, 237,* 475–479.

Fiorelli, M., Blin, J., Bakchine, S., Laplane, D., & Baron, J. C. (1991). PET studies of cortical diaschisis in patients with motor hemi-neglect. *Journal of Neurological Science, 104,* 135–142.

Freund, H. J. (1996, 21 June). Remapping the brain. *Science, 272,* 1754.

Ginsberg, M. D., Reivich, M., Giandomenico, A., & Greenberg, J. H. (1977). Local glucose utilization in acute focal cerebral ischemia: local dysmetabolism and diaschisis. *Neurology, 27,* 1042–1048.

Herold, S., Brown, M. M., Frackowiak, R. S. J., Mansfield, A. O., Thomas, D. J., & Marshall, J. (1988). Assessment of cerebral haemodynamic reserve: Correlation between PET parameters and CO_2 reactivity measured by the intravenous 133Xenon injection technique. *Journal of Neurology, Neurosurgery, and Psychiatry, 51,* 1045–1050.

Hetherington, H. P., Pan, J. W., Mason, G. F., Ponder, S. L., Twieg, D. B., Deutsch, G., Mountz, J. M., & Pohost, G. M. (1994). 2D Spectroscopic imaging of the human brain at 4.1T without field of view restriction. *Magnetic Resonance in Medicine, 32,* 530–534.

Kanno, I., Uemura, K., Higano, S., Murakami, M., Iida, H., Miura, S., Shishido, F., Inugami, A., & Sayami, I. (1988). Oxygen extraction fraction at maximally vasodilated tissue in the ischemic brain estimated from the regional CO_2 responsiveness measured by positron emission tomography. *Journal of Cerebral Blood Flow and Metabolism, 8,* 227–235.

Kinsbourne, M. (1971). The minor hemisphere as a source of aphasic speech. *Archives of Neurology, 25,* 302–306.

Kraft, G. H., Fitts, S. S., & Hammond, M. C. (1992). Techniques to improve function of the arm and hand in chronic hemiplegia. *Archives of Physical Medicine and Rehabilitation, 73,* 220–227.

Kwong, K., Belliveau, J. W., Chesler, D. A., Goldberg, I. E., Weisskoff, R. M., Poncelet, B. P., Kennedy, D. N., Hoppel, B. E., Cohen, M.S., Turner, R., Cheng, H. M., Brady, T. J., & Rosen, B. R. (1992). Dynamic magnetic resonance imaging of human brain activity during primary sensory stimulation. *Proceedings of the National Academy of Science USA, 89,* 5675–5679.

Lawrence, D. G., & Kuypers, H. G. J. M. (1968). The functional organization of the motor system in the monkey. I. The effects of bilateral pyramidal tract lesions. *Brain, 91,* 1–14.

Levine, R. L., Lagreze, H. L., Dobkin, J. A., Hanson, J. M., Satter, M. R., Rowe, B. R., & Nickles, R. J. (1989). Cerebral vasocapacitance and TIAs. *Neurology, 39,* 25–29.

Matsuda, H., Higashi, S., Kinuya, K., Tsuji, S., Nozaki, J., Sumiya, H., Hisada, K., & Yamashita, J. (1991). SPECT evaluation of brain perfusion reserve by the acetazolamide test using Tc-99m HMPAO. *Clinical Nuclear Medicine, 16,* 572–579.

Mountz, J. M. (1989). A method of analysis of SPECT blood flow image data for comparison with computed tomography. *Clinical Nuclear Medicine, 14,* 192–196.

Mountz, J. M. (1991). Quantification of the SPECT Brain scan. In L. M. Freeman (Ed.), *Nuclear medicine annual* (pp. 67–98). New York: Raven Press.

Mountz, J. M., Modell, J. G., Foster, N. L., DuPree, E. S., Ackermann, R. J., Petry, N. A., Bluemlein, L. A., & Kuhl, D. E. (1990). Prognostication of recovery following stroke using the comparison of CT and technetium-99m HM-PAO SPECT. *Journal of Nuclear Medicine 31,* 61–66.

Mountz, J. M., Deutsch, G., & Khan, S. H. (1993). An atlas of regional cerebral blood flow changes in stroke imaged by Tc-99m HMPAO SPECT with corresponding anatomic image comparison. *Clinical Nuclear Medicine, 18,* 1067–1082.

Mountz, J. M., Wilson, M. W., Wolff, C. G., Deutsch, G., & Harris, J. M. (1994a). Validation of a reference method for correlation of anatomic and functional brain images. *Computerized Medical Imaging and Graphics, 18,* 163–174.

Mountz, J. M., Zhang, B., Hong-Gang, L., & Inampudi, C. (1994b). A reference method for correlation of anatomic and functional brain images: Validation and clinical application. *Seminars in Nuclear Medicine, 24,* 256–271.

Mountz, J. M., Deutsch, G., Kuzniecky, R., & Rosenfeld, S. S. (1994c). Brain SPECT: 1994 update. In L. M. Freeman (Ed.), *Nuclear medicine annual 1994* (pp. 1–54). New York: Raven Press.

Mountz, J. M., San Pedro, E. C., Mason, G. F., Deutsch, G., & Hetherington, H. P. (1997). Diaschisis characterization in sub-acute stroke by combined rest and diamox rCBF brain SPECT and 4.1T 1H spectroscopy imaging. *Journal of Nuclear Medicine, 38,* 36P.

Muller, F., Kunesch, E., Binkofski, F., & Freund, H.-J. (1991). Residual sensorimotor functions in a patient after right sided hemispherectomy. *Neuropsychologia, 29,* 125–145.

Nudo, R. J., Wise, B. M., SiFuentes, F., & Milliken, G. W. (1996). Neural substrates for the effects of rehabilitative training on motor recovery after ischemic infarct. *Science, 272,* 1791–1794.

Ogawa, S., Lee, T. M., Kay, A. R., & Tank, D. W. (1990). Brain magnetic resonance imaging with contrast dependent on blood oxygenation. *Proceedings of the National Academy of Science USA, 87,* 9868–9872.

Ogawa, S., Menon, R. S., Tank, D. W., Kim, S. G., Merkle, H., Ellerman, J. M., & Ugurbil, K. (1993). Functional brain mapping by blood oxygenation level-dependant contrast magnetic resonance imaging. A comparison of signal characteristics with a biophysical model. *Biophysical Journal, 64,* 803–812.

Ohyama, M., Senda, M., Kitamura, S., Ishii, K., Mishina, M., & Terashi, A. (1996). Role of the nondominant hemisphere and undamaged area during word repetition in poststroke aphasics. *Stroke, 27,* 897–903.

Ottenbacher, K. J., & Jannell, S. (1993). The results of clinical trials in stroke rehabilitation research. *Archives of Neurology, 50,* 37–44.

Papanicolaou, A. C., Moore, B., Deutsch, G., Levin, H. S., & Eisenberg, H. M. (1988). Evidence for right hemisphere involvement in recovery from aphasia. *Archives of Neurology, 45,* 1025–1029.

Pedro-Cuesta, J., Widen-Holmquist, L., & Bach-y-Rita, P. (1992). Evaluation of stroke rehabilitation by randomized controlled studies: A review. *Neurologica Scandinavia, 86,* 433–439.

Raynaud, C., Rancurel, G., Samson, Y., & Baron, J. C. (1987). Pathophysiologic study of chronic infarcts: The importance of the periinfarct area. *Stroke, 18,* 21–29.

Reding, M. J., & McDowell, F. H. (1989). Focused stroke rehabilitation programs improve outcome. *Archives of Neurology, 46,* 700–701.

Rogers, R. L., Meyer, J. S., Mortel, K. F., Mahurin, R. K., & Thornby, J. (1985). Age-related reductions in cerebral vasomotor reactivity and the law of initial value: A 4-year prospective longitudinal study. *Journal of Cerebral Blood Flow and Metabolism, 5,* 79–85.

Sawner, K., & LaVigne, J. (Eds.). (1992). *Brunnstrom's movement therapy in hemiplegia: A neurophysiological approach* (2nd ed.). Philadelphia: Lippincott Raven.

Seitz, R. J., & Freund, H.-J. (1997). Plasticity of the human motor cortex. *Advances in Neurology, 73,* 321–333.

Seitz, R. J., Huang, Y., Knorr, U., Tellmann, L., Herzog, H., & Freund, H. J. (1995). Large-scale plasticity of the human motor cortex. *NeuroReport, 6,* 742–744.

Taub, E. (1995). Increasing behavioral plasticity following central nervous system damage in monkeys and man: A method with potential application to human developmental motor disability. In B. Julesz & I. Kovacs (Eds.), *Maturational windows and adult cortical plasticity* (pp. 201–215). Redwood City, CA: Addison-Wesley.

Vaughan, J. T., Hetherington, H. P., Otu, J. O., Pan, J. W., & Pohost, G. M. (1994). High frequency volume coils for clinical NMR imaging and spectroscopy. *Magnetic Resonance in Medicine, 32,* p. 206–218.

von Monakow, C. (1969). Diaschisis. In K. H. Pribram (Ed.), *Brain and behaviour I: Mood states and mind* (pp. 27–36). Baltimore: Penguin.

Voss, D. E., Ionta, M. K., & Myers, B. J. (1985). *Proprioceptive neuromuscular facilitation* (3rd ed.). Philadelphia: Harper & Row.

Wagenaar, R. C., Meijer, O. G., & van Wieringen, P. C. W. (1990). The functional recovery of stroke: A comparison between neuro-developmental treatment and the Brunnstrom method. *Scandinavian Journal of Rehabilitation Medicine, 22,* 1–8.

Weiller, C., Ramsay, S. C., Wise, R. S., Friston, K. J., & Frackowiak, R. S. J. (1993). Individual patterns of functional reorganization in human cerebral cortex after capsular infarction. *Annals of Neurology, 33,* 181–189.

Yudd, A. P. , Van Heertum, R. L., & Masdeu, J. C. (1991). Interventions and functional brain imaging. *Seminars in Nuclear Medicine, 21,* 153–158.

II

Neuropsychological Assessment

4

Nature, Applications, and Limitations of Neuropsychological Assessment following Traumatic Brain Injury

MURIEL D. LEZAK

Introduction

Neuropsychological assessment can provide information about the personality, behavior, mental abilities, learned skills, and rehabilitation potential of persons who have sustained traumatic brain injury (TBI). It is a psychological assessment procedure in that its primary data come from behavioral observations and its goal is to enhance understanding of behavior. It is neuropsychological in its use of specialized examination techniques requiring an educated appreciation of brain–behavior relationships and in its goal of elucidating behavioral manifestations of brain functions, both impaired and preserved. It is an assessment procedure in that it involves a comprehensive evaluation of the subject by means of a process that integrates test and other examination findings with information from other sources (e.g., data from the individual's social, educational, employment, and psychological history). Neuropsychological assessments will usually include direct observations of the subject but may or may not involve formal (i.e., standardized, published) tests (Lezak, 1995). The information obtained through neuropsychological assessment may help clinicians and research scientists to understand the nature of the underlying insult to the brain. In making apparent the neuropsychological competencies and deficiencies of TBI patients and the course of their neuropsychological functioning, appropriate assessments can guide the rehabilitation process.

MURIEL D. LEZAK • Department of Neurology, Oregon Health Sciences University, Portland, Oregon 97201.

International Handbook of Neuropsychological Rehabilitation, edited by Christensen and Uzzell.
Kluwer Academic/ Plenum Publishers, New York, 2000.

Neuropsychology's Tools

History

For neuropsychological assessment purposes, the relevant premorbid history for a TBI patient may include psychosocial information such as educational experiences, marriage dates and duration, psychosexual development and activity, vocational and avocational interests and achievements, and leisure pursuits (Sloan & Ponsford, 1995; Sohlberg & Mateer, 1989). The medical history, particularly that concerning the presenting condition, frequently contributes significantly to an understanding of the patient's neuropsychological status (Silver, Hales, & Yudofsky, 1997). Moreover, it is not unusual for medical problems predating the onset of the presenting condition to play an important role in its manifestations and the patient's reactions to the current disorder(s) as well. Thus, the medical history is important both for detailing the circumstances, nature, and course of the TBI and for indicating what premorbid medical circumstances may or may not be complicating the neurological picture.

For understanding the problems and needs of TBI patients, however, the importance of some kinds of historical information may vary with the severity of the injury. The psychosocial history of the most severely impaired patients, those who have lost much of their sense of identity and personhood, may not add greatly to comprehending their present neuropsychological status and needs: Patients who have minimal access to their past histories are less likely to appreciate their losses than those with keen awareness of their past, and examination evidence of the prior experiences and achievements of severely impaired patients may be scanty at best (Prigatano, 1991). In marked contrast are the mildly impaired TBI patients who can no longer perform complex tasks quickly or work in a noisy environment but who retain most premorbid abilities and personal characteristics along with an acute appreciation of premorbid competencies and goals. For these patients, knowledge of the psychosocial history in its broadest sense is necessary to understand their losses, as such an understanding is imperative if the examiner wants to comprehend their emotional reactions and how these reactions may be affecting other aspects of their neuropsychological status (Binder, 1986). Of course, when planning for all patients capable of benefitting from retraining and/or returning to work, educational and work history must be obtained, and information about premorbid social behavior and activities will also be useful.

Records

Whether or not the patient can report on past experiences, records from schools, employment, from military service, to name the most usual record sources, may flesh out or render more realistic the patient's self-report or information obtained from interested friends and relatives. Not only can these records be useful in themselves, but discrepancies between patient or family (e.g., parents, spouse) reports of achievements and what the actual records show can be a valuable source of information about the patient or about family expectations and pressures on the patient and the rehabilitation team.

Examination Observations

Observation Is the Foundation of All Psychological Assessment

Ultimately, all historical data and the content of records issue from someone's observation of the person being assessed. Most usually, more immediate observations make up the bulk of the assessment data.

Indirect Observations. These include current reports about the patient that do not come from formal assessments. They may be given by caregivers, employers, or family members. Sometimes invaluable observations are provided by receptionists or patient attendants who observe or work with patients in situations in which patients are not self-conscious about being observed. Other kinds of indirect observations include patient productions such as letters they have written or pictures they have drawn (Fig. 1).

Direct Observations: Informal. Some of the most valuable data acquired in a neuropsychological examination consist of observations made during the interview and as patients respond to the formal examination procedures. These observations provide qualitative information having to do with *how* the patient goes about answering questions, discussing issues, or solving problems, or *whether* the patient responds appropriately at all (see pp. 70, 71 below).

Direct Observations: Psychological Tests. A test is a set of observations made under standardized conditions for the purpose of measuring a characteristic or set of characteristics with dimensional or multivariate features. The key word in distinguishing observations made with tests from other (informal) observations is *standardized*; that is, test administration follows defined procedures that are replicable and that permit development of normative data. Standardization of procedures confines the observations obtained by testing to the features defined for testing (e.g., the number of words recalled from a word list; the time taken to draw a line through a set of numbered circles). Tests of behavioral phenomena, conditions, capacities, or states are *psychological* tests. Because of the standardization requirements, psychological testing rarely involves observations made in the natural setting.

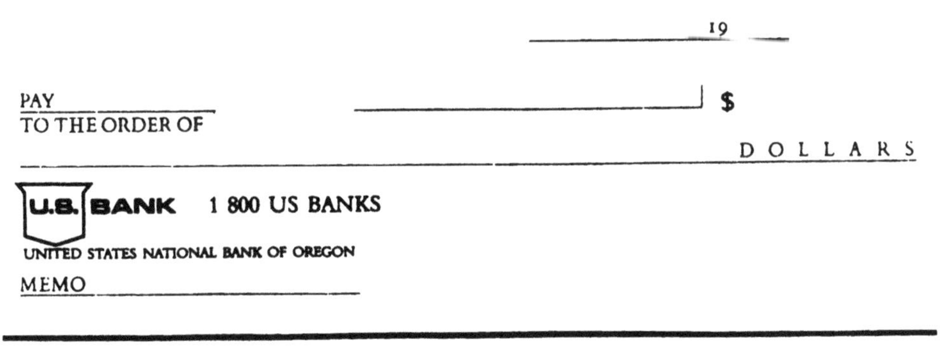

FIGURE 1. This 78-year-old retired history professor sustained head injuries when knocked down by a car as he crossed a street. Prior to the accident he had developed a mild hand tremor; following the accident the tremor had become more severe: (a) signature written shortly before the accident; (b) signature 6 months after the accident.

Why Test? Since psychological testing is typically conducted in artificial situations (e.g., a clinic office or testing laboratory), the examination findings may be biased, inapplicable to the patient's situation or needs, and thus a waste of time; or worse, the data may under- or overestimate the patient's capacities, resulting in poor and even damaging treatment, particularly if they are simply confined to scores and not enriched by qualitative observations:

> A 30-year-old man, who had sustained moderately severe brain damage in a car accident at age 16, had to live with his parents for several years, since every attempt at supporting himself independently had failed. He was examined by a psychologist who had had little experience with head trauma patients. On documenting Wechsler test scores in the 14 to 16 standard score range (i.e., percentile range, 91 to 98), he advised the parents to encourage their son to develop a career consistent with his abilities as indicated by test scores, rather than build wooden bird houses in the basement of the family home, an occupation the mother had found for her son.
>
> What the psychologist did not realize was that this man had significant frontal lobe damage, resulting in severely compromised abilities to initiate complex activities, plan for goals, or appreciate the subtleties of social conventions. Reliance on test scores alone led the psychologist to an inappropriate conclusion and recommendations that did not help the patient and confused the parents, adding to their already guilt-ridden sense of having somehow failed their son. When examined by a neuropsychologist who tested planning and judgment abilities and evaluated *how* the patient performed on traditional psychometric tasks, the patient's socially crippling deficits became immediately apparent. He was assisted in obtaining work requiring minimal judgment but a variety of technical skills, and finally could keep a job.

However, when the examiner takes into account the qualitative aspects of the test performances and includes in the examination those tasks and questions that call on the abilities most likely to be compromised by TBI, which are frequently the abilities necessary for social independence, the formal neuropsychological examination can facilitate the understanding and treatment of the TBI patient in three ways:

1. Important information is gained rapidly. Any trained observer who can spend several days with a TBI patient who has sustained relatively subtle impairment of executive abilities will be able to provide a fairly accurate description of what the patient can and cannot do spontaneously. However, it is uncommon for examiners to have the luxury of several days of observation time, or to have enough access to close and knowledgeable observers of the patient to be able to obtain a reasonably accurate picture of what the patient can and cannot do. A neuropsychologist who knows what to look for and how to do the examination can usually develop a fairly accurate description of the patient's behavior, treatment potential, and education/career prospects in a few hours.

2. In addition, a formal neuropsychological examination can elicit a practically accurate description of the patient's cognitive strengths and weaknesses, relatively free of observer bias, as is necessary for treatment and career planning. Excepting patients who are grossly impaired, it is typically not possible to describe a patient's cognitive status accurately without using standardized and normed test instruments. This is the case for cognitively intact persons, which is why testing is performed throughout the school years. It is even more relevant for TBI patients who may have attentional deficits, executive disorders, and/or memory problems that obscure their cognitive strengths when observed informally. For example, Gronwall, Wrightson, and Waddell (1990) point out that,

> There should be a system . . . where people who are likely to be at special risk after a mild head injury can be screened. . . . [O]lder people, as well as students and those who are in demanding jobs, should be referred for assessment of memory, concentration, and other problems that can follow closed head injury before they get back to work or school. (p. 94)

3. Moreover, because TBI is not a static condition, particularly when the patient has had the advantage of good treatment or the disadvantages of neglect, formal testing—and only formal testing—can document behavioral changes at a level of practical accuracy and in terms of their statistical (i.e., better than chance) significance. It thus enables patients and other interested persons to track patient progress or regression by comparing performances on the same behaviors (e.g., cognitive abilities, executive functions, personality and emotional characteristics) at different times. Without a formal assessment program, treatment effects or the impact of various social conditions can only be roughly estimated.

Integrating Assessment Data. Background information (history, reports) and descriptive examination observations provide the context for interpreting test scores. With this information, the examiner can develop an integrated picture of patients' current neuropsychological functioning, of their premorbid memories, skills, attitudes, and accomplishments, and how their past contributes to their present functioning and potential and may affect their future adaptation and accomplishments.

Theory and Practice of Neuropsychological Assessment

Dimensions of Behavior

The three dimensions of behavior are cognition, emotion–motivation, and the executive functions. Cognition concerns the information handling aspects of behavior, which include the acquisition of information (perception), its storage (memory), the processing of acquired and/or stored information (thinking, reasoning), and resulting actions (speaking, writing, building). Although conceptually separable, the inextricable linkage between emotion and motivation becomes evident when brain damage affects the emotion–motivation system, as changes in emotional capacity or control inevitably are paralleled by complementary motivational alterations. Executive functions have to do with whether activities are generated at all and how people go about their activities, including whether judgment is used, and if so, how appropriate it is. The executive functions include the capacity for volition, planning abilities, whether and how goals are carried out, and the self-regulating behavior necessary for effective activity (Lezak, 1982). In addition, two mental activity variables are not cognitive functions in themselves but provide the preconditions for self-serving, productive behavior: (1) attentional functions (on which cognitive efficiency depends), and (2) the level of awareness or consciousness.

A comprehensive neuropsychological examination will take all these aspects of behavior into account. Examination goals include identifying the patient's strengths and potentials and also the problem areas that either can benefit from remediation or may interfere with the remediation process or both.

Contributions of Tests

Formal tests provide information on mental abilities, learned skills, cognitive and executive functions, and on emotional status and personality characteristics. Formal tests generate this information in the form of scores or standardized classifications or categories (Anastasi, 1988). In addition, formal tests, because they are administered in a standardized manner, offer the almost unique opportunity of observing patient behavior in situations in which what are typical or usual responses is well known. Thus, deviations from the usual or expected pattern of response to a particular test may provide insights into the patient's behavioral repertoire or social understandings that may not be obtainable elsewhere.

> A 54-year-old woman sustained a mild head injury when her car ploughed into a car crossing in front of her. On several tests of immediate auditory span her performances were within normal limits. On a working memory test (consonant trigrams [Stuss *et al.,* 1985]) she performed at a borderline level. This test requires the subject to count backward from a given number. When counting backward (the interference task on the working memory test), she miscounted or lost her place several times (e.g., "181–179–176–172–169–168"; "82–81–87–181–182"; "50–58–57"). She also had difficulty performing serial subtractions. Her problems with counting backward coupled with several other indicators of difficulty with mental tracking helped to document a significant problem in this area, although the backward counting errors could not be taken into account by the scoring system.

Unscorable but distinctive deficits may show up on virtually any task given the patient:

> A 49-year-old university-educated high school instructor in automotive repairs had sustained a head injury in the Vietnam war when the helicopter in which he was riding suddenly dropped 1000 feet, propelling the top of his head up against the roof of the vehicle. Ten years later he sought help for complaints of memory deficit, but on formal testing his learning ability was excellent and he displayed no retrieval problems. He achieved a score at the 75th percentile on Raven's Progressive Matrices, which he had answered at his leisure. However, when he returned the test, he had completed only the first 48 of the 60 items (with no errors, hence his high score), leaving the last column of answer spaces untouched. He was surprised when this was brought to his attention. This lapse helped clarify his complaint of memory problems as due to impaired prospective memory. Again, no scoring procedure was available for documenting this important information, but it was not needed.

Kinds of Tests

Categorization by Functions Examined

Tests can be categorized in at least several ways. For neuropsychological purposes, it is often useful to identify tests in terms of the neuropsychological functions they examine (e.g., Sohlberg & Mateer, 1989; Trexler, Webb, & Zappala, 1994).

Cognitive Functions

Most of the tests that neuropsychologists give examine one or more of the cognitive functions directly. Most of these tests involve more than one function, and thus require a neuropsychologically sophisticated interpretation of a patient's performance: For example, many tests of visual memory examine both drawing ability and visual recall. In addition, appropriate examination of the cognitive functions always includes the study of attentional functions, either directly (as when requesting the subject to recite a number series or spell a word in reverse) or indirectly (as on tests of oral arithmetic, when impaired attention makes it difficult for a mathematically competent person to grasp, retain, or mentally juggle the arithmetic problem efficiently [see Lezak, 1995, pp. 136, 642–643]). Tests are available for examining all major aspects of cognition: sensation and perception, memory, thinking and reasoning, and tests of expressive abilities such as speaking, writing, drawing, and construction.

Executive Functions

Some part of the appraisal of executive functions will rely on qualitative aberrations appearing on the standardized cognitive and emotional status tests, the patient's responses in an open-ended interview, and the patient's examination behavior generally. A few tests with normative data provide direct measurements of particular aspects of executive functioning (Christensen, 1979; Lezak, 1993; Shallice & Berger, 1991). Those executive functions most amenable to formal examination and measurement are planning (e.g., mazes tests), ability to generate responses (e.g., word and design fluency tests), mental flexibility (sorting tasks), and ability to develop a structured response to an open-ended situation. Self-monitoring and self-correcting should be documented in the course of every neuropsychological examination, and while normative data are not available, this documentation is important in appraising self-awareness and active responsiveness aspects of executive functioning.

Emotional Status

Many tests and self-descriptive inventories are available to measure capacities for emotional behavior and the patient's current emotional state. Some are marketed as personality tests, others inquire into specific aspects of emotionality, such as anxiety or depression. Tests that have been normed on medically sound psychiatric populations present significant problems when given to brain injured patients, as their responses can be easily misinterpreted if the examiner is not fully conversant with the nature of the test norms, the content of the test, and the problems in attempting to impose psychiatric criteria onto neurologically impaired patients (e.g., the Minnesota Multiphasic Personality Inventory [Butcher *et al.*, 1989; Hathaway & McKinley, 1951]). This problem tends to be exacerbated by the use of computerized administration and interpretation methods, as the computer programs have not been adapted for the neuropsychologist's patients (e.g., see Matarazzo, 1986, for some of the problems that apply to computer interpretations generally). A second problem inherent in lengthy questionnaire type tests that can affect neurologically impaired patients lies in visually or grammatically complex formats, which can result in unintended responses by some cognitively compromised patients (Burke, Smith, & Imhoff, 1989; Krug, 1967).

Yet it is very useful to acquire documentation on patients' views of their emotional status at the time of examination. This information adds an important dimension to the context in which the performance of cognitive and executive functions can be best understood and can aid in determining what kind of assistance with emotional problems may help the patient. To this end, reasonably short inventories with appropriately clear formats are available to inquire into such issues as mood states, sense of well-being, and psychosocial adaptation. The knowledgeable neuropsychologist will know which of these will be most appropriate for which patients and for what purposes and will bring them into the examination selectively.

Categorization by Freedom of Response

Another difference among tests involves the degree to which the test is structured. A highly structured test limits subject responses. A good example of this would be a personality questionnaire that allows only "yes" or "no" responses, or a set of arithmetic problems for which only one answer is correct. A little more leeway is allowed in tests calling for a description or interpretation for which several ways of responding are acceptable. These tests

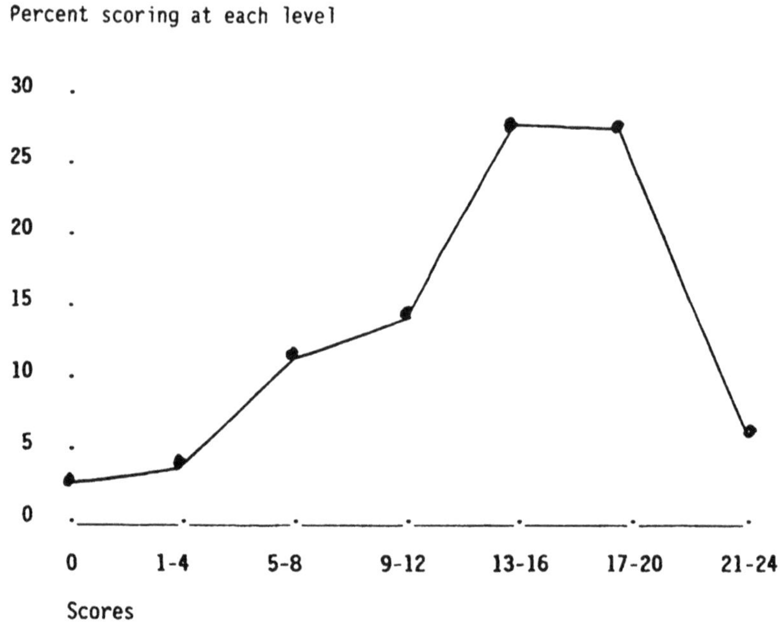

FIGURE 2. Serial Digit Learning (S9). Distribution of scores by percentages for 178 subjects (education range, 12–16; age range, 16–64).

are scored so that the most apt responses receive the highest score. Copying designs with pen or pencil is an example of an examination technique that not only has a range of acceptable scores (i.e., scores within the *average* range or better) but also provides the examiner opportunities to evaluate differences in *how* the drawing is approached (e.g., bit by bit in a piecemeal fashion? overall outline without regard to internal structure?) or how it is laid out on the page (too small or too large? cramped into a corner or stuck against a page edge? overlapping other drawings?).

Categorization by Data Handling and Reporting

Tests also differ in the kinds of data they generate and how these data can best be reported (Cronbach, 1984; Sattler, 1988). Tests involving complex and learned abilities (e.g., block construction, vocabulary, arithmetic) can produce relatively fine-grained scores ranging on a continuum. When these tests are given to an appropriately large sample of normal subjects, the scores tend to distribute into a classic bell-shaped curve, providing a set of scores that lend themselves to parametric statistical operations. These scores may then be converted into standard scores that enable reliable comparisons between scores obtained by a person in a single examination. Use of standard scores also permits comparisons between scores obtained over time to evaluate change (improvement, treatment effects, deterioration) and comparisons with normative or control populations.

Tests involving few functions or unlearned capacities (e.g., auditory span, finger-tapping rate, visuomotor tracking) are more likely to assume a nonparametric score distribution (see Fig. 2) (see also the discussion of the application of nonparametric statistics in clinical practice when distributions are not normal in Capitani, 1997). Practically, these distributions yield only three meaningful score categories: *within normal limits*, *borderline* (to normal limits), and *defective* (or impaired). For many of these tests, tables are available for converting raw scores into percentiles providing more refined data, but statistical transformations and evaluations must be made with caution.

Common Assessment Problems with Brain Damage

Typically, the neuropsychologist wants to see how patients perform at their best. Yet brain damage frequently compromises capacities required for giving a best performance or comprises the performance indirectly by affecting the patient's physiological state.

Attentional Deficits

Attentional problems can interfere with effective performance in a number of ways (Sloan & Ponsford, 1995): Patients with a reduced auditory span may mishear problems and thus produce an erroneous answer that belies their actual ability. This problem occurs frequently when giving oral arithmetic problems. For example, when asked questions of the type: "If you buy eight 3-cent stamps and give the clerk a half-dollar, how much change will you receive," these patients are likely to say "76 cents," as they performed the task correctly but omitted the "half." Errors such as this should alert the examiner to a possible problem with auditory span, in which case they need to test for it directly (with sentence repetition type tests) and, if the problem is present, to speak slowly and in short phrases. Other attentional problems include difficulty with mental tracking, which also tends to show up on oral arithmetic. These patients will confuse elements of what they heard and may require several repetitions of a problem. Their ability to solve the problem can usually be demonstrated when given paper and pencil. Distractibility also makes patients vulnerable to errors. These patients lose their train of thought or their place on a page when a phone rings or a door slams. Appropriate assessment requires a second opportunity to perform the interrupted task.

Memory Disorders

Memory impairments can also interfere with effective test performance (Sohlberg & Mateer, 1989). Besides the obvious compromise created by inability to recall information accurately for more than a few minutes, if at all, more subtle deficits can also obscure patients' potential.

Defective Working Memory

Defective working memory (the ability to keep something in mind while concentrating momentarily on something else) may appear as loss of set; that is, in the course of responding to the task patients forget the instructions. This problem can show up particularly when a patient is performing a series of items according to instructions given at the beginning of the test. For example, when asked to tell what is missing from a set of pictures with a missing part, these patients may respond correctly for the first five or ten items, but then begin telling what is "wrong" rather than what is "missing." In these instances, the examiner can ask the patient to repeat the instructions to determine whether they were actually forgotten. If forgotten, the examiner can then repeat them. In this process, the examiner will have also acquired useful information about the patient's practical memory. On some tests, vulnerability to loss of set is one of the characteristics being examined; some scoring systems for the Wisconsin Card Sorting Test even score for this problem (Heaton *et al.*, 1993).

Defective Retrieval

This is a very common problem among brain injured persons, and one that appears and increases with aging (Goodglass, 1980). It appears most typically as inability to recall verbal information, both old information, such as the capital of France, and recent information given in the course of a verbal learning test. Yet, when given cues or a recognition format, these subjects correctly identify the answers, demonstrating that they had stored the information. Thus it is important when examining for learning and memory to provide subjects who have difficulty with recall with a cuing system or recognition format (e.g., see the *WAIS-R NI* [Kaplan, Fein, Morris, & Delis, 1991]). Without this, the examiner cannot determine the nature of the recall problem.

Fatigue

Many TBI patients fatigue easily and, when fatigued, their performance level drops (Gronwall *et al.*, 1990). Some of these patients, particularly in the first few months after injury, will begin showing signs of fatigue after only an hour or two of testing. With fatigue, response speed drops, concentration weakens, failure rate increases, and self-aware patients may experience the examination as threatening to self-esteem and a painful reminder of their cognitive deficits. Examining patients beyond their stamina limit runs the risk of making them antagonistic to future examinations and enhancing any depressive reactions that may already be developing.

Optimal versus Realistic Conditions

For most neuropsychological examination purposes, the examiner strives to provide conditions that will allow patients to perform at their very best, for only then can a useful understanding of patient strengths and weaknesses be obtained. Moreover, a best-possible performance usually results in at least some scores at levels at or near where they would have been premorbidly. When highest levels are documented, then the extent of deficit can be realized for those functions that have been adversely affected. This comparison permits the examiner to appreciate the losses the patient has sustained and to guage the patient's self-awareness vis-à-vis these losses. Thus, by virtue of optimal examination conditions, the examiner can obtain information about what functions need remediation or would benefit from compensatory training. Under optimal conditions the examiner can also determine what functions can be utilized to aid the rehabilitation process, and how realistic the patient is about his or her losses (Prigatano, 1991).

On the other hand, conditions in which patients are held to time constraints, examined for periods of time consistent with normal work schedules, or in a noisy worklike setting can be useful in determining whether the patient is ready to return to the workplace or the classroom, or what kinds of changes would be required to facilitate this return. For this latter evaluation, a comparison between optimal and realistic conditions can demonstrate some of the problems that could arise in a classroom or on the job and what steps are needed to ameliorate them.

Putting Assessment to Work for the Patient

Whenever possible and to whatever extent possible, examination findings must be given to patients in as constructive a manner as possible. When the examiner does not have much good news for a TBI patient, it is still possible to emphasize residual capacities and skills before indicating what areas would benefit from retraining or learning of compensatory techniques. The skilled examiner appreciates that patients whose capacity for self-awareness and abstract conceptualization has been compromised will not be able to comprehend some of their most important deficits. This self-knowledge may come only over time with skilled intervention in a sophisticated rehabilitation program. However, most patients will be aware that something is amiss, and most are relieved to understand what it is, and that it is not "craziness."

Whenever possible these findings should be given to the patient with significant family member(s) present so that they too can understand the problems with which the patient has had to cope. In some situations the family needs to hear information that the patient may not be ready to tolerate, and then a family or caregiver meeting can be arranged. In short, the maximum possible use should be made of examination information: The neuropsychological assessment is not for the purpose of making a record or merely for the purpose of advising clinical staff, but rather it is information about the patient and for the patient. When used wisely, it can greatly enhance rehabilitation efforts as well as the quality of life for patient and family.

Three Practical Assessment Rules

The following rules presuppose a patient-focused examination in which the purpose of the examination is to gain clinically and practically relevant information that can be used to treat the patient as effectively as possible. Examinations that simply generate a set of descriptive numbers or unquestioningly and rigidly follow procedures defined by test developers are out of place in the clinical rehabilitation setting. The former kind of examination may occasionally be necessary when legal issues are in dispute; the latter may be required when gathering research data. Neither provides the multidimensional, in-depth, and individualized information each patient requires. Thus, these three rules:

1. *Treat each patient as an individual.* No two TBI patients will be alike, even though many will share similar patterns of competencies and deficits. Not only must each examination be individualized to take into account testable strengths and weaknesses, treatment possibilities, and reasonable long-term goals, but the examination must be experienced by the patient, insofar as possible, as a personalized inquiry in which his or her interests are foremost.
2. *Think about what you are doing.* At each step in the examination, that is, at each test item being administered and at each interview question and discussion, the examiner needs to question the appropriateness of the question or item, whether—and if so, what—further development of that particular issue or ability is needed, and what other directions the examination should take.
3. *Control the examination to enhance understanding of the patient while minimizing negative examination experiences.* The examiner, not the test developer, is in charge of the examination. It is up to the examiner to decide whether all the tests in a battery are necessary, whether some are mostly redundant for this particular patient, or

whether some other test will bring out the needed information more effectively or less tiresomely. The examiner can also decide at what level to begin testing and when to stop, using clinical experience, knowledge of the tests and the functions they examine, and sensitivity to the patient being examined.

When the goal of assessment is the identification and description of the patient's competencies and deficits, attitudes, and emotional capacities that are relevant for rehabilitation, tests and the testing procedures become just one of the means to achieve this goal. The examiner who can use interview procedures and test material creatively, flexibly, and appropriately will be able to obtain maximally useful information with minimal patient distress. The neuropsychological examination should not be a frightening, demeaning, or exhausting experience, but rather works best when the examiner enables the patient to be an interested coparticipant in this search for understanding.

References

Anastasi, A. (1988). *Psychological testing* (6th ed.). New York: Macmillan.

Binder, L. M. (1986). Persisting symptoms after mild head injury: A review of the postconcussive syndrome. *Journal of Clinical and Experimental Neuropsychology, 8,* 323–346.

Burke, J. M., Smith, S. A., & Imhoff, C. L. (1989). The response styles of post-acute brain-injured patients on MMPI. *Brain Injury, 3,* 35–40.

Butcher, J. N., Dahlstrom, W. G., Graham, J. R., Tellegen, A., & Kaemmer, B. (1989). *Minnesota Multiphasic Personality Inventory-2: Manual for Administration and Scoring.* Minneapolis: Univeristy of Minnesota Press.

Capitani, E. (1997). Normative data and neuropsychological assessment. Common problems in clinical practice and research. *Neuropsychological Rehabilitation, 7,* 295–309.

Christensen, A.-L. (1979). *Luria's neuropsychological investigation* (2nd ed.). Copenhagen: Munksgaard.

Cronbach, L. J. (1984). *Essentials of psychological testing* (4th ed.). New York: Harper & Row.

Goodglass, H. (1980). Disorders of naming following brain injury. *American Scientist, 68,* 647–655.

Gronwall, D., Wrightson, P., & Waddell, P. (1990). *Head injury. The facts.* Oxford, UK: Oxford University Press.

Hathaway, S. R., & McKinley, J. C. (1951). *The Minnesota Multiphasic Personality Inventory Manual* (Revised). New York: Psychological Corporation.

Heaton, R. K., Chelune, G. J., Talley, J. L., Kay, G. G., & Curtiss, G. (1993). *Wisconsin Card Sorting Test. Manual.* Odessa, FL: Psychological Assessment Resources.

Kaplan, E., Fein, D., Morris, R., & Delis, D. (1991). *The WAIS-RNI.* San Antonio, TX: The Psychological Corporation.

Krug, R. S. (1967). MMPI response inconsistency of brain damaged individuals. *Journal of Clinical Psychology, 23,* 366.

Lezak, M. D. (1982). The problem of assessing executive functions. *International Journal of Psychology, 17,* 281–297.

Lezak, M. D. (1993). Newer contributions to the neuropsychological assessment of executive functions. *Journal of Head Trauma Rehabilitation, 8,* 24–31.

Lezak, M. D. (1995). *Neuropsychological assessment* (3rd ed.). New York: Oxford University Press.

Matarazzo, J. D. (1986). Computerized clinical psychological test interpretation. Unvalidated plus all mean and no sigma. *American Psychologist, 41,* 14–24.

Prigatano, G. P. (1991). Disturbances of self-awareness of deficit after traumatic brain injury. In G. P. Prigatano & D. L. Schachter (Eds.), *Awareness of deficit after brain injury* (pp. 111–126). New York: Oxford University Press.

Sattler, J. M. (1988). *Assessment of children* (3rd ed.). San Diego: J. M. Sattler.

Shallice, T., & Burgess, P. (1991). Higher-order cognitive impairments and frontal lobe lesions in man. In H. S. Levin, H. M. Eisenberg, & A. L. Benton (Eds.), *Frontal lobe functions and dysfunction* (pp. 125–138). New York: Oxford University Press.

Silver, J. M., Hales, R. E., & Yudofsky, S. C. (1997). Neuropsychiatric aspects of traumatic brain injury. In S. C. Yudofsky & R. E. Hales (Eds.), *American Psychiatric Press textbook of psychiatry* (pp. 521–560). Washington, DC: American Psychiatric Press.

Sloan, S., & Ponsford, J. (1995). Assessment of cognitive difficulties following TBI. In J. Ponsford (Ed.), *Traumatic brain injury. Rehabilitation for everyday adaptive living* (pp. 65–102). Hove, UK: Lawrence Erlbaum.

Sohlberg, M. M., & Mateer, C. A. (1989). *Introduction to cognitive rehabilitation.* New York: Guilford Press.

Stuss, D. T., Ely, P., Hugenholtz, H., Richard, M. T., LaRochelle, S., Poirier, C. A., & Bell, I. (1985). Subtle neuropsychological deficits in patients with good recovery after closed head injury. *Neurosurgery, 17,* 41–47.

Trexler, L. A., Webb, P. M., & Zappala, G. (1994). Strategic aspects of neuropsychological rehabilitation. In A.-L. Christensen & B. P. Uzzell (Eds.), *Brain injuiry and neuropsychological rehabilitation* (pp. 99–124). Hillsdale, NJ: Lawrence Erlbaum.

5

The European Brain Injury Questionnaire

Patients' and Families' Subjective Evaluation of Brain-Injured Patients' Current and Prior to Injury Difficulties

GÉRARD DELOCHE, GEORGES DELLATOLAS, AND ANNE-LISE CHRISTENSEN

Introduction

The European Brain Injury Questionnaire (EBIQ) study reported here formed part of the 4-year BIOMED1 EU Concerted Action project entitled "European Standardized Computerized Assessment Procedure for the Evaluation and Rehabilitation of Brain-Damaged Patients." The project included nine groups focusing on assessment and rehabilitation in the traditional cognitive areas (i.e., memory, language, attention, visual neglect, etc.). Such a reductionist approach toward cognitive functioning was adopted in order to simplify the experimental protocols and designs, but it resulted in fractionating the study of persons with brain injury. To counter this, an "integration" work group was established by Professor Christensen, whose aim was to study emotional, personality, and social aspects of patients' daily lives, in combination with the consequences and sequelae of cognitive dysfunction. This international work group developed and researched a unified questionnaire for tapping the subjective experience of patients across these areas.

The EBIQ was administered to a large group ($n = 905$) of brain-injured patients and their close relatives. From the study, the main findings were the following: (1) responses from patients and their relatives showed very similar patterns in terms of the factor structure of the areas of patients' difficulties; and (2) relatives generally rated patients' difficulties as being

GÉRARD DELOCHE • CIRLEP and INSERM U472, F-51096 Reims Cedex, France. **GEORGES DELLATOLAS** • INSERM U169, F-94807 Villejuif Cedex, France. **ANNE-LISE CHRISTENSEN** • Center for Rehabilitation of Brain Injury, University of Copenhagen, 2300 Copenhagen S, Denmark.

International Handbook of Neuropsychological Rehabilitation, edited by Christensen and Uzzell. Kluwer Academic/ Plenum Publishers, New York, 2000.

more severe than did the patients themselves. Moreover, the validity of the questionnaire was shown by the elevated ratings of patients' difficulties, as compared to ratings obtained from a control group of non-brain-injured subjects (Teasdale *et al.*, 1997).

In France, the EBIQ questionnaire has been the source of a number of studies. Depending on the particular research objectives, different populations of subjects received distinct EBIQ versions (Deloche *et al.*, 1996). Regarding the difficulties of patients, data were collected on a group of 489 brain-injured subjects, and the questionnaire evaluating patients' difficulties was also completed by a close relative (465 cases) and by a clinician responsible for the patient (230 cases). A subgroup of 232 subjects out of the 489 patients also completed the questionnaire regarding their status prior to injury and the corresponding information was obtained from relatives in 215 cases. A group of 306 neurologically normal subjects have also received the EBIQ. This control group provided the reference norms for the preinjury status of brain-damaged patients.

In addition to presenting a description of the structure and content of the EBIQ questionnaire, the purpose of this chapter is twofold. First, the evaluations of patients' present difficulties, independently provided by patients themselves, relatives, and clinicians will be compared. The literature contains conflicting reports regarding the degree of agreement among the three perceptions. On the one hand, some authors have found similar patterns of symptoms most frequently indicated in patients' and relatives' reports (Oddy & Humphrey, 1978; Fordyce, Roueche, & Prigatano, 1983). On the other hand, some have suggested that there exist three different types of families: ones where patients and their relatives agree; ones where the relatives rate problems more highly than patients; and one where the reverse is true (Cavallo, Kay, & Ezrachi, 1992). The clinicians have been found to score aphasics' communicative difficulties higher than the spouses (Helmick, Watamori, & Palmer, 1976). The direct comparisons of data from the three points of view, recorded using the same EBIQ evaluation tool, should shed some light on these debated issues.

Our second purpose is to study the preinjury status of patients, as they view it now, and compare their responses to those of their relatives evaluating the same period of time. The question of changes in patients' cognitive, emotional, and social dimensions has generally been addressed only from one side: either the experience reported by the patients (Finset, Dyrnes, Krogstad, & Berstad, 1995), or the complaints expressed by their close relatives (Gray, Sheperd, McKinlay, Robertson, & Pentland, 1994). This issue deserves some clarification, since patients have been found to minimize their changes of temperament, whereas it is precisely such changes that relatives report as the main source of their burden (Fahy, Irving, & Millac, 1967). As a supplement to this approach, we will compare the preinjury status of patients to that currently reported by non-brain-injured "normal" subjects. By definition, patients were also normal prior to injury; therefore, the EBIQ profiles should logically be the same in the two groups. However, it is a clinically common phenomenon that patients and their relatives appear to idealize their lives prior to injury. It therefore might be the case that reports on the preinjury period would significantly differ from the expected normal level.

Method

The EBIQ Questionnaires

There were several kinds of methodological problems encountered in the development of the EBIQ questionnaire by the integration work group. Regarding its content, the scope had to be wide enough to encompass cognition, emotion, and social life. The questions were in part carefully selected and adapted from the Symptom Checklist (SCL-90-R) (Derogatis, 1983) and the Katz Adjustment Scales (KAS) (Hogarty & Katz, 1971). These psychiatric questionnaires could not be used directly with the brain-damaged patients because some questions have definitely different meanings for the two populations. For instance, feeling unsatisfied with one's own body is a symptom that does not convey the same information in the case of hemiplegic patients and in subjects showing psychiatric disorders. Other items were added from the activities of daily living (ADL) questionnaire used at Professor Christensen's Copenhagen center and others again were suggested by the members of the integration work group.

Taken together, the questions thus cover the broad areas of personal activities (e.g., needing to be reminded about personal hygiene); family activities (e.g., problems with household chores); economic activities (e.g., difficulties managing finances); social relationships (e.g., losing contact with friends); cognitive and executive functions (e.g., memory—trouble remembering things; attention—trouble concentrating; planning—being unable to plan activities; orientation in time and space—difficulty finding one's way in new surroundings; language and communication—difficulty participating in conversations); somatic factors (e.g., having sleep problems); depression (e.g., feeling hopeless about the future); obsessiveness (e.g., difficulty making decisions), and other dimensions. There are 66 questions in all (see Appendix). As can be seen, the first 63 concern patients' subjective experience (i.e., difficulties, feelings, reactions to their situations). The last three items are not included in the present study because they do not refer to patients' difficulties, but to difficulties that relatives themselves may have as a result of the situation.

Given that a significant proportion of patients had language comprehension disorders, the phrasing of questions was carefully controlled. Only very simple syntactical formulations were employed, and double negatives were particularly avoided. In order to bypass possible language production impairments, patients indicated their responses simply by pointing to a response panel. Three black circles were shown, increasing in size from left to right. Each circle symbolized a different level of difficulties experienced by patients with respect to the particular question area. The quantification of difficulties was: 1 = not at all, 2 = a little, and 3 = a lot, for the small, medium, and large circles, respectively.

In addition to the EBIQ administered to the patients, two other strictly parallel versions of the questionnaire were developed. Both aimed at collecting information on patients' difficulties on the same 63 questions, but one from the point of view of close relatives and the other from that of responsible clinicians. Finally, the 63 questions of the patients' form were also administered to non-brain-injured control subjects for the purpose of the EBIQ standardization.

Populations

The group of 489 brain-injured subjects in France comprised adult patients engaged in some type of rehabilitation. They were drawn from diverse establishments, mainly rehabilitation facilities and hospital departments. About two thirds of the patients were male. This gender ratio discrepancy might be due to the high proportion of aphasics in the sample, this being a consequence of the number of speech therapists having collaborated to the study (see below). Demographic, medical, and neuropsychological information concerning the patients' status at the time of testing is shown in Table 1.

Most cases (47% of the total) were outpatients attending neuropsychological and/or motor rehabilitation departments in hospitals; other patients received treatments from speech therapists, physiotherapists, and/or psychologists working either in their private offices (31%) or visiting patients at home (22%). Rehabilitation was either speech therapy (53%), physiotherapy

TABLE 1. Demographic and Clinical Information on the 489 Brain-Damaged Patients

Gender
- Males: 64.6%
- Females: 35.4%

Age (years)
- 17–30: 19.9%
- 31–40: 14.5%
- 41–50: 17.8%
- 51–60: 17.8%
- 61–70: 14.7%
- 71–80: 10.8%
- 81–93: 4.5%

Education level
- Low: 15%
- Intermediate: 51.4%
- High: 33.6%

Employment postinjury
- None: 88.8%
- Yes: 11.2%

Marital status
- Partners living together: 64.2%
- Others: 35.8%

Time since injury
- 1–6 months: 13%
- 7 months–1 year: 18.3%
- 13 months–2 years: 25.2%
- 25 months–23 years: 43.5%

Etiology[a]
- CVA: 61.7%
- TBI: 28.1%
- Others: 10.2%

Lesion side
- Left: 64.6%
- Right: 16.5%
- Bilateral: 18.9%

Aphasia
- Yes: 68%
- No: 32%

Attention disorders
- Yes: 51.1%
- No: 49.9%

Memory disorders
- Yes: 52%
- No: 48%

Hemiplegia
- Yes: 55.6%
- No: 44.4%

Type of rehabilitation
- Only speech therapy: 53%
- Only physiotherapy: 1%
- Only psychotherapy: 1%
- Combination: 45%

Place of rehabilitation
- Hospital: 47%
- Private office: 31%
- Home: 22%

[a] CVA, cerebrovascular accident; TBI, traumatic brain injury.

(1%), psychotherapy (1%) alone, or a combination of the three (45%). Age varied from 17 to 93 years, with a mean of 49.7 years and standard deviation of 18.5 years. Education level was low (i.e., below 9 years of formal schooling) in one sixth of the population, at university level (high) in one third, and intermediate in half of the cases. The large majority of patients (89%) was unemployed postinjury. In addition to the cases of subjects already retired at the time of injury, the high proportion of unemployed might be due to the selection procedure that recruited only patients who were still engaged in some formal rehabilitation process. About two thirds of the patients were married or cohabiting with a partner. The remaining 36% of subjects were living at home with their parents or, conversely, were parents living at the home of their children (70% and 30%, respectively).

The time since injury varied from 1 month to 23 years, with a median of 35 months. The minimum delay was set to 1 month in order to allow patients to be discharged from the hospital neurological departments and to have returned home for a 2-week period of time, thereby allowing sufficient time to experience difficulties in daily life activities. Etiology was mainly vascular or traumatic (62% and 28%, respectively). The remaining cases were mainly due to tumors, anoxia, and infections. Two thirds of the lesions were localized to the left hemisphere, one sixth to the right hemisphere, and the remainder were bilateral. The same proportion of patients (two thirds) showed language disorders, with a predominance of Broca's aphasia over Wernicke's, anomic, conduction, and global aphasias. On the basis of local clinical criteria, about one half of the patients were evaluated as presenting with attention and/or memory disorders. Patients with hemiplegia accounted for 56% of the total sample.

The 465 close relatives were recruited as those family members who best knew the patients and their daily life activities. For a given patient, the relative was either his or her spouse (two thirds of the cases), one of his or her own parents (one fifth) or child (8%), or someone else providing care on a daily basis and familiar with the patient prior to injury. There were 24 patients without close relatives.

The 306 control subjects were in fact 153 couples living together and free from any known history of neurological or psychiatric impairments. The gender distribution (50% males and 50% females) thus differed from that of the patients group (65% and 35%, respectively; $P < 0.01$). A statistically significant difference was also found regarding employment, with 54% of the controls being active versus only 12% of the patients ($P < 0.01$). The two groups were comparable regarding to age (means: 49.2 and 49.7 for controls and patients, respectively) and the proportion of intermediate education levels (46% and 51%, respectively). However, there was a tendency for controls to be more educated than patients (41% of controls had a university education against 34% of patients; $P < 0.05$).

Measures and Data Analyses

The relevant EBIQ version was administered depending on the population group (i.e., patients, relatives, clinicians, and controls) and the time period concerned (i.e., difficulties experienced by patients and controls during the preceding month, or the status of patients prior to injury). In each case, the same 63 questions were included. Any missing responses were re-

TABLE 2. The Three Dimensions of Patients' Dysfunctions as Identified by Factor Analysis

Factor 1: Executive Functions 13 representative items	Factor 2: Depression 10 representative items	Factor 3: Irritability/impulsivity 11 representative items
Being unable to plan activities	Feeling sad	Getting into quarrels easily
Forgetting the day of the week	Feeling life is not worth living	Reacting too quickly to what others say or do
Trouble concentrating	Feeling lonely, even when together with other people	Having temper outbursts
Failing to get things done on time	Feelings of worthlessness	Shouting at people in anger
Forgetting appointments	Feeling isolated	Feeling anger against other people
Difficulty making decisions	Feeling hopeless about your future	Feeling annoyed or irritated
Trouble remembering things	Feeling inferior to other people	Mood swings without reasons
Acting inappropriately in dangerous situations	Lack of interest in hobbies at home	Feeling critical of others
Having to do things slowly in order to be correct	Being confused	Being obstinate
Difficulty finding your way in new surroundings	Feeling uncomfortable in crowds	Being "bossy" or dominating
Problems with household chores		Throwing things in anger
Difficulties managing your finances		
Being unsure what to do in dangerous situations		

placed with appropriate means. From each completed questionnaire, difficulty scale scores were constructed from the simple average of responses to groups of items (see below) among the 63 questions.

Comparisons between the three different points of view (patients, relatives, and clinicians) on the difficulties experienced by patients' during the last month are based on the data collected on these populations (with $N = 489$, 465, and 230, respectively). For each of these three groups separately, a factor analysis (principal components followed by varimax rotation) was performed using the Statistical Analysis System (SAS) statistical package. This was done in order to determine the factor structure of the EBIQ and to define scales to be derived from the separate items. These calculated scales were then compared both within and between the three groups.

The issue of the preinjury state was addressed by several comparisons performed on four sets of data. Patients ($N = 232$) and their relatives ($N = 215$) independently rated the levels of difficulties shown prior to patients' injuries. Comparing the values of the index of difficulties scored by the two groups indicates their level of agreement on the past situation. For controls, each member of the 153 couples responded twice to the questionnaire: once about him- or herself, and once about his or her spouse. In this way, the self-questionnaires of the control subjects ($N = 306$) represented a baseline by which the judgments indicated by patients ($N = 232$) can be compared. Similarly, the questionnaires concerning the spouses ($N = 306$) served as reference to the set of data collected on the relatives ($N = 215$) of the patients.

The Factor Analytic Structure of Reported Subjective Difficulties

The principal component analyses separately performed on the EBIQ data obtained from the patients, relatives and clinicians revealed three statistically significant factors (i.e., with eigenvalues greater than unity). Considering only those items that contributed strongly to a given factor (i.e., with factor weight coefficients ≥ 0.5), it was found that the three-factor solutions were quite similar across the patients', relatives', and clinicians' questionnaires. The questions that were common to the same factors are listed in Table 2. It is clear that these three factors, emerging independently from the three sources, can be readily categorized as concerning (1) executive–cognitive functions, (2) depression, and (3) difficulties in adaptation to social relations (irritability–impulsivity). On the basis of these analyses, three scale scores therefore were calculated from each questionnaire. These represented the average score (ranging from 1.0 to 3.0) for the items listed in Table 2, and the following statistical analyses employ these three scales—executive, depression and irritability–impulsivity—together with a total scale score derived as the average of all responses in a given questionnaire.

TABLE 3. Correlation Coefficients between Patients', Relatives', and Clinicians' Judgments on the Three Dimensions of Patients' Dysfunctions

	Patients/ relatives $N = 465$	Patients/ clinicans $N = 230$	Relatives/ clinicians $N = 230$
Executive functions	.48	.44	.58
Depression	.51	.46	.46
Irritability/impulsivity	.47	.43	.44

Results

Comparisons between Patients, Relatives, and Clinicians on the Degrees of Subjective Difficulties Currently Experienced by Patients

For each of the three scales concerning patients' difficulties, there was moderate to good agreement between the three sources: patients, relatives, and clinicians. Taken pairwise, the correlation coefficients ranged from .44 to .58 (see Table 3). Thus among patients tending to report relatively high levels of difficulties, their relatives and clinicians also reported relatively higher levels of difficulties, and vice versa.

Mean scores for the three groups on the four scales also showed differences (Table 4). In the case of the total score and the three scale scores, the relatives reported the highest levels of difficulties. Clinicians did not differ from patients in their ratings of executive functions and depression, but were lower in their ratings of irritability–impulsivity ($t = 3.93$, $P < 0.001$). Relatives were higher than patients in their ratings of patients' difficulties regarding executive functions ($t = 5.44$, $P < 0.001$), depression ($t = 2.42$, $P < 0.05$) and irritability–impulsivity ($t = 4.34$, $P < 0.001$) and also in the total score ($t = 7.07$, $P < 0.001$). Relatives were similarly higher than clinicians with respect to the three dimensions: executive functions ($t = 3.80$, $P < 0.001$), depression ($t = 2.49$, $P < 0.05$), and irritability–impulsivity ($t = 7.06$, $P < 0.001$), and also in the total score ($t = 7.14$, $P < 0.001$). In the three groups, the rank order of specific difficulties was the same. Patients, relatives, and clinicians rated executive function difficulties highest; thereafter, depression and the lowest scores were recorded for the irritability–impulsivity factor.

Comparisons of Present and Preinjury Status

Evaluations of difficulties experienced by patients prior to their injury were independently obtained from patients and their close relatives. Comparing those data to the evaluation of patients' present difficulties indicated three interesting results. First, it was found that uniformly for all scales and for both patients and their relatives, present difficulties of patients were rated as greater than their difficulties before injury. Second, the tendency for relatives to rate present patients' difficulties higher than patients did (see Table 4) was not observed on the preinjury

TABLE 4. Means and Standard Deviations of Patients' Dysfunction Scores in Three Dimensions as Indicated by Patients, Their Relatives, and Clinicians

	Patients $N = 489$	Relatives $N = 465$	Clinicians $N = 230$
Executive functions	1.76 (.43)	1.92 (.47)	1.78 (.45)
Depression	1.73 (.49)	1.81 (.51)	1.71 (.49)
Irritability/impulsivity	1.61 (.41)	1.74 (.50)	1.47 (.46)
Mean total score of 63 items	1.68 (.24)	1.79 (.24)	1.64 (.27)

period (see Table 5). Third, the rankings of the three dysfunction factors considered prior to and after injury were exactly in reverse orders. The impact of injury was thus a differential increase in dysfunction levels. The effect was greatest in the area of executive functions and least for irritability–impulsivity. The effect in depression was in between the two other dimensions.

The comparison of scores derived from the non-brain-injured control subjects revealed no quantitative differences between self-evaluations and evaluations performed by relatives (Table 6). Furthermore, the ranking of the three factors was the same in the two groups: normal subjects showed some difficulties that were very discrete in executive functions, moderate on irritability–impulsivity, and intermediate for depression. It was exactly the rank order observed in the patients' and relatives' evaluations of the preinjury situation of patients (Table 5). However, patients and relatives revealed the expected idealized view of the preinjury situation in that their ratings concerning that time (see Table 5) are consistently lower than those of the noninjured controls (see Table 6) as regards the three domains: executive functions (patients, $t = 8.12$, $P < 0.001$, and relatives, $t = 6.23$, $P < 0.001$), depression (patients, $t = 5.62$, $P < 0.001$, and relatives, $t = 3.43$, $P < 0.001$), and irritability–impulsivity (patients, $t = 2.69$, $P < 0.01$, and relatives, $t = 2.22$, $P < 0.05$), and in the total score also (patients, $t = 9.18$, $P < 0.001$, and relatives, $t = 6.55$, $P < 0.001$).

Discussion

Having identified and characterized three main dimensions in patients' dysfunction, namely, impaired executive functions, depression, and problems in the adaptation to social interactions (irritability–impulsivity), our results and findings provide some interesting information on currently debated issues in the area of the evaluation of subjective difficulties experienced by brain-injured patients.

The Agreement between Patients, Relatives, and Clinicians on Patients' Current Subjective Difficulties

The factor-analysis-derived areas of dysfunction that emerged from the independent statistical analyses showed no real differences between the three evaluations performed by pa-

TABLE 5. Means and Standard Deviations Prior-to-Injury Dysfunction Scores on the Three Dimensions

	Patients' judgments on patients $N = 232$	Relatives' judgments on patients $N = 215$
Executive functions	1.17 (.26)	1.19 (.28)
Depression	1.21 (.32)	1.24 (.31)
Irritability/impulsivity	1.51 (.37)	1.54 (.45)
Mean total score of 63 items	1.30 (.20)	1.32 (.18)

TABLE 6. Means and Standard Deviations Dysfunction Scores on the Three Dimensions in Control Subjects

	Controls: self-reports $N = 306$	Controls: reports on relatives $N = 306$
Executive functions	1.37 (.31)	1.35 (.30)
Depression	1.38 (.38)	1.34 (.35)
Irritability/impulsivity	1.60 (.40)	1.63 (.46)
Mean total score of 63 items	1.46 (.20)	1.43 (.20)

tients, relatives, and clinicians. This result thus supports previous reports on the agreement between patients and relatives (Fordyce *et al.,* 1983). However, some discrepancies may exist in their internal structure of the dysfunction factors. For instance, it needs to be clarified whether different questions contribute to the "executive functions" dimension in precisely the same manner in the factor analyses from the three data sources.

Patients' dysfunctions were scored lower by clinicians than by patients and higher by relatives than by patients. This result is at variance with the report of clinicians rating difficulties higher than relatives (Helmick *et al.,* 1976) and with the identification of diverse patterns of families (Cavallo *et al.,* 1992). Some items might account for these discrepancies between the studies, and thus should be considered as variables with possible significant effects on the consensus between the different judgments. Due to particular selection criteria, there were differences in the characteristics of patients between our study and that of Cavallo *et al.* (1992). In the latter study, most subjects were not participating in rehabilitation programs, and a significant proportion were employed. By contrast, only 11% of the patients in the present study were employed, and they were all engaged in rehabilitation. Moreover, the issue of agreement between different groups (e.g., patients and relatives) is not a simple question but depends on factors of consensus (Cavallo *et al.,* 1992) and individual characteristics (e.g., gender) (Willer, Allen, Liss, & Zicht, 1991). Psychological variables such as patients' lack of insight might account for some part of disagreements, but other clinical variables implicated in communication efficiency should also be considered (e.g., presence–absence of aphasia).

Regarding the lower scoring of patients' difficulties by clinicians, it tentatively might be hypothesized that it was related to the experienced clinicians' personal scale that could be adjusted with reference to the extremely bad cases they met once or simply the cases they heard about during their academic training. Thus, the finding of rating disagreements also points to the critical issue of the internal references used by the different subjects (patients, relatives, clinicians) when evaluating degree of difficulties. Indeed, such references may vary according to individual, medical, clinical, and also personal factors, among which are the experience of brain injury and its consequences in daily life situations.

Another source of difference between the evaluations of patients' difficulties might be due to the particular assessment instrument. At a psychometric level, it has been shown that the degree of consensus between patients and relatives can depend on the scales that are used. In a study by Kinsella, Moran, Ford, and Ponsford (1988), the statistical relations between the two judgments varied considerably, with correlation coefficients ranging from a high of .66 to a low of .18 (for the Leeds Scale of Depression and the Leeds Scale of Anxiety, respectively). Two arguments in our study exist against such bias. First, the standardization of EBIQ showed no statistically significant difference between control subjects evaluating their present situation and the judgments indicated by their relatives. Second, EBIQ ratings of the preinjury status did not differ among relatives and patients.

The Idealized View of the Preinjury Status of Patients

Perceptions by patients and their relatives of the changes that occurred in patients' psychosocial, cognitive, and affective situations following brain injury were not directly evaluated in the present study. Rather, this issue was indirectly addressed in two ways. Patients and relatives ratings of the preinjury status of the patients were compared first to their ratings of their present status, and second, to the "normal" status as indicated by controls.

According to patients, changes since injury occurred in all three dimensions under study. The most important impact was on executive functions ($P < 0.001$) and the least important on irritability–impulsivity ($P < 0.01$). This finding is in agreement with other studies reporting that patients ranked their temperament changes as low and cognitive changes as high (Fahy *et al.*, 1967; Hendryx, 1989). There are, however, some discrepancies with the study by Hendryx (1989) regarding the evaluations performed by relatives. Whereas we found a pattern of differentially increased difficulties that paralleled the one observed in patients, the latter study reported no differences in the degrees of changes on cognition, emotion, and physical areas.

Our finding of the idealized view of the preinjury status by both patients and relatives who rated difficulties significantly below the normal level was the more important. The precise nature of this phenomenon needs to be further clarified, since it may bear on setting realistic goals for rehabilitation (Christensen, Pinner, Moller Pedersen, Teasdale, & Trexler, 1992). As long as returning to the performance level of the preinjury status is the common goal of patients and relatives, there is little chance for success of evaluating of this status when it is biased toward some idealized situation that never really existed.

Further research is needed to clarify differences in subjective feelings about the impact of brain injury on patients and their families. Some studies have indicated that the evaluation of changes was more related to the actual situations than to the objective comparisons between pre- and postinjury (Finset *et al.*, 1995). In another domain, Gerin, Dazord, Cialdella, Leizorovicz, and Boissel (1991) observed that the degree of changes was mainly related to the value attached by patients to the area investigated.

ACKNOWLEDGMENTS Thanks are due to Mrs. C. Martin for technical support, and to the European Union for a grant (BMH1-CT 92-0218).

Appendix

EBIQ 1*: Subjective Difficulties Experienced by Patients since Last Month

01 Headaches
02 Failing to get things done on time

*EBIQ versions in other European languages are available from the Copenhagen Centre.

03 Reacting too quickly to what others say or do
04 Trouble remembering things
05 Difficulty participating in conversations
06 Others do not understand your problems
07 Everything is an effort
08 Being unable to plan activities
09 Feeling hopeless about your future
10 Having temper outbursts
11 Being confused
12 Feeling lonely, even when together with other people
13 Mood swings without reasons
14 Feeling critical of others
15 Having to do things slowly in order to be correct
16 Faintness or dizziness
17 Hiding your feelings from other people
18 Feeling sad
19 Being "bossy" or dominating
20 Needing to be reminded about personal hygiene
21 Difficulties managing your finances
22 Trouble concentrating
23 Failing to notice other people's moods
24 Feeling anger against other people
25 Having your feelings easily hurt
26 Feeling unable to get things done
27 Feeling annoyed or irritated
28 Problems with household chores
29 Lack of interest in hobbies at home
30 Feeling isolated
31 Feeling inferior to other people
32 Sleep problems
33 Feeling uncomfortable in crowds
34 Shouting at people in anger
35 Difficulty communicating what you want to
36 Being unsure what to do in dangerous situations
37 Being obstinate
38 Lack of interest in your surroundings
39 Thinking only of yourself
40 Mistrusting other people
41 Crying easily
42 Difficulty finding your way in new surroundings
43 Being inclined to eat too much
44 Getting into quarrels easily
45 Lack of energy or being slowed down
46 Forgetting the day of the week
47 Feelings of worthlessness
48 Lack of interest in hobbies outside of home
49 Needing help with personal hygiene
50 Restlessness

51 Feeling tense
52 Acting inappropriately in dangerous situations
53 Feeling life is not worth living
54 Forgetting appointments
55 Leaving others to take the initiative in conversations
56 Loss of sexual interest or pleasure
57 Throwing things in anger
58 Preferring to be alone
59 Difficulty making decisions
60 Losing contact with your friends
61 Lack of interest in current affairs
62 Behaving tactlessly
63 Having problems in general
64 Do you think that your relative's life has changed after you had the injury?
65 Do you think that your relative is having problems due to your present situation?
66 Do you think that your relative's mood has changed due to your present situation?

References

Cavallo, M. M., Kay, T., & Ezrachi, O. (1992). Problems and changes after traumatic brain injury: Differing perceptions within and between families. *Brain Injury, 6,* 327–335.

Christensen, A. L., Pinner, E. M., Moller Pedersen, P., Teasdale, T. W., & Trexler, L. E. (1992). Psychosocial outcome following individualized neuropsychological rehabilitation of brain damage. *Acta Neurologica Scandinavica, 85,* 32–38.

Deloche, G., North, P., Dellatolas, G., Christensen, A. L., Cremel, N., Passadori, A., Dordain, M., & Hannequin, D. (1996). Le handicap des adultes cérébro-lésés: Le point de vue des patients et de leur entourage. *Annales de Réadaptation et de Médecine Physique, 39,* 1–9.

Derogatis, L. R. (1983). *SCL-90-R, administration, scoring and procedures.* Towson, MD: Clinical Psychometric Research.

Fahy, T. J., Irving, M. H., & Millac, P. (1967). Severe head injuries: A six-year follow-up. *Lancet, 3,* 475–479.

Finset, A., Dyrnes, S., Krogstad, J. M., & Berstad, J. (1995). Self-reported social networks and interpersonal support 2 years after severe traumatic brain injury. *Brain Injury, 9,* 141–150.

Fordyce, D. J., Roueche, J. R., & Prigatano, G. P. (1983). Enhanced emotional reactions in chronic head trauma patients. *Journal of Neurology, Neurosurgery and Psychiatry, 46,* 620–624.

Gerin, P., Dazord, A., Cialdella, P., Leizorovicz, A., & Boissel, J. P. (1991). Le questionnaire "Profil de la Qualité de la Vie Subjective" (PQVS). *Thérapie, 46,* 131–138.

Gray, J. M., Shepherd, M., McKinlay, W. W., Robertson, I., & Pentland, B. (1994). Negative symptoms in the traumatically brain-injured during the first year post discharge, and their effect on rehabilitation status, work status and family burden. *Clinical Rehabilitation, 8,* 188–197.

Helmick, J. W., Watamori, T., & Palmer, J. (1976). Spouses' understanding of the communication disabilities of aphasic patients. *Journal of Speech and Hearing Disorders, 41,* 238–243.

Hendryx, P. M. (1989). Psychosocial changes perceived by closed-head-injured adults and their families. *Archives of General Psychiatry, 70,* 526–530.

Hogarty, G. E., & Katz, M. M. (1971). Norms of adjustment and social behavior. *Archives of General Psychiatry, 25,* 470–480.

Kinsella, G., Moran, C., Ford, B., & Ponsford, J. (1988). Emotional disorder and its assessment within the severe head injured population. *Psychological Medicine, 18,* 57–63.

Oddy, M., & Humphrey, M. (1978). Subjective impairment and social recovery after closed head injury. *Journal of Neurology, Neurosurgery and Psychiatry, 41,* 611–616.

Teasdale, T. W., Christensen, A. L., Willmes, K., Deloche, G., Braga, L., Stachowiak, F., Vendrell, J., Castro-Caldas, A., Laaksonen, R. K., & Leclercq, M. (1997). Subjective experience in brain-injured patients and their close relatives: A European Brain Injury Questionnaire study. *Brain Injury, 11,* 543–563.

Willer, B. S., Allen, K. M., Liss, M., & Zicht, M. S. (1991). Problems and coping strategies of individuals with traumatic brain injury and their spouses. *Archives of Physical Medicine and Rehabilitation, 72,* 460–468.

6

Novel Approaches to the Diagnosis and Treatment of Frontal Lobe Dysfunction

ELKHONON GOLDBERG AND DMITRI BOUGAKOV

Introduction

When people talk about the frontal lobes, they often mean prefrontal cortex, which is conventionally composed of Brodmann cytoarchitectonic areas 8, 9, 46, 10, 44, 45, 47, 11, and 12. Other definitions of the prefrontal cortex are based on its subcortical projections: the prefrontal cortex is that which receives projections from dorsomedial thalamic nucleus. Yet other definitions are based on its biochemical projections: the prefrontal cortex is that which receives dopamine (DA) through mesocortical projections.

The status of the prefrontal cortex in neuropsychology and behavioral neurology has been elevated from Cinderella to the princess. According to some old texts, the prefrontal cortex is a silent part of the brain, which does not serve any purpose. This misconception was abandoned gradually and over the last 15–20 years there has been a surge of interest in the prefrontal cortex. A number of recent discoveries indicate that, contrary to the old beliefs, the prefrontal cortex is particularly vulnerable in a very broad number of conditions and it has a very pivotal role in the neural control over cognition.

It is common to talk about the prefrontal cortex as if it were a unitary structure. In reality, however, it consists of several subdivisions. It is common to distinguish between dorsolateral, medial, and orbital prefrontal cortex, each endowed with their own properties (Goldberg, 1985). While recognizing functional heterogeneity of the prefrontal cortex, one also should recognize its unity in the sense that all these subdivisions can be characterized in some invariant terms. The prefrontal cortex is unique in a variety of ways.

ELKHONON GOLDBERG • New York University School of Medicine, and the Fielding Institute, New York, New York 10019. **DMITRI BOUGAKOV** • The Graduate School and University Center, City University of New York, New York, New York 10036.

International Handbook of Neuropsychological Rehabilitation, edited by Christensen and Uzzell.
Kluwer Academic/ Plenum Publishers, New York, 2000.

It is phylogenetically the youngest addition to the ensemble of structures of which the brain is comprised. Indeed, it begins to assume the differentiation comparable with the humans only in the great apes, which means that it is indeed a very late addition to the brain. The prefrontal cortex ontogenetically is also very young, at least according to some criteria, such as pathway myelinization. The prefrontal cortex is among the last structures to complete its myelinization; according to the recent studies this process is barely completed by the age of 18.

The prefrontal cortex is embedded in a uniquely rich pattern of pathways, richer than any other part of the brain. This was described very poetically, almost romantically, by Nauta (1971). The prefrontal cortex is connected monosynaptically with virtually every distinct functional system in the brain: with the posterior association cortex; the dorsomedial thalamus; premotor cortex; the basal ganglia; cerebellum; parahippocampal and entorhinal cortices and the hippocampi; the amygdala; hypothalamus; and, very interestingly, with various reticular nuclei in the ventral brain stem at a pontine and in particular mesencephalic level (Goldberg & Bilder, 1987). There is no other part of the brain so richly and so directly interconnected with virtually every processing station in the brain.

The brain structure, which is so richly endowed in terms of its anatomical pathways and is so phylogenetically and ontogenetically young, can be expected to serve commensurately advanced functions in cognition. However, our efforts to identify these functions have met with limited success. In describing the functions of the prefrontal cortex, it is not unusual to lapse into poetic metaphors for the lack of more precise concepts.

It is presumed that the prefrontal cortex is involved in the formulation of plans, in intentionality, in the formulation of goals and the plans subordinate to the goals, in the identification of the goal-appropriate cognitive routines, in sequential access to these routines, and in the editorial evaluation of the outcome of our actions (Luria, 1980). All these functions can be thought of as metacognitive rather than cognitive, in that they do not support any specific cognitive skills but provide an organizing role for all of them. This is why some authors refer to the functions of the prefrontal cortex as "executive," by analogy with the corporate chief executive officer. An analogy with the orchestra conductor might be even more appropriate. The conductor does not play any instrument but stays on the podium with a baton in his or her hands and calls on specific players, setting the order and pace of their involvement: "Now you . . . now you . . . now you." Without the conductor, the orchestra disintegrates into chaos, even when it consists of perfectly competent individual musicians.

Components of Executive Control

Guiding Behavior by Internal Representations

In the literature, two types of cognitive operations often are linked to the prefrontal cortex. The first is the organism's ability to guide its behavior by internal representations (Goldman-Rakic, 1987). This is not a trivial thing. We are able to guide our behavior according to internal representations and we take this ability for granted. Yet this ability arises quite late in evolution. Imagine a dog whose attention is attracted to some object, then there is a distractor, and the dog's attention is diverted toward this distractor. Unless the original object is food, the likelihood that the dog will return to the exploration of the first object is close to zero.

Patricia Goldman-Rakic, a prominent researcher of the frontal lobes, likes to characterize this type of "afrontal behavior" as "out of site–out of mind." In order for the animal to return to the exploration of the original object, its behavior must be guided by the internal representation of the previously situation. This ability appears to be quite limited in the canines. It appears to be quite developed, however, in apes. Even a gibbon, a lesser ape, is able to return to the previous activity after an introduction of a distracting stimulus. This means that its behavior is effectively guided by the internal representation, which is a very fundamental evolutionary change arising relatively late in evolution. There is a reason to believe that the emergence of this cognitive ability parallels the development of the frontal lobes.

To refer to this function of the prefrontal cortex, Ingvar (1976) coined the peculiar notion of the "memories of the future." What is a memory about the future? Memories are supposed to be about the past. The frontal lobes are the structure central for the formulation of plans and then guiding behavior according to these plans. Once a plan has been formulated, it is delegated to memory. But this memory is about what the future should be like, and this memory of the future guides the behavior of the organism. It is a very elegant way to capture the role of the frontal lobes in planning behavior and guiding it by the internal representations of the plans. This function of the frontal lobes has been studied very extensively in a rather pioneering way by Goldman-Rakic (1987).

Field-dependent behavior occurs when subject's behavior is guided by some incidental stimuli in the external environment as opposed to an internally generated plan. An example of verbal field-dependent behavior is represented in the transcript of the patient's story recall. A patient with a bilateral prefrontal trauma and subsequent removal of the fractured frontal bone and frontal pole resection bilaterally listens to the story, "A hen and golden eggs," which reads as follows: "A man owned a hen which was laying golden eggs. The man was greedy and wanted to get more gold at once. He killed the hen and cut it open hoping to find a lot of gold inside, but there was none." The patient's recall proceeds as follows:

> A man was living with a hen . . . or rather the man was the hen's owner. She was producing gold. . . . The man . . . the owner . . . wanted more gold at once . . . so he cut the hen into pieces but there was no gold. . . . No gold at all . . . he cuts the hen more, . . . no gold . . . the hen remains empty. . . . So he searches again and again. . . . No gold . . . he searches all around in all places. The search is going on with the tape recorder . . . they are looking here and there, nothing new around. They leave tape recorder turned on, something is twisting there . . . what the hell are they recording there . . . some digits . . . 0,2,3,0, . . . so, they are recording all these digits . . . not very many of them . . . that's why all the other digits were recorded . . . turned out to be not very many of them either . . . so, everything was recorded. . . . (monologue continues). (Goldberg & Costa, 1986, p. 48)

The introduction of the tape recorder into the recall is triggered by the fact that the examiner had a tape recorder placed before the subject.

Shifting Cognitive Sets

An organism must be capable not only of guiding its behavior by internal representations, but also "switching gears" when something unanticipated happens. To deal effectively with such situations, another ability is needed: mental flexibility, the capacity to respond rapidly to unanticipated environmental contingencies. Milner (1982) was particularly instrumental in advancing this notion.

One can think of these cognitive operations as acting in dynamic balance in the normal brain (Goldberg, Podell, Harner, Lovell, & Riggio, 1994). But in various forms of brain pathology this balance can be upset and then two extreme types of cognitive symptoms arise: perseveration and field-dependent behavior.

Although in many cases of frontal lobe pathology we see these symptoms intertwined, we are just as likely to encounter them separately; some cases are predominantly characterized by the perseverations and others by field-dependent behavior. By perseveration we mean any situation when events of prior behavior find their way maladaptively in the ongoing behavior. Various kinds of perseveration exist. Perseveration is not unique to the frontal lobe pathology. One can see them in many other forms of brain damage, but what is unique about the frontal lobe pathology is the pervasiveness and severity of perseveration.

The analysis of perseveration reveals the interaction between the prefrontal cortex and other parts of the brain. Dysfunction of the prefrontal cortex may interfere with the outputs from other parts of the brain, even when the latter are not themselves affected by a lesion. In its simplest form, perseverating behavior may be limited to a single motor act. We know that motor cortex controls single motor acts (Brodmann area 4). Yet the lesion in this case was restricted to the frontal poles with no direct damage to motor cortex.

Figure 1(a,b) represents a different type of perseveration. Here, the perseverating behavior constitutes a whole motor sequence. Premotor cortex is responsible for generating motor sequences (Brodmann area 6). Again, the actual lesion is in the Brodmann area 44 and 46, but one of the net effects of this lesion is the malfunctioning of Brodmann area 6.

Another type of perseveration is represented in Fig. 1(c,d). It is different since it lacks the additive quality of the previous ones. One can argue that this type of perseveration occurs at the level of retrieval from semantic memory; it is a perseveration between different contents of semantic memory. This implies that the areas whose functioning is affected are posterior association regions of the left hemisphere, but the actual lesion is again restricted to the frontal lobes. Yet another type of perseveration is depicted in Fig. 1(e,f). Here, entire types of cognitive activities perseverate: writing versus drawing.

Perseverations and field-dependent behavior could be thought of as two opposites. Maintaining dynamic balance between the ability to guide behavior by internal representation and the ability to respond rapidly to changing environmental contingencies is an important function of the frontal lobes.

When this balance is upset and behavior becomes too strongly dependent on the internal representation and unable to change because the tasks change, then perseveration develops. If, on the other hand, the behavior becomes too weakly controlled by the internal representation and totally responsive to incidental environmental events, then field-dependent behavior develops. Although perseverations and field-dependent behavior often co-occur in parallel in the same patient case, it is not uncommon for a patient to have one but not the other.

Resolving Ambiguity

Another very interesting role of the frontal lobes is its role in dealing with inherent ambiguity. In psychology and neuropsychology, we are used to the notion that tasks have correct responses. Usually, only one response is right and the rest are wrong. We deal with the highly constrained, deterministic situation. But this have little to do with the real life. In most real-life situations, the choices are not what is right and what is wrong. Should one put on a blue suit or a gray suit in the morning? Should one have omelet for breakfast or yogurt? Should one take a cab or walk? Should one go to law school or medical school? These real-life questions have no intrinsically wrong or right answers. Saying that wearing a blue suit is intrinsically correct and wearing a gray one is intrinsically wrong would be an inane statement.

In most real-life situations there are no intrinsically correct or incorrect choices. There are more adaptive and less adaptive decisions, but the situations are usually intrinsically ambiguous. What is correct and what is incorrect depends on the interplay of the properties of the situation and the properties of the actor; the actor's goals, motives, personal history, idiosyncratic

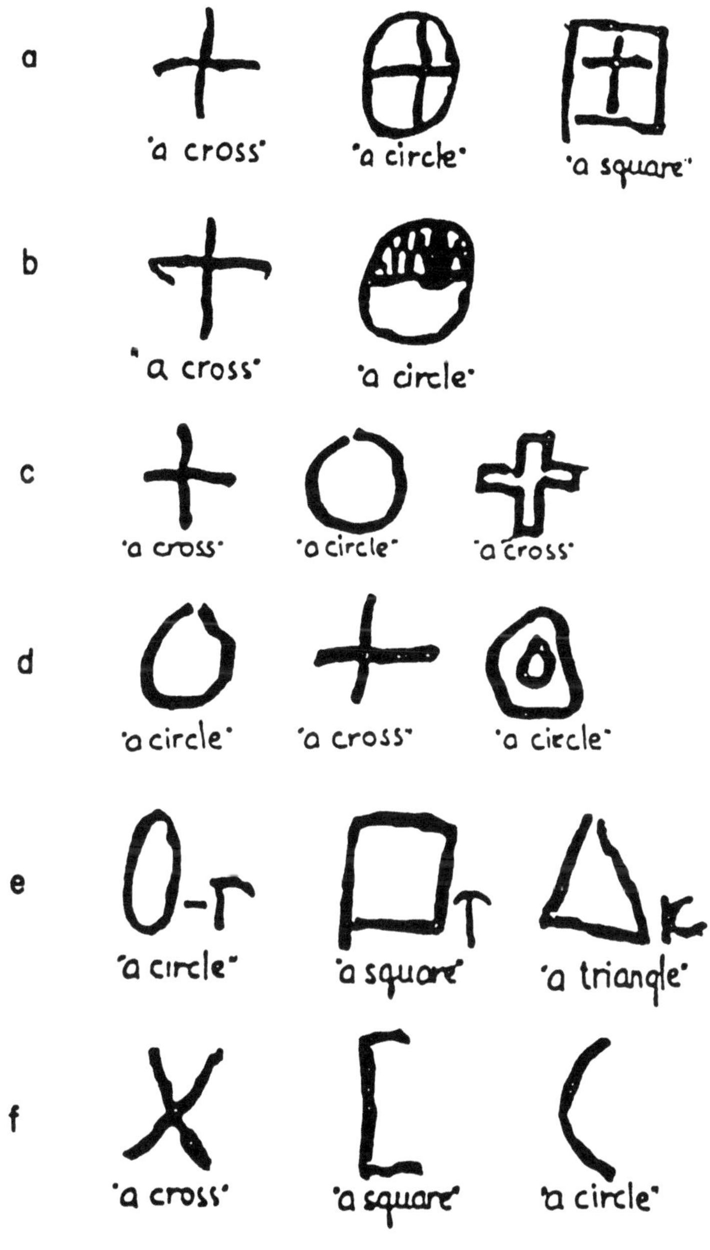

FIGURE 1. Types of perseveration. (a,b) Perseveration of elements; (c,d) perseveration of features; (e) perseveration of activities; and (f) perseveration of semantic categories. a,b,e, and f are from patient K. who suffered head trauma with prefrontal site of impact and fracture of the frontal bone. The operation consisted of removal of the fractured bone and resection of the frontal poles. Pronounced symptoms of convexital and mediobasal frontal dysfunction were observed. The experimental data were obtained 2 weeks to $3\frac{1}{2}$ months after operation. In f, the patient's choice of items in wrong semantic category was facilitated by the similarity of verbal labels (see text for explanation). Figures c and d are from patient S., who had cystic tumor of the third ventricle. The operation consisted of the removal of the cyst, with the approach through the premotor zone and the body of the third ventricle. Postoperative edema was observed, with the prevailing dysfunction of deep and medial areas of the premotor zone and ventral areas of the brainstem. The data were obtained 8 to 12 days after the operation. (From Goldberg & Bilder, 1987, p. 165. Reprinted by permission.)

predilections, and so forth. In our life, we spend more time making decisions about the ambiguous situations than we do making decisions about situations where there are intrinsically wrong and right answers.

We were taught in our professional training that in the experimental situation we have to know what the subject is doing, but by creating these highly constraining conditions, we are taking our subjects away from the real-life situations and totally ignoring the way humans really operate in life. We designed the Cognitive Bias Task (CBT) (Goldberg *et al.*, 1994; Podell, Lovell, Zimmerman, & Goldberg, 1995), which requires the subject to look at the stimulus and then pick between two other stimuli according to the subject's liking (Fig. 2). There is no in-

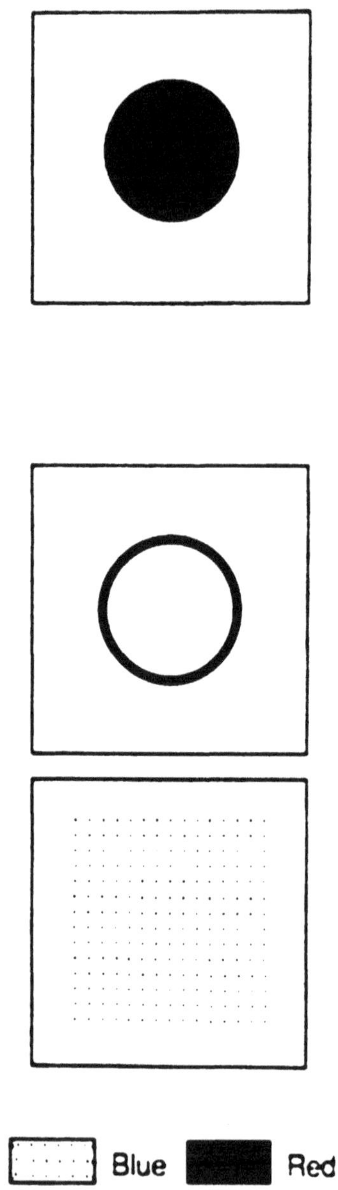

FIGURE 2. Example of CBT trial. (From Goldberg *et al.*, 1994, p. 277. Reprinted by permission.)

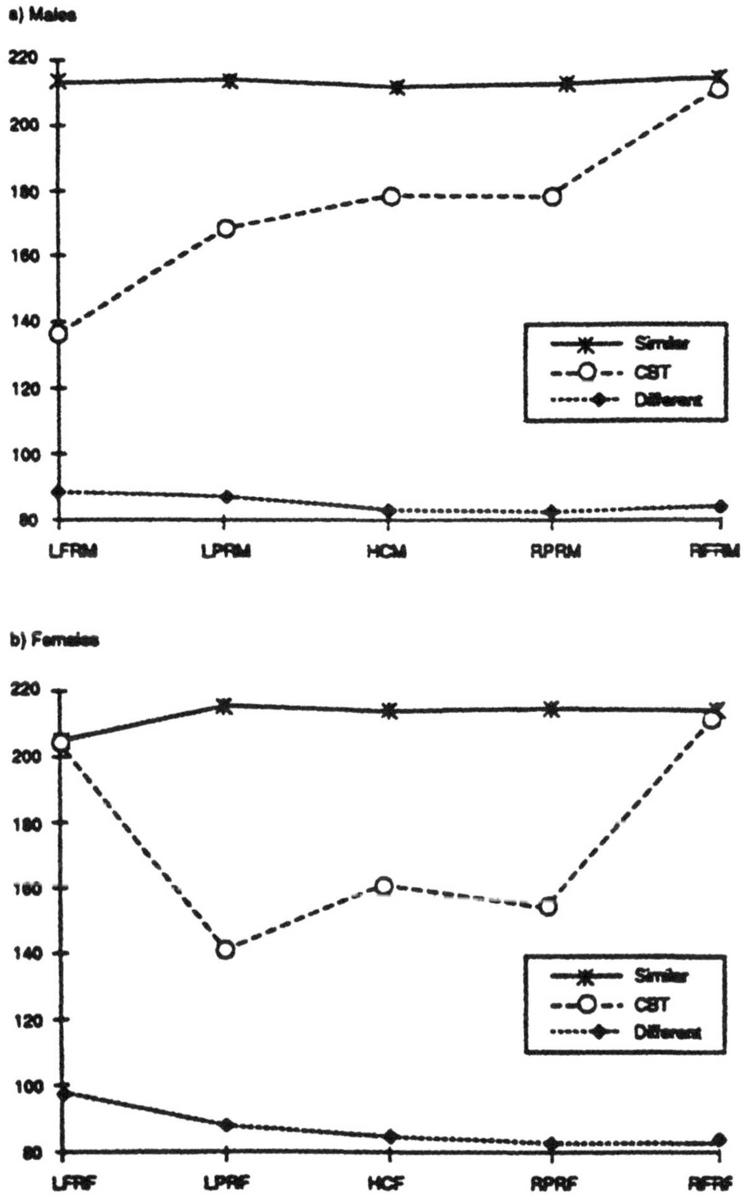

FIGURE 3. Mean group scores for CBT and the control task with explicit instructions in strictly right-handed subjects: (a) males: (b) females. LFRM, left frontal right-handed males; LPRM, left posterior right-handed males; HCM, healthy control males; RPRM, right posterior right-handed males; RFRM, right frontal right-handed males: LFRF, left frontal right-handed females; LPRF, left posterior right-handed females; HCF, healthy control females; RPRF, right posterior right-handed females; RFRF, right frontal right-handed females. (From Goldberg *et al.*, 1994, p. 282. Reprinted by permission.)

trinsically correct or incorrect response in this task. It is an intrinsically ambiguous situation that is left up to the subject to disambiguate. We can think of it as a cognitive projective task.

In Fig. 3, we present the data from right-handed males and females: neurologically intact, with right frontal lesions, left frontal lesions, left parietal lesions, and right parietal lesions.

Scores range from 80 to 220: normal subjects score on the average 180; patients with left and right parietal lesions attain similar scores; but patients with right and left frontal lesions attain significantly different scores from that of normal subjects and patients with parietal lesions. The data suggest that frontal cortex helps us to deal with intrinsic ambiguity.

When we disambiguate the situation by asking the subjects to choose the stimuli that are more similar to the target, we introduce intrinsically correct and incorrect responses. Nothing is changed in the task itself, but by the nature of our instruction we disambiguate it. Finally, we asked our subjects to choose the stimuli that are the most dissimilar to the target. So, in our experiment we have one ambiguous task and two control tasks where there is no ambiguity. In the nonambiguous situation the effect of frontal lobe lesion disappears; frontal lobe patients behave exactly like normal controls. That means the prefrontal cortex appears to be uniquely critical in dealing with inherent ambiguity. To disambiguate the intrinsically ambiguous situation is cardinal to the human decision-making process.

In order to study the functions of the frontal lobes we need the instruments that can measure how an organism deals with ambiguous situations. As it stands today, there are very few such instruments available. The CBT is one of them.

In a recent study we administered the CBT to various groups of the elderly: normal subjects, patients with mild Alzheimer's-type dementia (AD), and patients with moderate AD (Goldberg *et al.,* 1997). We found that there is a drastic change in the performance on the critical (ambiguous) CBT between normal subjects and AD patients, but there was no significant change between mild and moderate AD patients. But when we gave our patients the control disambiguated task, we found that there is no difference between normal subjects and the mild AD patients but there is a difference between normal subjects and moderate AD patients. This means that cognitive changes that interfere with performance on the ambiguous task are affected much earlier in the disease process than the processes that interfere with the subjects' ability to perform on the control task. It appears that the ability to deal with intrinsic ambiguity fails very early in the AD process. We can speculate that the frontal lobes were affected by AD very early in the disease process.

Novelty

Another important property of the frontal lobes is its relationship to novelty. It appears than when an organism is faced with a novel, unexpected situation, then the frontal lobes are very critically engaged, but when the organism encounters the routine situation, the role of the frontal lobes is less prominent. Neuroimaging studies with positron emission tomography (PET) show prominent activation in the prefrontal cortex with an introduction of the novel task (Raichle *et al.,* 1994). Once the subjects become more proficient in the task, the role of the frontal lobes diminishes.

To summarize, the frontal lobes appear to be important in guiding an organism by internal representations, in ensuring the mental flexibility necessary for responding to the unanticipated environmental events, in dealing with intrinsic ambiguity, and in dealing with novelty.

Frontal Lobe Vulnerability to Disease

Prefrontal cortex is afflicted in an inordinately broad range of conditions (Goldberg, 1992). Historically, it was thought that in order to find prefrontal dysfunction one has to look for various esoteric, low-prevalence focal conditions like rupture of the anterior communicating artery, or surgery requiring resection of the frontal lobes bilaterally. As the arena of neuropsychology began to expand and as neuroscientists started to apply neuropsychological methods to various nonfocal conditions, it became clear that, contrary to the old assumption, the frontal lobes are particularly vulnerable.

Today, schizophrenia is thought of as a frontal lobe disease (Ingvar & Franzen, 1974). Mild head trauma often produces frontal lobe syndrome accompanied by pronounced hypofrontality (reduction in the frontal cerebral activation relative to other regions of the cortex) (Deutsch & Eisenberg, 1987). Particularly revealing is a study of the effects of scopolamine in normal volunteers (Honer, Prohovnik, Smith, & Lucas, 1988). Normal volunteers were treated with cholinergic antagonist scopolamine to create a reversible model of AD based on the assumption that AD is a cholinergic disorder. Cholinergic pathways are distributed throughout the cortex and they do not tend to favor prefrontal cortex in particular. Nonetheless, a pattern of hypofrontality was found using regional cerebral blood flow (rCBF) technique. That means the function of the prefrontal cortex was disrupted despite the fact the cholinergic pathways are not particularly prevalent in the frontal lobes.

It appears that it is not necessary to have a frontal lobe lesion to have a frontal lobe syndrome. There are many conditions where based on the physiological studies there is frontal lobe dysfunction but there is no evidence of structural damage to the frontal lobes. These are conditions that are characterized by frontal lobe dysfunction in the absence of morphological damage. There is no other part of the brain to which a statement like that could be applied. This mysterious divergence implies that the functional breakdown threshold of the frontal cortex is lower than that of other parts of neocortex. The classical neurological view was that all cortical regions have similar breakdown thresholds and that the extent of the lesion would predict the extent of the deficit. Classical neuropsychology would predict, for instance, that brain atrophy equally and diffusely distributed throughout the brain would cause an equal amount of cognitive dysfunction as measured by regionally sensitive neuropsychological tests. In reality, however, equal amount of cortical atrophy is likely to produce unequal cognitive effects, performance on the frontal lobe tests being particularly impaired. The challenge is to find the mechanism responsible for the particularly low functional breakdown threshold of the frontal lobes.

The Reticulofrontal Disconnection Syndrome

Many years ago we described a victim of a horse-riding accident. The patient developed a flagrant frontal lobe syndrome with all its textbook attributes: disinhibition, lack of interest in anything that used to be of high significance to him before the accident, and lack of insight. However, his performance on nonfrontal types of measures was relatively spared. The puzzle for us was that no frontal lobe lesion was evident. There was damage to the temporoparietal structures, bilaterally enlarged ventricles, but no frontal lobe damage. Instead, we found a lesion in the ventral tegmentum (Goldberg *et al.*, 1981; Goldberg, Bilder, Hughes, Antin, & Mattis, 1989). The ventral tegmental area (VTA) contains nuclei that are points of origin of massive mesocortical DA projections via the medial forebrain bundle to the prefrontal cortex. DA projections mostly target the prefrontal cortex. We called this syndrome the *reticulofrontal disconnection syndrome.* Originally, the notion of the disconnection syndrome was introduced by Geshwind (1965), but he was talking about horizontal, corticocortical disconnection syndromes. We introduced the notion of the "vertical" disconnection syndrome: midbrain to the frontal cortex disconnection syndrome.

By interfering with the DA system in monkeys, one can produce a syndrome indistinguishable from that which is produced by the lesions in the frontal lobes proper (Brozoski *et al.*, 1979). Oades (1982) created an animal model where he destroyed VTA nuclei in rats, and the effects of the VTA lesions were indistinguishable from the effects of frontal lobe lesions. It appears that both in humans and animal models by interfering with the projections (DA mostly but not exclusively) from mesencephalon to the frontal lobes we can produce a frontal lobe syndrome without a frontal lobe lesion.

We believe that the reticulofrontal disconnection syndrome can serve as a model for many etiologies of frontal dysfunction. This model might bring together conditions as diverse as traumatic brain injury (TBI) and schizophrenia. Etiologically, TBI is an acute, acquired damage and schizophrenia is a neurodevelopmental disorder, but physiologically both involve frontal lobe dysfunction. Current thinking of schizophrenia links it to abnormalities in the mesocortical and mesolimbic DA pathways (Roberts, Leigh, & Weinberger, 1993a). Mesolimbic and mesocortical pathways both originate in the VTA. On the other hand, it long has been thought that closed head injury particularly affects long myelinated fiber structures, particularly the projections coming out of upper brain stem and ultimately going to the frontal lobes (Roberts, Leigh, & Weinberger, 1993b). It has been thought that the acceleration effects of the closed head injury exert their disruptive effect predominantly on the long myelinated pathways emanating from the upper brain stem and projecting into the cortex. Until recently, this type of damage had to remain a hypothetical construct, supported by the animal studies but not directly demonstrable in human victims of TBI. In our case of reticulofrontal disconnection syndrome we had a macroscopic model of damage that in many cases happens on a more microscopic level, but presumably in the same anatomical location. In our case the lesion was large enough to be visualized. In many other cases the lesion is too small to be visualized but presumably is nonetheless present.

We believe that the mechanism of the reticulofrontal disconnection syndrome is a very pervasive mechanism in mild head injury, and because of the trajectory of these projections the frontal lobes are particularly susceptible to the effects of this syndrome.

The Pharmacology of Frontal Lobe Syndromes

Pharmacology has been used in TBI cases for some time, but it has been an ancillary pharmacology of anticonvulsants, antidepressants, stimulants, and sedatives. With the demonstration that frontal lobe dysfunction may be caused by a remote lesion comes an opportunity to design some pharmacological regiments to target the core of the cognitive problems in the TBI patients. Increasingly, scientists talk about cognotropic medications. Great effort is underway to design medications (usually cholinergic agonists) to address the core of the cognitive deficit in the Alzheimer's type dementia patients. It would be extremely tempting and extremely powerful to design pharmacological interventions that would directly address the cognitive deficit of the closed head injury.

In mild TBI (which often affects relatively young people who are medically healthy), frequently the only deficit is the executive deficit. It is plausible to think that DA pharmacology would be a fruitful ground for such intervention. Prefrontal cortex depends on the DA transmission.

In cases when there is a structural lesion in the prefrontal cortex, there is not much hope for using any kind of pharmacology because the receptor sites are likely to be damaged. But in the frontal lobe syndrome due to the disconnection of the DA pathway to the prefrontal cortex the receptor sites in the frontal lobes are still intact.

This opens an opportunity for the pharmacological treatment that will address the cognitive deficit of the mild TBI patients. Very recently, there have been a surge of publications in the scientific journals describing the attempts of pharmacological treatment of the TBI patients to address their cognitive deficits. Because the frontal lobes are the predominant DA target sites, it is reasonable to use various dopaminergic agonists in attempts to treat cognitive deficits in patients with mild TBI.

Currently, a great deal of interest exists in identifying specific DA receptors and developing receptor-specific pharmacology. But the thrust of current research is driven by the needs of schizophrenic patients. Therefore, the thrust of the current effort is to develop DA receptor-specific antagonists. For the selective treatment of TBI, DA and norepinephrine (NE) receptor-specific agonists are needed. This poses a new challenge to behavioral pharmacology research.

We think that the mechanism of the frontal lobe dysfunction in mild TBI is related to the reticulofrontal disconnection syndrome, and that the pharmacological intervention directly addressing cognitive deficits in such patients is possible. Indeed, there has been some preliminary work (mostly case reports) suggesting that such treatment may be beneficial. If this is so, then for the first time we are at the threshold of pharmacological treatment of mild brain injury, which of course should be used in conjunction with cognitive approaches to address the core of the problem of the frontal lobe injury.

Current Pharmacological Approaches in Traumatic Brain Injury

The possibility of pharmacological treatment in TBI is extremely attractive, since out of 2,000,000 people sustaining TBI in the United States yearly, 90,000 will acquire chronic disability that will prevent them from successful social and occupational reintegration (Interagency Head Injury Task Force Report, 1989). Symptoms consistent with dysfunction of the frontal lobes following TBI include problems with working memory, attention, problem solving, impulsivity, disinhibition, poor motivation, and other behavioral and cognitive problems.

These symptoms may respond to certain drugs, such as DA-enhancing drugs (levodopa, carbidopa, amantadine, bromocriptine, selegiline, pergolide), classic stimulants (pemoline, methylphenidate, dextroamphetamine), tricyclic antidepressants (TCAs) (desipramine, protriptyline), selective serotonin reuptake inhibitors (SSRIs) (fluoxetine, sertraline, paroxetine), and dopaminergic antidepressants (bupropion) (Wroblewski & Glenn, 1994). Increase in cerebral concentration of DA and NE has been shown to improve general arousal, alertness, attention, and memory (Smith, 1976; Cope, 1986). Conversely, reduced concentration of homovanillic acid (HVA), the main metabolite of DA, are known to accompany unconsciousness after chronic TBI (Barregi, Porta, & Selanati, 1975; Vecht, Van Woerkom, Teelkan, & Minderhoud, 1975a; Vecht *et al.*, 1975b; Van Woerkom, Teelkan, & Minderhoud, 1977; Hyyppa, Langvik, Nieminen, & Vapalhti, 1977; Minderhoud, Van Woerkom, & VanWeerdon, 1976; Van Woerkom, Miderhoud, Gottschal, & Nicolai, 1982).

The effects of levodopa are linked to NE activity, since levodopa is a metabolic precursor of NE (Eames, 1989). Chandra (1978) reported statistically and clinically significant improvement in arousal after administration of levodopa in a double-blind, placebo-controlled study in 39 patients with measles encephalitis and disturbed consciousness.

Haig and Ruess (1990) reported subjective improvement in consciousness, verbalization, ability to follow command, and pointing to objects after administration of levodopa–carbidopa to a patient with TBI who remained in the vegetative state for 6 months. Levodopa has been shown to improve long-term memory in normal subjects, depressed subjects, and patients with parkinsonism, cerebrovascular accident, and TBI (Lal, Merbitz, & Grip, 1988; Newmann, Weingartner, & Smallberg, 1984; Murphy, Henry, & Weingartner, 1972; Mohr, Fabbrini, & Ruggieri, 1987).

Other researchers report increase in the level of arousal and alertness in patients with TBI after treatment with amantadine (Gualtieri, Chandler, Coons, & Brown, 1989; Chandler, Barnhill, & Gualtieri, 1988). Amantadine was originally introduced as an antiviral agent (Herrman, Grabliks, & Engle, 1960), and later was found to be effective in treating parkinsonism (Schwab, England, & Postkanzer, 1969). Amantadine is thought to facilitate DA release and delay DA reuptake (Aoki & Sitar, 1988). Amantadine also may increase the number of postsynaptic receptors (Gianutsos, Stewart, & Dunn, 1985) or alter their conformation (Allen, 1983). In addition, amantadine is an *N*-methyl-D-aspartate (NMDA) glutamate receptor antagonist and might provide protection against secondary damage by this excitotoxic neurotransmitter (Weller & Kornhuber, 1992). Gualtieri *et al.* (1989) treated 30 TBI patients with extensive frontal and temporal lesions (ranging 2 to 144 months postinjury) and severe neurobehavioral symptoms with amantadine in an uncontrolled study. Nineteen patients (63%) showed reductions in agitation, physical agressivenes, distractibility, and mood swings. Other researchers report improvement of apathy, amotivation, slowness, perseveration, visual attention, speed of information processing, attentional span, learning, and alertness (Van Reekum, Bayley, & Garner, 1995; Andersson, Berstad, & Finset, 1992).

In summary, case studies or small controlled studies of treatment with amantadine show improvement in cognitive functioning, electroencephalograph records, activity levels, or depressive symptoms in patients with TBI (Kraus & Maki, 1997a).

Recently, Kraus and Maki (1997b) have conducted a pharmacological intervention using a combination of dopaminergic agents to treat a 50-year-old woman who showed persistent frontal dysfunction 5 years postinjury. Amantadine alone produced an improvement in memory, attentiveness, concentration, motivation, motor abilities, generativity, and cognitive flexibility and a decrease in expression of such symptoms as impulsivity, perseveration, and dysarthria. The addition of levodopa and carbidopa (peripheral inhibitor of dopa decarboxylase) has led to further improvement in alertness, divided attention, and constructional ability.

Bromocriptine, a postsynaptic dopamine agonist with a particular affinity to D_2 receptors, has been utilized for speech and language disorders and hemispatial neglect in TBI patients. It is believed, however, that it also may be effective in treatment of abulic TBI patients (Ross & Stewart, 1981; Catsman-Berrevoets & Harskamp, 1988; Kneale & Eams, 1991; Barret, 1991).

Powell, Al-Adawi, Morgan, and Greenwood (1996) administered bromocriptine to 11 brain-injured patients with abulia and found an increase in motivation, cognition, and responsiveness to incentive measures. Interestingly, after withdrawal from the drug there was a moderate deterioration on these measures followed by some recovery, which allowed authors to speculate that a short period of administration may have effectively "kick-started" the dopaminergic system in these patients. Also, bromocriptine has been reported to improve verbal memory, functional memory, and early recall on formal neuropsychological tests in a single-case study of a patient with a mediobasal forebrain injury and amnestic syndrome (Ross & Stewart,1981; Dobkin & Hanlon, 1993).

Dextroamphetamine (AMP) has been shown to increase arousal, mood, and attention according to global assessment reports and improve performance on formal neuropsychological tests in the patients with TBI (Lipper & Tuchman, 1976; Evans, Gualtieri, & Patterson, 1987; Bleiberg, Garmo, & Cederquist, 1993). Evans *et al.* (1987) and more recently Bleiberg *et al.* (1993) report an improvement in verbal naming, learning skills, sustained and selective attention, and simple and complex reaction time on formal neuropsychological tests in patients with TBI after treatment with AMP. Evans *et al.* (1987) obtained similar results in double-blind, placebo-controlled single-case study using methylphenidate (MP). In addition, Evans *et al.* (1987) found improvement in memory after treatment with AMP and MP.

These studies indicate that pharmacological treatment of cognitive impairment in TBI is possible and has been investigated for some time. However, most of the catecholaminergic agents have a general effect on a wide spectrum of mental functions through an increase in the level of arousal and alertness. Since many patients with mild TBI and frontal lobe dysfunction need more specific approach to their deficits, there is a need for more specific pharmacological agents. Among available agents, bromocriptine seems to be the most appropriate for treatment of patients with mild TBI and frontal lobe dysfunction. Since bromocriptine has been reported to improve spatial working memory (Luciana, Depue, Arbisti, & Leon, 1992) (a mental function thought to be primarly mediated by the frontal lobes) and executive functions (Kimberg, D'Esposito, & Farah, 1994) in young normal subjects, it is plausible to use bromocriptine in mild TBI patients to improve cognitive functions mediated by frontal lobes.

Subtyping the Frontal Lobe Syndromes

The frontal lobes are a very extensive system. Our ability to design more selective pharmacological interventions and cognitive remedial therapies will be greatly enhanced by the knowledge of distinct variants of the frontal lobe executive syndromes. In the future, cognitive assays will be used to guide theraputic interventions in specific and selective ways.

Lateralization

It has been suggested by animal studies that the distribution of the catecholamine pathways in the frontal lobe is somewhat asymmetric. The DA pathways tend to favor the left frontal lobe and the NE pathways tend to favor the right frontal lobe (Tucker & Williamson, 1984).

It has been shown that patients with mild frontal lobe dysfunction that appears to be structurally intact on magnetic resonance imaging (MRI) are likely to exhibit hypofrontality on physiological studies such as single photon emission tomography (SPECT) (Masdeu, Van Heertu, & Abdel-Dayem, 1995). While hypofrontality is presumed to be bilateral, bilaterality itself is a statistical abstraction (resulting from averaging data across large numbers of patients). In any given patient the pattern of hypofrontality is more likely to affect one hemisphere than the other. Unfortunately, PET, functional MRI (fMRI), and even SPECT examinations are quite expensive and not always readily available. It would be useful to design cognitive tasks that would enable us to classify these patterns of the frontal lobe dysfunction as predominantly left or right. This, in turn, would guide the choice of pharmacology (dopaminergic or norepinephrinergic, depending on the involved hemisphere) to treat the patient.

Earlier, we outlined the types of cognitive operations for which the frontal lobes appear to be critical. Among them are the ability to guide behavior by internal representation and the ability to alter the cognitive context in response to unanticipated contingencies. We hypothesized that these two classes of cognitive operations are differentially controlled by the left and the right prefrontal cortices (Goldberg *et al.*, 1994). We decided to test this hypothesis with CBT. The test is composed of 60 independent trials of simultaneous presentation of the target stimulus on the top of the screen and two response stimuli on the bottom of the screen. Stimuli are designed along five binary dimensions: shape (circle or square), size (small or large), color (blue or red), number of items in the frame (two or one), and the way shapes are drawn (outline or solid). Each dimension can assume two values and one can construct 32 different items. For any given stimulus one can compute a "perceptual similarity index." Similarity index between target stimulus and response stimulus can carry from 0 to 5, where 5 means that two items are similar in all five dimensions and 0 that they are disparate in all five dimensions. For every trial the similarity index is never the same for two response stimuli and the subject is "forced" to choose between the stimulus that is more similar to the target and the stimulus that is less similar to the target. Three distinct strategies are possible: (1) the subject consistently picks the more similar responses, which will yield high cumulative score; (2) the subject consistently picks the more different target, which will yield a low cumulative score; or (3) the subject makes the choices in the way that is oblivious of the target, which will yield an intermediate score. The extent to which the subjects' choice is driven by the target, regardless whether the subject picks the most similar or most dissimilar response, is of a particular interest. This is why we converted scores in such a way that the high scores reflect behavior guided by internal representation and low scores represent the responses that are consistently oblivious of the target.

We hypothesized that response selection guided by the left prefrontal system will produce a very high score and that response selection guided by the right prefrontal system will produce a very low score. This test shows high test–retest reliability for males. In normal subjects we found significant gender differences even though the original hypothesis was stated in the gender-agnostic way. It appears that response selection in males is much more context dependent and response selection in females much more context independent (Goldberg *et al.*, 1994).

In view of these findings, we also decided to analyze the data separately for males and females in patient samples. Our data were acquired from normal controls, left parietal, right parietal, left frontal, and right frontal patients. All the patients with the frontal lobe damage had well-lateralized acquired lesions, affecting mostly dorsolateral structures.

In males, the findings were consistent with our hypothesis: patients with a right frontal lesion had a high score and patients with a left frontal lesion had a low score. Our data are interesting in two respects. First, the scores for the normal subjects are in the middle of the range, whereas the scores for the left frontal lobe patients are low and scores for the right frontal lobe patients are high. This gives us a graphic representation of the dynamic balance of activity between the two types of control presumably executed by the frontal lobes in normals. Second,

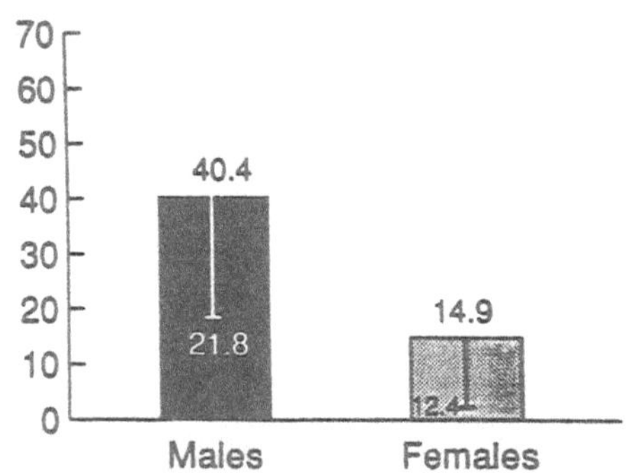

FIGURE 4. Means and standard deviations for converted CBT scores in strictly right-handed healthy subjects. (From Goldberg *et al.*, 1994, p. 278. Reprinted by permission.)

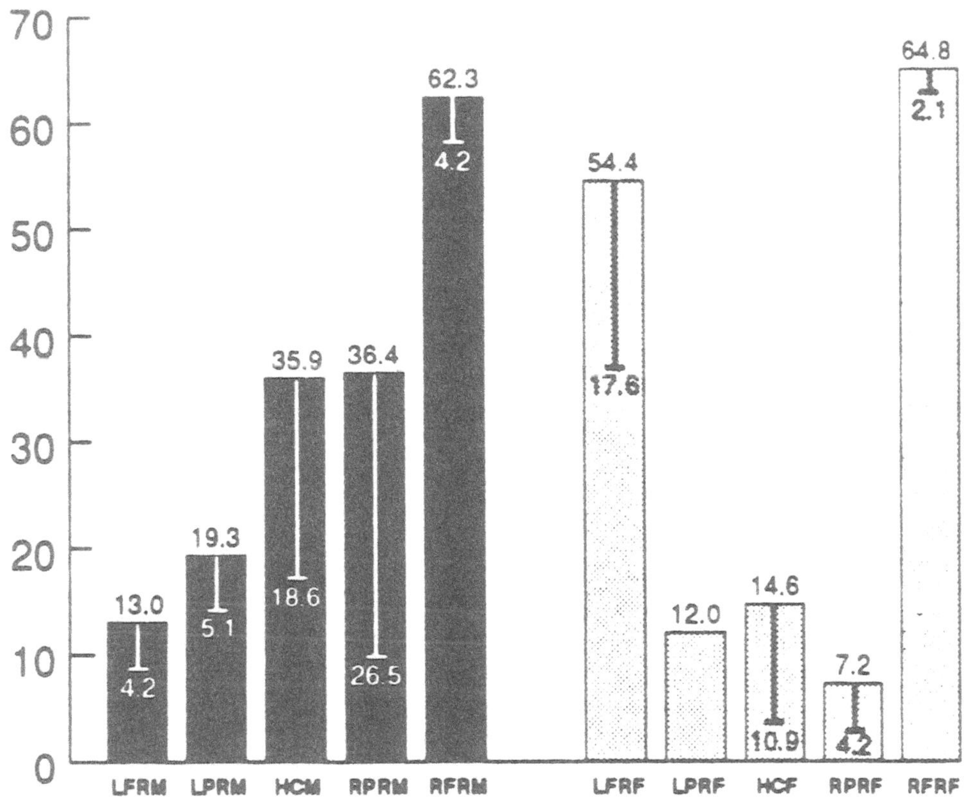

FIGURE 5. Mean converted CBT score in male and female lesion groups. LFRM, left frontal right-handed males ($n = 5$); LPRM, left posterior right-handed males ($n = 3$); HCM, healthy control males ($n = 21$); RPRM, right posterior right-handed males ($n = 8$); LFRF left frontal right-handed females ($n = 5$); LPRF, left posterior right-handed females ($n = 1$); NCF, healthy control females ($n = 14$); RPRF, right posterior right-handed females ($n = 4$); RFRF, right frontal right-handed females ($n = 4$). (From Goldberg *et al.*, 1994, p. 282. Reprinted by permission.)

the variability of scores in the frontal lobe patients is decreased relatively to normal subjects and this supports the notion that unilateral damage to the prefrontal cortex produces extreme, marginal conditions of imbalance.

We conclude that for the right-handed males we can use the CBT to determine the side of the impairment of the prefrontal system and that we can use this test to guide therapies in the absence of the PET technique. Aside from pharmacology, these cognitive assays can be used to guide remediation, because they identify two distinct types of impairment: a perseverative type and a field-dependent type. Clearly, one should apply different remedial strategies to address these two different types of impairment.

Sexual Dimorphism

When we administered CBT to females with right and left prefrontal lesions, a totally different pattern emerged (Goldberg *et al.*, 1994). No functional lateralization of the frontal lobes is evident in females based on CBT scores. Both left and right prefrontal lesions drive the scores up, toward context dependence (Goldberg *et al.*, 1994) (Fig. 5).

We have demonstrated robust functional sexual dimorphism of the prefrontal cortex . This by itself is very useful information, because it implies that one might need different strategies for cognitive rehabilitation in males and females. What are these differences? In males, there is a strong asymmetry between the effects of the left and right prefrontal lesion, and in females it is absent. Left and right prefrontal lesions in females both drive the CBT score up, making behavior more context dependent.

If we look at the cases of the mild closed head injury from the perspective of our data, we can predict that in males there is an equal occurrence of the predominantly perseverative type of impairment and predominantly field-dependent type of impairment, whereas in females there are many more cases of the predominantly perseverative type of impairment than predominantly field-dependent type of impairment. Therefore, one should be prepared to design different strategies of cognitive remediation for males and females.

We hypothesize that the sexual dimorphism of the prefrontal cortex also might be expressed in terms of the biochemical pathways, and that the principles of functional cortical geometry are somewhat different in males and females. The long-standing assumption has been that the principles of functional cortical neuroanatomy organization are the same in males and females, but are better articulated in males. Therefore, the tendency in mainstream neuropsychological research has been to study right-handed males, on the assumption that whatever one learns from right-handed males is also applicable to right-handed females. That might not be the case. It would not be surprising if a careful examination of the biochemical pathways were to reveal that the catecholamine asymmetries (more extensive dopaminergic innervation of the left frontal cortex and more extensive norepinephrinergic innervation of the right frontal cortex) are present in males but not in females. In females the pattern may be different, with a greater preponderance of norepinephrinergic pathways in both hemispheres. This would mean that pharmacological interventions should be gender dependent.

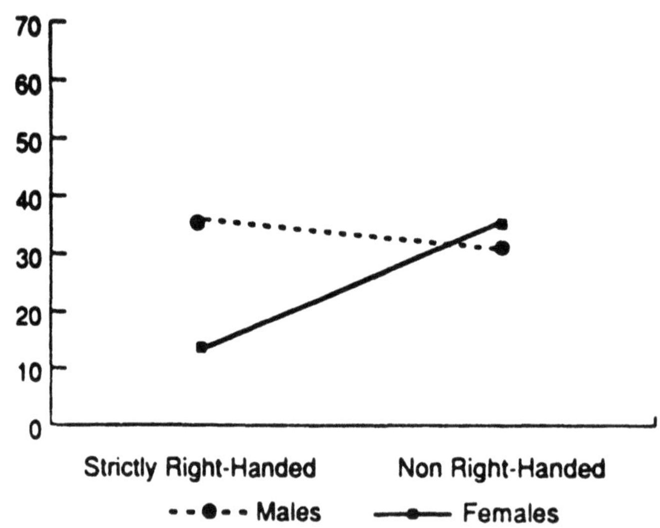

FIGURE 6. Converted CBT scores in strictly right-handed and non-right-handed healthy males and females. Strictly right-handed: males (n = 19) and females (n = 19); non-right-handed: males (n = 7) and females (n = 11). (From Goldberg *et al.*, 1994, p. 285. Reprinted by permission.)

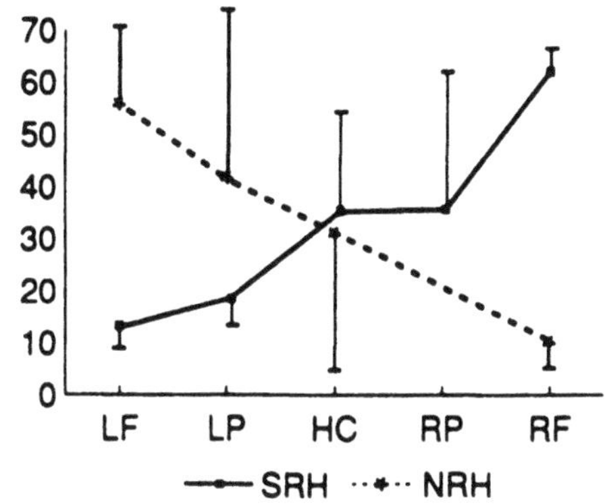

FIGURE 7. Converted CBT scores in strictly right-handed (SRH) and non-right-handed (NRH) lesioned males. SRH-LF, left frontal (*n* = 5); LP left posterior (*n* = 3); HC, healthy control (*n* = 21); RP, right posterior (*n* = 5); RF, right frontal (*n* = 8). NRH-LF, left frontal (*n* = 2); LP, left posterior (*n* = 3); HC, healthy control (*n* = 7); RP, right posterior (*n* = 0); RF, right frontal (*n* = 2). (From Goldberg *et al.*, 1994, p. 287. Reprinted by permission.)

Both morphological and biochemical evidence exist that male and female frontal lobes are different. They are different in the patterns of cortical growth. Cortical thickness, especially in the frontal lobes, is asymmetric in males (right hemisphere is thicker than the left one), but symmetric in females. The distribution of various neurohormonal receptor sites is lateralized in males, but not in females. The existence of these differences further suggests that pharmacotherapy should be different for males and females.

Handedness

Attempts to relate hemispheric specialization to handedness generally have been unsuccessful. Strong relationship between hemispheric specialization and handedness would imply that in the right-handed individuals language is mediated predominantly by the left hemisphere and in the left-handed individuals by the right hemisphere. But this is not the case, and in 60–70% of the left-handed population language is still mediated by the left hemisphere. The failure to find this crossover, the mirror symmetry between right-handers and left-handers, occurred on a number of tasks. This made many researchers conclude that there is no strong relationship between handedness and hemispheric specialization.

We compared right-handed and non-right-handed normal individuals of both genders on the CBT and found a very strong interaction between behavior on our task and handedness (Fig. 6). Non-right-handed females behave like right-handed males on CBT. Morphometric studies of Williamson, Habib, and others parallel our findings (Goldberg *et al.*, 1994).

When we administered CBT to patients who were premorbidly non-right-handed and suffered lateralized brain lesions, we saw a virtual mirror inverse crossover relative to the right-handed data (Goldberg *et al.*, 1994).

This shows that, at least in terms of the frontal lobe cognitive assays that we designed, a strong relationship exists between handedness and response selection bias both in males and in females. It appears that handedness also should be considered in the selection of cognitive and pharmacological remedial strategies. Thus, the side of the prefrontal damage, gender, and handedness are all important in designing remediation strategies. All these variables should be

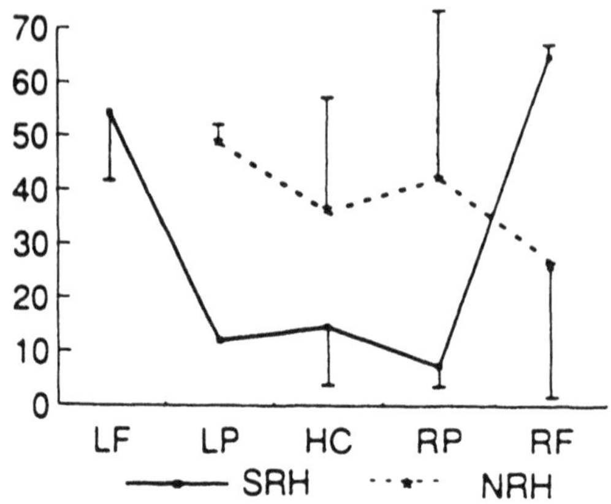

FIGURE 8. Converted CBT scores in strictly right-handed (SRH) and non-right-handed (NRH) lesioned females. SRH-LF, left frontal ($n = 5$); LP, left posterior ($n = 3$); HC, healthy control ($n = 21$); RP, right posterior ($n = 5$); RF, right frontal ($n = 8$). NRH-LF, left frontal ($n = 0$); LP, left posterior ($n = 2$); HC, healthy control ($n = 7$); RP, right posterior ($n = 2$); RF, right frontal ($n = 3$). (From Goldberg *et al.*, 1994, p. 287. Reprinted by permission.)

considered for both pharmacological and cognitive remediation with CBT-like cognitive assays to guide them.

ACKNOWLEDGMENTS The work on this chapter was supported by the East–West Foundation for Science and Education.

References

Allen, R. M. (1983). Role of amantadine in the management of the neuroleptic-induced extrapyramidal syndromes: Overview and pharmacology. *Clinical Neuropharmacology, 6*(Suppl.), S64–S73.

Andersson, S., Berstad, J., & Finset A. (1992). Amantadine in cognitive failure in patients with traumatic head injuries. *Tidsskrift for den Norske Lageforening, 112,* 2070–2072.

Aoki, F., & Sitar, D. (1988). Clinical pharmacokineticsof amantadine hydrochloride. *Clinical Pharmacokinetics, 14,* 35–51.

Barregi, S. R., Porta, M., & Selenati A. (1975). Homovanillic acid and 5-hydroxyindolacetic acid in the CSF of patients after severe head injury. *European Neurology, 13,* 528–544.

Barret, K. (1991). Treating organic abulia with bromocriptine and lisuride: four case studies. *Journal of Neurology, Neurosurgery and Psychiatry, 54,* 718–722.

Bleiberg, J., Garmo, W. M., & Cederquist, J. (1993). Effects of dexedrine on performance consistency following brain injury. *Neuropsychiatry, Neuropsychology and Behavioral Neurology, 6,* 245–248.

Brozoski, T. J., Brown, R. M., Rosvold, H. E., Waters, R. N., Cappelletti, J., & Goldman, P. S. (1979). Cognitive deficit caused by regional depletion of dopamine in prefrontal cortex of rhesus monkey. *Science, 205,* 929–932.

Catsman-Berrevoets, C. E., & Harskamp, F. (1988). Compulsive pre-sleep behavior and apathy due to bilateral thalamic stroke: Response to bromocriptine. *Neurology, 38,* 647–649.

Chandler, M. C., Barnhill, J. L., & Gualtieri, C. T. (1988). Amantadine for the agitated head-injury patient. *Brain injury, 2*(4), 309–311.

Chandra, B. (1978). Treatment of disturbance of consiousness caused by measles encephalitis with levodopa. *European Neurology, 17,* 265–270.

Cope, D. N. (1986). The pharmacology of attention and memory. *Journal of Head Trauma Rehabilitation, 1*(3), 34–92.

Deutsch, G., & Eisenberg, H. M. (1987). Frontal blood flow changes in recovery from coma. *Journal of Cerebral Blood Flow and Metabolism, 7,* 29–34

Dobkin, B. H., & Hanlon, R. (1993). Dopamine agonist treatment of anterograde amnesia from mediobasal forebrain injury. *Annals of Neurology, 33,* 313–316.

Eames, P. (1989). The use of Sinemet and bromocriptine. *Brain injury, 3*(3), 319–320.

Evans, R. W., Gualtieri, C. T., & Patterson, D. R. (1987). Treatment of closed head injury with psychostimulant drugs: A controlled case study and appropriate evaluation procedure. *Journal of Nervous and Mental Diseases, 175*(2), 106–110.

Geshwind, N. (1965). Disconnection syndromes in animals and man. *Brain, 88,* 237–294, 585–644.

Gianutsos, G., Stewart, C., & Dunn, J. P. (1985). Pharmacological changes in dopaminergic systems induced by long-term administration of amantadine. *European Journal of Pharmacolology, 110,* 357–361.

Goldberg, E. (1985). Akinesia, tardive dysmentia, and frontal lobe disorder in schizophrenia. *Schizophrenia Bulletin, 11,* 255–263.

Goldberg, E. (1992). Introduction: The frontal lobes in neurological and psychiatric conditions. *Neuropsychiatry, Neuropsychology, and Behavioral Neurolology, 5*(4), 231–232.

Goldberg, E., & Bilder, R. M. (1987). The frontal lobes and hierrarchical organization of cognitve control. In E. Perecman (Ed.), *The frontal lobes revisited* (pp. 159–187). New York: IRBN Press.

Goldberg, E., & Costa, L. D. (1986). Qualitative indices in neuropsychological assessment: An extension of Luria's approach to executive deficit following prefrontal lesions. In I. Grant & K. M. Adams (Eds.), *Neuropsychological assessment of neuropsychiatric disorders* (pp. 48–64). New York: Oxford University Press.

Goldberg, E., Antin, S. P., Bilder, R. M., Gerstman, L. J., Hughes, J. E. O., & Mattis, S. (1981). Retrograde amnesia: Possible role of mesencephalic reticular activation in long-term memory. *Science, 213,* 1392–1394.

Goldberg, E., Bilder, R. M., Hughes, J. E. O., Antin, S. P., & Mattis, S. (1989). A reticulo-frontal disconnection syndrome. *Cortex, 25,* 687–695.

Goldberg, E., Podell, K., Harner, R., Lovell, M., & Riggio, S. (1994). Cognitive bias, functional cortical geometry, and the frontal lobes: Laterality sex, and handedness. *Journal of Cognitive Neuroscience, 6*(3), 276–296.

Goldberg, E., Kluger, A., Griesing, T., Malta, L., Shapiro, M., & Ferris, S. (1997). Early diagnosis of frontal lobe dementias. *Presentation given at the Eighth Congress of the International Psychogeriatric Association.* Jerusalem, Israel.

Goldman-Rakic, P. S. (1987). Circuitry of primate prefrontal cortex and representation of behavior by representational memory. In F. Plum (Ed.), *Handbook of physiology—The nervous system V* (pp. 46–92). Betheseda, MD: American Physiological Society.

Gualtieri, C. T., Chandler, M., Coons, T. B., & Brown, L. T. (1989). Amantadine: A new clinical profile for traumatic brain injury. *Clinical Neuropharmacology, 12*(4), 258–270.

Haig, A. J., & Ruess, J. M. (1990). Recovery from vegetative state of six months' duration associated with Sinemet (levodopa/carbidopa). *Archives of Physical Medicine and Rehabilitation, 71,* 1081–1083.

Herrman, E. C., Grabliks, J., & Engle, C. (1960). Antiviral activity of L-adamantamine (amantadine). *Proclaims of Society of Experimental Biology and Medicine, 106,* 625–630.

Honer, W. G., Prohovnik, I., Smith, G., & Lucas, L. R. (1988). Scopolamine reduces frontal cortexperfusion. *Journal of Cerebral Blood Flow and Metabolism, 8,* 635–641.

Hyyppa, M. T., Langvik, V., Nieminen, V., & Vapalhti, M. (1977). Tryptophan and monoamine metabolites in ventricular cerebrospinal fluid after severe cerbral trauma. *Lancet, 1,* 1367–1368.

Ingvar, D. H. (1976). Functional landscape of the dominant hemisphere. *Brain Research, 107,* 181–197.

Ingvar, D. H., & Franzen, G. (1974). Abnormalities of the cerebral blood flow distribution in patients with chronic schizophrenia. *Acta Psychiatrica Scandinavica, 50,* 425–462.

Interagency Head Injury Task Force Report: National Institute of Neurological Disorders and Stroke (1989). Bethesda, MD, National Institute of Health.

Kimberg, D., D'Esposito, M., & Farah, M. (1994). The effects of bromocriptine, a D-2 receptor agonist, on the cognitive abilities of human subjects with different working memory capacities. *Society of Neuroscience Abstracts, 20,* 1271.

Kneale, T. A., & Eames, P. (1991). Pharmacology and flesxibility in the rehabilitation of two brain-injured adults. *Brain, 5*(3), 327–330.

Kraus, M. F., & Maki, P. M. (1997a). The combined use of amantadine and L-dopa/carbidopa in the treatment of chronic brain injury: Case report. *Brain Injury, 11,* 455–460.

Kraus, M. F., & Maki, P. M. (1997b). Effect of amantadine hydrochloride on symptoms of frontal lobe dysfunction in brain injury: Case studies and review. *Journal of Neuropsychology and Clinical Neuroscience, 9,* 222–230.

Lal, S., Merbitz, C. P., & Grip, J. C. (1988). Modification of function in head-injured patients with Sinemet. *Brain Injury, 2*(3), 225–233.

Lipper, S., & Tuchman, M. M. (1976). Treatment of chronic posttraumatic organic brain syndrome with dextroamphetamine: First reported case. *Journal of Nervous and Mental Diseases, 162*(5), 366–371.

Luciana, M., Depue, R., Arbisi, P., & Leon, A. (1992). Facilitation of working memory in humans by a D2 dopamine receptor agonist. *Journal of Cognitive Neuroscience, 107,* 394–404.

Luria, A. R. (1980). *Higher cortical functions in man* (2nd ed., pp. 373–417). New York: Basic Books.

Masdeu, J. C., Van Heertu, R. L. M., & Abdel-Dayem, H. (1995). Head trauma: Use of SPECT. *Journal of Neuroimaging, 5,* s53–s57

Milner, B. (1982). Some cognitive effects of frontal lesion in man. In D. E. Broadbent & L. Weiskranzt (Eds.), *The neuropsychology of cognitive function* (pp. 211–226). London: The Royal Society.

Minderhoud, J. M., Van Woerkom, T. C. A. M., & VanWeerdon, T. W. (1976). On the nature of the brainstem disorder in sever head injured patients. *Acta Neurochirurgica, 34,* 23–35.

Mohr, E., Fabbrini, G., & Ruggieri, S. (1987). Cognitives concomitants of dopamine system stimulation in parkinsonian patients. *Journal of Neurology, Neurosurgery and Psychiatry, 50*(1), 192–196.

Murphy, D. L., Henry, G. M., & Weingartner, H. (1972). Catecholamines and memory: Enhanced verbal learning during L-dopa administration. *Psychopharmacologia, 27,* 319–326.

Nauta, W. J. H. (1971). The problem of the frontal lobe: A reinterpretation. *Journal of Psychiatric Research, 8,* 167–187.

Newmann, R. P., Weingartner, H., & Smallberg, S. A. (1984). Effortfull and automatic memory: Effects of dopamine. *Neurology, 34,* 805–807.

Oades, R. D. (1982). Search strategies on a hole-board are impaired in rats with ventral tegmental damage: Animal models for tests of thought disorders. *Biological Psychiatry, 2,* 243–258.

Podell, K., Lovell, M., Zimmerman, M., & Goldberg, E. (1995). The cognitive bias task and lateralized frontal lobe functions in males. *Journal of Neuropsychiatry and Clinical Neuroscience, 7,* 491–501.

Powell, J. H., Al-Adawi, S., Morgan, J., & Greenwood, R. J. (1996). Motivational deficits after brain injury: Effects of bromocriptine in 11 patients. *Journal of Neurology, Neurosurgery and Psychiatry, 60,* 416–421.

Raichle, M. E., Fiez, J. A., Videen, T. O., MacLeod, A. K., Pardo, J. V., Fox, P. T., & Petersen, S. E. (1994). Practice-related changes in human brain functional anatomy during nonmotor learning. *Cerebral Cortex, 4,* 8–26.

Roberts, G. W., Leigh, P. N., & Weinberger, D. R. (1993a). *Neuropsychiatric disorders* (pp. 14.1–14.8). London: Wolfe Publishing.

Roberts, G. W., Leigh, P. N., & Weinberger, D. R. (1993b). *Neuropsychiatric disorders* (pp. 5.1–5.16). London: Wolfe Publishing.

Ross, E. D., & Stewart, R. M. (1981). Akinetic mutism from hypothalamic damage: Successful treatment with dopamine agonists. *Neurology, 31,* 1435–1439.

Schwab, R. S., England, A. C., & Postkanzer, D. C. (1969). Amantadine in the treatment of Parkinson's disease. *Journal of the American Medical Association, 208,* 1168–1170.

Smith, G. P. (1976). The arousal function of central catecholamine neurons. *Annals of New York Academy of Science, 270,* 45–55.

Tucker, D. M., & Williamson, P. A. (1984). Assymetric neural control systems in human self-regulation. *Psychological Review, 91,* 185–215.

Van Reekum, R., Bayley, M., & Garner, S. (1995). *N* of one 1 study: Amantadine for the amotivational syndrome in a patient with traumatic brain injury. *Brain Injury, 9,* 49–53.

Van Woerkom, T. C. A. M., Minderhoud, J. M., Gottschal, T., & Nicolai, G. (1982). Neurotransmitters in the treatment of patients with severe head injuries. *European Neurolology, 21,* 227–234.

Van Woerkom, T. C. A. M., Teelkan, A. W., & Minderhoud, J. M. (1977). Difference in neurotransmitter metabolism in frontotemporal-lobe contusion and diffuse cerebral contusion. *Lancet, 1,* 812–813.

Vecht, C. J., Van Woerkom, T. C. A. M., Teelkan, A. W., & Minderhoud, J. M. (1975a). 5-Hydroxyindolacetic acid (5-HIAA) levels in the cerbral spinal fluid in consiousness and unconsiousness after head injury. *Life Sciences, 16,* 1179–1186.

Vecht, C. J., Van Woerkom, T. C. A. M., Teelkan, A. W., & Minderhoud, J. M. (1975b). Homovanillic acid and 5-hydroxyindolacetic acid cerebral spinal fluid levels. *Archives of Neurolology, 32,* 792–797.

Weller, M., & Kornhuber, J. (1992). A rationale for NMDA receptor antagonist therapy of the neuroleptic malignant syndrome. *Medical Hypotheses, 38,* 329–333.

Wroblewski, B. A., & Glenn, M. B. (1994). Pharmacological treatment of arousal and cognitive deficits. *Journal of Head Trauma Rehabilitation, 9*(3), 19–42.

III

Neuropsychological Rehabilitation

7

A Brief Overview of Four Principles of Neuropsychological Rehabilitation

GEORGE P. PRIGATANO

Introduction

Throughout the United States and Europe, economic support for various health-related services is diminishing. As part of this economic tidal wave, rehabilitation services for persons with an acquired brain injury likewise have been reduced. The failure to clarify which types of rehabilitation services are efficacious for specific patient groups has further compounded this problem. Too often, no clear scientific database is available to counter decisions based more on economic concerns than on the needs of patients (Prigatano, 1996b).

The field of neuropsychological rehabilitation needs such guidelines and underlying principles to orchestrate the work of clinicians. This chapter is partially based on a forthcoming book entitled *Principles of Neuropsychological Rehabilitation* (Prigatano, in press), which presents 13 principles of neuropsychological rehabilitation. These principles have evolved from clinical and scientific observations of persons who have attempted to regain a productive lifestyle and to reestablish meaning in their life after sustaining significant disturbances of their higher cerebral functioning. Four of these principles are discussed here. Readers are referred to the original text for a more detailed discussion of each of the 13 principles and the observations from which they emerged.

GEORGE P. PRIGATANO • Section of Clinical Neuropsychology, Barrow Neurological Institute, St. Joseph's Hospital and Medical Center, Phoenix, Arizona 85013.

International Handbook of Neuropsychological Rehabilitation, edited by Christensen and Uzzell.
Kluwer Academic/ Plenum Publishers, New York, 2000.

Thirteen Principles of Neuropsychological Rehabilitation*

In this chapter, a principle is defined as an initial formulation that guides decisions about actions or the interpretation of events. The following principles, which were greatly influenced by the work of a number of individuals (see Chapter 1, Prigatano, in press), emerged from my own clinical and scientific work in the course of directing two clinical neuropsychological rehabilitation programs:

Principle 1. The clinician must begin with patients' subjective or phenomenological experience to reduce their frustrations and confusion in order to engage them in the rehabilitation process.

Principle 2. The patients' symptom picture is a mixture of premorbid cognitive and personality characteristics as well as neuropsychological changes directly associated with brain pathology.

Principle 3. Neuropsychological rehabilitation focuses on both the remediation of higher cerebral disturbances and their management in interpersonal situations.

Principle 4. Neuropsychological rehabilitation helps patients observe their behavior and thereby teaches them about the direct and indirect effects of brain injury.

Principle 5. Failure to study the intimate interaction of cognition and personality leads to an inadequate understanding of many issues in cognitive (neuro)sciences and neuropsychological rehabilitation.

Principle 6. Little is known about how to retrain a brain dysfunctional patient systematically because the nature of higher cerebral functions is not fully understood.

a. General guidelines for cognitive remediation, however, can be specified.

Principle 7. Psychotherapeutic interventions often are an important part of neuropsychological rehabilitation because they help patients (and families) deal with their personal losses.

a. The process, however, is highly individualized.

Principle 8. Working with brain dysfunctional patients produces affective reactions in both the patient's family and the rehabilitation staff. Appropriate management of these reactions facilitates the rehabilitative and adaptive process.

Principle 9. Each neuropsychological rehabilitation program is a dynamic entity. It is either in a state of development or decline.

a. Ongoing scientific investigation helps the rehabilitation team learn from their successes and failures and is needed to maintain a dynamic, creative rehabilitation effort.

Principle 10. Failure to identify which patients can and cannot be helped by different (neuropsychological) rehabilitation approaches creates a lack of credibility for the field.

Principle 11. Disturbances in self-awareness after brain injury are often poorly understood and mismanaged.

Principle 12. Competent patient management and planning innovative rehabilitation programs depend on understanding mechanisms of recovery and deterioration of direct and indirect symptoms after brain injury.

Principle 13. The rehabilitation of patients with higher cerebral deficits requires both scientific and phenomenological approaches. Both are necessary to maximize recovery and adaptation to the effects of brain injury.

---

*Permission to reprint these 13 principles and introductory comments was obtained from Oxford University Press.

Due to space limitations, only four principles are discussed below. Principles 1, 3, 11, and 12 were chosen because they highlight issues involved in engaging patients in rehabilitation, conceptualize the important problem of impaired self-awareness after brain injury, and reconsider the efficacy of past interventions and what neuropsychological rehabilitation programs may wish to consider in the future.

Principle 1: The Clinician Must Begin with Patients' Subjective or Phenomenological Experience to Reduce Their Frustrations and Confusion in Order to Engage Them in the Rehabilitation Process

After brain injury, patients' eagerness to engage rehabilitation therapies varies. During the acute phase (the first 30 to 90 days after brain insult), some patients passively participate in various rehabilitation processes but are perplexed and frustrated about why they must perform different tasks, which seem unnecessary to them. Some patients may be too tired or confused to engage tasks aimed at helping their cognitive and physical recovery. During the intermediate (6 to 12 months after lesion onset) and the postacute phases (at least 1 year after lesion onset), the insight of patients with severe traumatic brain injuries (TBIs) or other diffuse cerebral injuries into their cognitive and personality disturbances may be limited. Consequently, they do not know why it is difficult for them to function independently or to return to work.

At each stage of the rehabilitation process, it is the neuropsychologist's responsibility to examine patients in a manner that helps clarify the nature of their higher cerebral disturbances. As this information is obtained, the implications for rehabilitation need to be communicated to the patient, family, rehabilitation physician, and various rehabilitation team members in a manner that facilitates the rehabilitation enterprise. Consequently, the neuropsychologist must not just "test" patients. He or she must examine patients in a way that helps them to understand what has "gone wrong" with their higher cerebral functioning, without overwhelming the patients.

Repeatedly, I have found that neuropsychologists are quite competent at testing but have a difficult time understanding what patients are actually experiencing during testing or outside the testing session. Without such knowledge, however, it is difficult for the therapist to communicate with patients adequately and even more difficult to engage them in various rehabilitation activities. Thus, entering the phenomenological field of patients helps reduce their frustration and associated confusion and is the first major principle of neuropsychological rehabilitation.

Goldstein (1942, 1952) was one of the first clinicians to recognize that patients often become overwhelmed when their cognitive deficits result in daily failures that they had not anticipated. In some instances, such repeated failures lead to the emergence of a catastrophic reaction (Goldstein, 1952). Helping patients understand and manage their catastrophic reactions is a major contribution of neuropsychological rehabilitation (Prigatano *et al.,* 1986).

Although everyone experiences frustrations, the confusion that patients experience after brain injury is atypical. Brain dysfunctional patients often fail to solve problems but do not understand their failure. Moreover, their failures often have an especially disorganizing effect (Chapman & Wolf, 1959). Consequently, they may be unable to reapproach a problem in a productive way. Thus, their confusion removes them from the "problem-solving" loop and renders them inactive as well as ineffective. Patients then may become belligerent or angry, or they may simply withdraw. By understanding patients' confusion and helping them better understand how to reapproach problems when disorganized by their failures, clinicians can substantially assist patients in the process of rehabilitation.

In the context of understanding patients' phenomenological experiences, clinicians frequently encounter patients' mental fatigue (Brodal, 1973). Many brain dysfunctional patients report that they tire easily even after doing the simplest cognitive tasks. Rehabilitation activities are seldom planned with adequate consideration of this factor. Rehabilitation activities must be developed that help patients to increase their level of mental energy. Rehabilitation activities also should be modifiable if patients become too fatigued by the task. As straightforward as these observations are, seldom do even experienced neurorehabilitation therapists ask patients, "How can I help reduce your frustration? What is it that seems to be most confusing to you? Are you too tired or fatigued by the activities that we are doing?"

There are numerous barriers to entering the phenomenological field of patients. At times, rehabilitation therapists themselves may be confused by the nature of a patient's higher cerebral dysfunction (Prigatano, 1989). If therapists cannot provide a reasonable (let alone accurate) definition of higher cerebral functions, how can they begin to conceptualize the higher cerebral dysfunctions exhibited by patients? Many therapists know little about brain–behavior relations. Consequently, they may misinterpret why patients behave in a certain manner.

In addition to their lack of technical knowledge, therapists may become angry with patients precisely because they act in a brain dysfunctional way. Many therapists want patients to respond logically and appropriately when, in fact, their brain injury precludes such behavior. Still other therapists find it difficult to maintain their own mental energy and psychological resources when treating brain dysfunctional patients. This problem can reflect several factors, including pressures placed on therapists to see more and more patients within shorter and shorter intervals.

Patients' artistic expressions can be especially helpful to therapists attempting to enter their phenomenological field, particularly when patients cannot clearly articulate their experiences. By attending to the spontaneous drawings of brain dysfunctional patients, their choice of music, and the poetry they may compose, clinical neuropsychologists are in a better posi-

FIGURE 1. Drawing by a patient who suffered a brain injury. Reprinted with permission from Barrow Neurological Institute.

tion to sense what patients experience. This dialogue may help clinicians initiate a working alliance with patients and to engage them in the rehabilitation effort.

For example, a young woman who suffered a gunshot wound to the head initially presented with subtle verbal memory and language difficulties. During the early stages of her rehabilitation, she was quite cooperative but often appeared depressed. At one point in her neuropsychological rehabilitation, she refused to participate in a rehabilitation exercise that required videotaping. The patient could not verbally explain her position, but she was adamant that she would not participate. With the help of a drawing, her clinical neuropsychologist better appreciated her feelings. As her drawing showed (see Fig. 1), she literally had no mouth to express her ideas in words. Yet, the drawing revealed much about how this patient actually felt and what she experienced. Like many other patients, she had a variety of feelings that were difficult to articulate. She also experienced a fair amount of confusion. By entering this patient's phenomenological field via her drawings, the clinical neuropsychologist was in a better position to guide her and the rehabilitation team during a difficult time. Eventually, the patient was able to complete her rehabilitation experience precisely because she felt understood and was not forced to participate in an activity that was not necessary for her rehabilitative care. No neuropsychological tests that I am aware of could have captured the complexity of this patient's experience as well as her drawing. Despite their scientific training, clinical neuropsychologists should not avoid obtaining such information to improve their understanding of patients' experiences. Such attempts often facilitate neuropsychological assessments and rehabilitation outcomes.

Principle 3: Neuropsychological Rehabilitation Focuses on Both the Remediation of Higher Cerebral Disturbances and Their Management in Interpersonal Situations

Modern efforts at conducting systematic neuropsychological rehabilitation are typically dated to the early work of Goldstein (1942), Zangwill (1947), and Luria (1948/1963). Each of their approaches was based on some conceptualization of how brain activity is altered when the cerebral hemispheres or brain stem is damaged. Goldstein (1942) noted, for example, that the loss of abstract attitude was associated with an extremely concrete approach to problem solving. This attitude, in turn, created behavioral adaptations that sometimes resulted in a catastrophic reaction or condition (Goldstein, 1952). Restructuring the environment and placing patients in a work setting that they could handle substantially improved their psychosocial adjustment.

In contrast, Luria (1948/1963) and his colleagues (Luria, Naydin, Tsvetkova, & Vinarskaya, 1969) were impressed that impaired higher cerebral functions apparently could be restored by deinhibiting or "deblocking" temporarily disturbed higher cerebral functional systems. Von Monakow's (1885) theory of "diaschisis" could account for such phenomena. Interestingly, Luria cites an example where "special psychotherapeutic suggestive measures, aimed at modifying the orientation of the personality" (p. 431) actually seemed to facilitate rate of recovery (Luria *et al.,* 1969).

The later work of Ben-Yishay and Diller (1993) emphasized the concept of remediation in neuropsychological rehabilitation (also see Ben-Yishay and Prigatano, 1990). Remediation can mean relieving the pain of a disorder or actually curing it (*American Heritage Dictionary,* 1976, p. 1045). The milieu-oriented, holistic approach championed by these investigators clearly demonstrated that selected postacute TBI patients could increase their level of psychosocial adjustment by systematic retraining (i.e., reduce the pain of the disorder). In a few cases, their "remediational" exercises were associated with greater than expected cognitive improvements in patients (Rattok *et al.*, 1992). Overall, however, no type of therapy can return a damaged higher cerebral function to "normal."

Clinical experience with a milieu-oriented approach suggests that it helps many patients to adjust to their disturbances, and their psychosocial adjustment thereby improves. Prigatano *et al.* (1984), for example, demonstrated that patients treated within the context of this model had a high incidence of regaining a productive lifestyle. The finding was later replicated (Prigatano *et al.*, 1994). The quality of the working alliance between the rehabilitation staff and the patient and family also correlates with better psychosocial outcomes. Prigatano therefore has argued that it can be crucial to incorporate a psychotherapeutic approach in neuropsychological rehabilitation (Prigatano *et al.*, 1986; Prigatano, 1991b; 1995, in press).

The psychotherapeutic approach emphasizes helping patients to engage rehabilitation exercises and thereby to reenter society despite the suffering caused by their brain damage (see Fig. 2). It has become progressively clearer that a psychotherapeutic approach improves the management of disturbances of higher cerebral functioning and therefore can lead to improved interpersonal relationships for patients. For the field to continue to grow, however, Luria's (1948/1963) concept of developing methods of restoring disturbed higher cerebral function must again be emphasized.

The study of the components underlying disturbed higher cerebral functioning greatly helps in this regard. For example, Diamond, DeLuca, and Kelley (1997) helped to illuminate the nature of memory disorders after ruptured aneurysms of the anterior communicating artery (ACoA). Their study showed that some of these patients had trouble with the initial organization of information (an executive function?). It also showed that systematically teaching patients how to overcome this organizational defect could improve their performance on memory tasks. This study follows the spirit of Luria's (1948/1963) vision and message. Further work is needed to rekindle this approach in contemporary efforts at neuropsychological rehabilitation. Thus, principle 3 posits that new techniques for the remediation of disturbed higher cerebral functioning should constantly be under development, while still attending to patients' personal experiences and helping them adjust to their neuropsychological deficits in the context of interpersonal situations.

PHILOSOPHICAL PATIENCE IN THE FACE OF SUFFERING

SOCIAL RE-INTEGRATION

CONTROL

MASTERY

AWARENESS

ENGAGEMENT

FIGURE 2. Global components of neuropsychologically oriented rehabilitation. Adapted with permission from Ben-Yishay and Prigatano (1990).

Principle 11: Disturbances in Self-Awareness after Brain Injury Are Often Poorly Understood and Mismanaged

Many patients with a history of severe TBI exhibit disturbances in self-perception and awareness that have been difficult to define. Early literature suggested that many of these patients had some insight into their impairments but were simply denying the disturbances (Weinstein & Kahn, 1955). The opportunity to study these patients in the context of neuropsychological rehabilitation has revealed that this conjecture may be oversimplified (Prigatano, 1991a, 1996b). Disorders of self-awareness are quite complex. Some aspects of these disorders seem to reflect unequivocal brain dysfunction. In other instances, the impairments seem to reflect individuals' attempts to cope with painful self-perceptions.

A historical perspective on the problem of impaired self-awareness provides fruitful observations for contemporary conceptualizations. As Bisiach and Geminiani (1991) reminded us, Seneca observed impaired awareness during antiquity:

> You know that Harpastes, my wife's fatuitous companion, has remained in my home as an inherited burden. . . . this foolish woman has suddenly lost her sight. Incredible as it might appear, what I am going to tell you is true: she does not know that she is blind. Therefore, again and again, she asks her guardian to take her elsewhere. She claims that my home is dark.

Disorders of self-awareness related to cortical blindness were thus recorded long before the advent of the scientific method. This lack of insight seems unequivocally related to brain dysfunction. Whether this lack of awareness reflects pure cognitive dysfunction has been the subject of considerable debate.

Whenever consciousness is disturbed, residual disturbances may persist weeks, months, or years later, much like with aphasia. After an individual experiences a global aphasia, persistent signs of anomia, difficulties with repeating lengthy sentences, and difficulties understanding complex verbal narratives would be expected even after the best recovery. So, an individual who has had a prolonged period of unconsciousness should be expected to show subtle disturbances of consciousness.

It is beyond the scope of this discussion to consider this phenomenon in detail (see Chapter 12 in Prigatano, in press), but Mesulam's (1985) concept of the heteromodal cortex suggests a model of impaired self-awareness. That is, different forms of impaired awareness may occur depending on the region of the brain that has been compromised. Theoretically, complete and partial heteromodal cortical syndromes of unawareness would exist. Clinically, four syndromes are seen: frontal heteromodal disorder syndrome, parietal heteromodal disorder syndrome, temporal heteromodal disorder syndrome, and occipital heteromodal disorder syndrome. Whether these syndromes are complete or partial depends on the passage of time and the diffuseness of the cerebral injury.

It is important to recognize that a disorder of awareness is a disorder of (subjective) experience. Experience, by definition, implies an integration of thinking and feeling. Thus, both dimensions are disrupted in patients with disorders of self-awareness. In fact, patients who have impaired self-awareness perform poorly on tests involving the perception and expression of emotion (Cutting, 1978; Starkstein, Fedoroff, Price, Leiguarda, & Robinson, 1992). Moreover, the initial level of disturbed consciousness relates to ratings of impaired awareness months or years after injury (Sherer *et al.*, 1998; Prigatano *et al.*, 1998).

An important issue in disorders of self-awareness is raised by patients who have partial knowledge of their disorder but who seem to use methods of coping that reflect some effort at "denial." Therefore, it may be useful to conceptualize methods of coping as defensive or nondefensive. Denial of disability is present when patients who have partial awareness use defensive methods to cope with their deficits. Many patients who have partial knowledge of their disability, however, use nondefensive methods of coping. Thus, the simple dichotomy of impaired self-awareness versus denial of disability (Prigatano & Klonoff, 1998) that was recently suggested already appears to be inadequate.

The speed of finger tapping is often slow bilaterally in patients with impaired self-awareness (Prigatano & Altman, 1990). This finding has been cross validated in a study with Japanese TBI patients (Prigatano, Ogano, & Amakusa, 1997), where the patients who tended to overestimate their behavioral competency compared to relatives' and physical therapists' reports of their competency also tended to tap their fingers slowly.

Finger tapping may be mediated by both cerebral hemispheres. Both the contralateral and ipsilateral sensorimotor strips are activated by rapid finger movements. Furthermore, the ipsilateral cerebellum and the supplementary motor cortex may be activated (Roland, 1993). These findings are especially interesting in the context of evidence that suggests that patients who have experienced a unilateral cerebrovascular accident tend to achieve their rehabilitation goals if their speed of finger tapping in the "unaffected" hand approaches a normal range within 30 days of their inpatient rehabilitation (Prigatano & Wong, 1997). It appears that neurobehavioral markers sensitive to impaired awareness may relate to rehabilitation outcomes.

In another study (Prigatano & Wong, 1999), patients were first asked to predict if they could recall three words with distraction. Typically, at admission, only one of five patients can perform this task accurately. Patients who achieved their rehabilitation goals also tended to predict their memory performance at discharge accurately. Thus, the ability to show a realistic level of self-awareness soon after brain injury may be a useful predictor of outcome of even acute rehabilitation after brain injury. Patients who could display spontaneous affect and who could perceive facial affect accurately also had a greater incidence of achieving their rehabilitation goals. Thus, both early and late forms of neuropsychological rehabilitation (Prigatano *et al.*, 1986) emphasize the role of cognitive and affective variables in predicting progress and outcome.

Principle 12: Competent Patient Management and Planning Innovative Rehabilitation Programs Depend on Understanding Mechanisms of Recovery and Deterioration of Direct and Indirect Symptoms after Brain Injury

The brain is a dynamic organ that is constantly changing for the "better" or "worse." Geschwind (1985) made this point when he commented, ". . . one can probably never speak of a fixed neurological lesion" (p. 2). In this context, the clinical follow-up of postacute TBI patients who have undergone extensive neuropsychological rehabilitation has taught some sobering lessons, among which are two important facts. First, patients can show continued recovery and/or deterioration of both direct and indirect effects of brain damage after such rehabilitation. Second, patients who are not helped to deal adequately with their disturbances of self-awareness may be at risk for developing late onset psychosis.

Placing acutely impaired TBI patients in milieu-oriented neuropsychological rehabilitation programs developed for postacute patients may be a mistake. For example, a patient who had undergone such intensive rehabilitation (Prigatano *et al.*, 1986) just 4 months after injury continued to have very poor insight and judgment about his impairments and their implications for his adjustment at discharge 1 year later. At that time, his wife also noted that he had angry outbursts increasingly often. Three years later he was reexamined. His cognitive status after rehabilitation had continued to improve, but he was also much quicker to anger and was experiencing major psychosocial adjustment problems. In retrospect, the patient appeared to have entered the rehabilitation program prematurely (in part due to fiscal pressures) and his psychosocial outcome was not positive. (For a more detailed discussion of this patient, see Chapter 13, Prigatano, in press.)

As Thomsen (1984) noted, some patients develop psychotic reactions several years after injury. Clinically, these patients seem to have extremely severe disturbances of self-awareness that are not remediated by neuropsychological rehabilitation. For example, a patient who has been followed for 18 years after his injury failed to understand his repeated failures at work and interpersonal relationships. Eventually, he developed a psychotic reaction with clear signs of delusions and hallucinations. Whether his psychotic reaction reflects a true deterioration in brain function or the cumulative effects of years of impaired self-awareness is unclear.

Corkin, Rosen, Sullivan, and Clegg (1989) followed World War II veterans 10 and 40 years after injury. They demonstrated that some of these patients showed a decline in their higher cerebral functioning 40 years after injury that was not observed when they were evaluated 10 years after injury. Their data clarify that neuropsychological functions can worsen in some patients as they age. Understanding the mechanisms of this deterioration and conversely the mechanisms of maintained function will become extremely important in developing innovative rehabilitation programs for the future.

Recent work on the role of genetic factors in influencing recovery and deterioration also offers some interesting ideas for neuropsychological rehabilitation. The apolipoprotein e (APOE) gene may be an important genetic marker for the emergence of Alzheimer's disease (Roses & Saunders, 1997). Individuals who are positive for the e4 allele have a high risk of developing Alzheimer's disease, which may have an early age of onset. After various brain insults, patients with other brain disorders who are positive for the APOE gene type with the e4 allele may show less recovery than those who do not have this genotype. For example, individuals who suffer intracranial hemorrhage have high rates of mortality and morbidity. Individuals who are positive for the APOE gene type with the e4 allele not only have a threefold higher incidence of death but poor rehabilitation outcomes as measured by the Barthel Index score (Table 1). The neuropsychological recovery of individuals undergoing cardiac surgery can also vary, depending on whether patients are positive for the e4 allele. Citing a study by Tardiff *et al.* (1997), Roses and Saunders (1997) noted "that patients with an e4 allele did not recover neuropsychological parameters as well as did patients without an e4 allele" (p. 197).

Is it possible that the subgroup of patients whose condition deteriorated with the passage of time were positive for the e4 allele? Could patients with mild head injury who do not show the expected "good" neuropsychological recovery have a different genotype than patients who do? These questions need further investigation, as does the role of genetic markers in determining recovery and deterioration after brain injury. Depending on the findings, future neuropsychological rehabilitation may well include some form of "gene therapy."

TABLE 1. Mortality and Recovery as a Function of APOE Genotype in Intracerebral Hemorrhage[a]

Genotype	Number	Mortality	Barthel
$\epsilon2/\epsilon3$, $\epsilon3/\epsilon3$	26	19%	88
$\epsilon3/\epsilon4$	16	68%	60

[a] From Roses & Saunders (1997). Reprinted with permission of New York Academy of Sciences.

Future Perspectives

The field of neuropsychological rehabilitation needs guidelines for care and principles to help guide clinicians dealing with the formidable problems encountered in rehabilitating individuals with impaired higher cerebral functions. This chapter highlights 4 of 13 such principles recently described elsewhere (Prigatano, in press).

Work with brain dysfunctional patients in neuropsychological rehabilitation emphasizes three important facts. First, patients' premorbid psychological adjustment and cognitive status vary greatly. Second, brain lesions interact with premorbid status to produce various patterns of recovery soon after brain injury. Thus, recovery reflects at least two important variables: the severity of brain injury and an individual's premorbid state (Luria, 1948/1963). From this observation emerges the third point. Following patients for many years after their brain injury has revealed that some individuals show a precipitous decline in higher cerebral functioning that cannot be accounted for by the aging process per se, while others do not. Understanding the mechanisms responsible for these changes (both recovery and deterioration) is crucial for developing innovative programs of neuropsychological rehabilitation. Future programs of neuropsychological rehabilitation should have two aims: facilitating recovery during the first few years after a brain injury and preventing long-term deterioration. Combining both scientific and phenomenological approaches to develop such rehabilitation programs will likely be the most practical venue for helping patients.

References

American Heritage Dictionary. (1976). Boston: Houghton Mifflin, p. 1045.

Ben-Yishay, Y., & Diller, L. (1993). Cognitive remediation in traumatic brain injury: Update and issues. *Archives of Physical Medicine Rehabilitation, 74,* 204–213.

Ben-Yishay, Y., & Prigatano, G.P. (1990). Cognitive remediation. In E. Griffith, M. Rosenthal, M. R. Bond, & J. D. Miller (Eds.), *Rehabilitation of the adult and child with traumatic brain injury* (pp. 393–409). Philadelphia: F. A. Davis.

Bisiach, E., & Geminiani, G. (1991). Anosognosia related to hemiplegia and hemianopia. In G. P. Prigatano & R. R. Schacter (Eds.), *Awareness of deficit after brain injury. Clinical and theoretical issues* (pp. 17–39). New York: Oxford University.

Brodal, A. (1973). Self-observations and neuro-anatomical considerations after a stroke. *Brain, 96,* 675–694.

Chapman, L. F., & Wolf, H. G. (1959). The cerebral hemispheres and the highest integrative functions of man. *Archives of Neurology, 1,* 357–424.

Corkin, S., Rosen, T. J., Sullivan, E. V., & Clegg, R.A. (1989). Penetrating head injury in young adulthood exacerbates cognitive decline in later years. *Journal of Neuroscience, 9,* 3876–3883.

Cutting, J. (1978). Study of anosognosia. *Journal of Neurology, Neurosurgery, and Psychiatry, 41,* 548–555.

Diamond, B. J., DeLuca, J., & Kelley, S. M. (1997). Memory and executive functions in amnesic and non-amnesic patients with aneurysms of the anterior communicating artery. *Brain, 120,* 1015–1025.

Geschwind, N. (1985). Mechanisms of change after brain lesions. In F. Nottebohm (Ed.), *Hope for a new neurology* (pp. 4–11). New York: New York Academy of Sciences.

Goldstein, K. (1942). *Aftereffects of brain injury in war.* New York: Grune & Stratton.

Goldstein, K. (1952). The effect of brain damage on the personality. *Psychiatry, 15,* 245–260.

Luria, A.R. (1948/1963). *Restoration of function after brain trauma* (in Russian). Moscow: Academy of Medical Science (London: Pergamon, 1963).

Luria, A. R., Naydin, V. L., Tsvetkova, L. S., & Vinarskaya, E. N. (1969). Restoration of higher cortical function following local brain damage. In P. J. Vinken & G. W. Bruyn (Eds.), *Handbook of clinical neurology* (Vol. 3, pp. 368–433). Amsterdam: North-Holland.

Mesulam, M. M. (1985). *Principles of behavioral neurology.* Philadelphia: F. W. Davis.

Prigatano, G. P. (1989). Bring it up in milieu: Toward effective traumatic brain injury rehabilitation interaction. *Rehabilitation Psychology, 34,* 135–144.

Prigatano, G. P. (1991a). Disturbances of self-awareness of deficit after traumatic brain injury. In G. P. Prigatano & D. L. Schacter (Eds.), *Awareness of deficit after brain injury: Theoretical and clinical implications* (pp. 111–126). New York: Oxford University.

Prigatano, G. P. (1991b). Science and symbolism in neuropsychological rehabilitation after brain injury. The Tenth Annual James C. Hemphill Lecture, November 7, 1991, Rehabilitation Institute of Chicago.

Prigatano, G. P. (1995). 1994 Sheldon Berrol, MD, Senior Lectureship: The problem of lost normality after brain injury. *Journal of Head Trauma Rehabilitation, 10,* 87–95.

Prigatano, G. P. (1996a). Behavioral limitations TBI patients tend to underestimate: A replication and extension to patients with lateralized cerebral dysfunction. *The Clinical Neuropsychologist, 10,* 191–201.

Prigatano, G. P. (1996b). Neuropsychological rehabilitation after brain injury: Scientific and professional issues. *Journal of Clinical Psychology in Medical Settings, 3,* 1–10.

Prigatano, G. P. (in press). *Principles of neuropsychological rehabilitation.* New York: Oxford University Press.

Prigatano, G. P., & Altman, I. M. (1990). Impaired awareness of behavioral limitations after traumatic brain injury. *Archives of Physical Medicine Rehabilitation, 71,* 1058–1063.

Prigatano, G. P., & Klonoff, P. S. (1998). A clinician's rating scale for evaluating impaired self-awareness and denial of disability after brain injury. *The Clinical Neuropsychologist, 12*(1), 56–67.

Prigatano, G. P., & Wong, J. L. (1997). Speed of finger tapping and goal attainment after unilateral cerebral vascular accident. *Archives of Physical Medicine and Rehabilitation, 78,* 847–852.

Prigatano, G. P., & Wong, J. L. (1999). Cognitive and affective improvement in brain dysfunctional patients who achieve inpatient rehabilitation goals. *Archives of Physical Medicine and Rehabilitation, 80*(1), 77–84.

Prigatano, G. P., Fordyce, D. J., Zeiner, H. K., Roueche, J. R., Pepping, M., & Wood, B. (1984). Neuropsychological rehabilitation after closed head injury in young adults. *Journal of Neurology, Neurosurgery, and Psychiatry, 47,* 505–513.

Prigatano, G. P., Fordyce, D. J., Zeiner, H. K., Roueche, J. R., Pepping, M., & Wood, B. (1986). *Neuropsychological rehabilitation after brain injury.* Baltimore: Johns Hopkins University.

Prigatano, G. P., Klonoff, P. S., O'Brien, K. P., Altman, I., Amin, K., Chiapello, D. A., Shepherd, J., Cunningham, M., & Mora, M. (1994). Productivity after neuropsychologically oriented, milieu rehabilitation. *Journal of Head Trauma and Rehabilitation, 9,* 91–102.

Prigatano, G. P., Ogano, M., & Amakusa, B. (1997). A cross-cultural study on impaired self-awareness in Japanese patients with brain dysfunction. *Neuropsychiatry, Neuropsychology, and Behavioral Neurology, 10,* 135–143.

Prigatano, G. P., Bruna, O, Mataro, M., Munoz, J. M., Fernandez, S., & Junque, C. (1998). Initial disturbances of consciousness and resultant impaired awareness in Spanish patients with traumatic brain injury. *Journal of Head Trauma Rehabilitation, 13*(5), 29–38.

Rattok, J., Ben-Yishay, D., Lakin, P., Piasetsky, E., Ross, B., Silver, S., Vakil, E., Zide, E., & Diller, L. (1992). Outcome of different treatment mixes in a multidimensional neuropsychological rehabilitation program. *Neuropsychology, 6,* 3395–3414.

Roland, P. E. (1993). *Brain activation.* New York: Wiley-Liss.

Roses, A. D., & Saunders, A. M. (1997). ApoE, Alzheimer's disease, and recovery from brain stress. *Annals of the New York Academy of Sciences, 826,* 200–212.

Sherer, M., Boake, C., Levin, E., Silver, B. V., Ringholz, G., & High, W. (1998). Characteristics of impaired awareness after traumatic injury. *Journal of International Neuropsychological Society, 4,* 380–387.

Starkstein, S. E., Fedoroff, J. P., Price, T. R., Leiguarda, R., & Robinson, R. G. (1992). Anosognosia in patients with cerebrovascular lesions. A study of causative factors. *Stroke, 23,* 1446–1453.

Tardiff, B. E., Newman, M. F., Saunders, A. M., Strittmatter, W. J., Blumenthal, J. A., White, W. D., Croughwell, N. D., Davis, R. D., Jr., Roses, A. D., & Reves, J. G. (1997). Preliminary report of a genetic basis for cognitive decline after cardiac operations. The Neurologic Outcome Research Group of the Duke Heart Center. *Annals of Thoracic Surgery, 64*(3), 715–720.

Thomsen, I. V. (1984). Late outcome of very severe blunt head trauma: A 10–15 year second follow-up. *Journal of Neurology, Neurosurgery, and Psychiatry, 47,* 260–268.

von Monakow, C. (1885). Experimentelle und pathologisch-anatomische Untersuchungen über die Beziehungen der sogentannen Sehsphäre zu den infracorticalen Opticuscentren und zum N. opticus. *Archives für Psychiatrie, 16,* 151–199.

Weinstein, E. A., & Kahn, R. L. (1955). *Denial of illness: Symbolic and physiological aspects.* Springfield, IL: Charles C Thomas.

Zangwill, O. L. (1947). Psychological aspects of rehabilitation in cases of brain injury. *British Journal of Psychiatry, 37,* 60–69.

8

Postacute Neuropsychological Rehabilitation

A Holistic Perspective

YEHUDA BEN-YISHAY

Introduction

The aim of this chapter is to articulate the key conceptual foundations of the holistic, therapeutic millieu approach to postacute neuropsychological rehabilitation. For a description of the structural, programmatic, and cognitive–psychotherapeutic remedial elements of such a program, the reader is referred to Chapter 12, this volume.

The holistic approach to postacute neuropsychological rehabilitation is in some respects a direct extension and in some respects derivative of Kurt Goldstein's view of human nature in normal and pathological states.

A View of Functional Impairments

Any consideration of Goldstein's notions about neuropsychological rehabilitation must begin with his unique view of impairments of functioning in brain-injured persons. Goldstein (1959) stated that an observed failure to function in a person with a head injury, at a given moment, can be the consequence of either one or a combination of three underlying causes: (1) It can be the direct result of an impaired or reduced capacity due to a brain lesion. (2) It can be the result of a disuse by the person of some still intact capacities, which the person does not apply; for although "he is in principle able to use undamaged capacities, he seems not to use those which may bring him—under some conditions—in spite of the protection—into catastrophe" (Goldstein, 1959, p. 9). This avoidance is not a conscious phenomenon. Rather, it is

---

YEHUDA BEN-YISHAY • Brain Injury Day Treatment Program, New York University Medical Center, New York, New York 10016.

International Handbook of Neuropsychological Rehabilitation, edited by Christensen and Uzzell.
Kluwer Academic/ Plenum Publishers, New York, 2000.

the expression of the protective mechanisms of the organism, which "in the brain-impaired person occurs passively through organismic adjustment" (Goldstein, 1952, p. 65).

In Goldstein's view, this organismic defense is the reason for the "conservative" tendencies of brain-injured persons. By avoiding seeking new challenges or new experiences and sticking to the familiar or the routine, they minimize the chances for experiencing catastrophic responses. The disuse of intact capacities is thus in the service of safety. (3) A third cause of a failure to function adequately is the actual occurrence of a major or minor catastrophic experience or condition. A catastrophic condition is a symptom "of disordered functioning of the whole organism, which shows all the characteristics of severe anxiety" (Goldstein, 1959, p. 8). It is the behavioral manifestation of a threat to the persons's very "existence," due to the failure to cope.

A View of the Rehabilitation Process

Goldstein maintained that when it is impossible to restore the organism to its full preinjury integrity "after we have arranged an environment where no demands are made on him which would lead him to catastrophe, then, he feels healthy; and one could say he is in a state of health" (Goldstein, 1959, p. 9). Thus, a state of "health" can be achieved if others order the patient's environment, thus rendering it predictable. The ordered environment makes it possible for the individual to cope and that produces a feeling that he or she is "healthy."

But, "becoming healthy demands a transformation of the individual's personality which enables him to bear restrictions . . . (and accepting these restrictions) to such a degree that life remains worth living in spite of restrictions" (Goldstein, 1959, p. 10). Hence, since the ordering of one's environment by necessity limits that person's choices, accepting restrictions, without feeling helpless and victimized by these restrictions, can be achieved only if the individual makes a conscious and voluntary choice to accept restrictions. And, "it is our task in therapy to help the patient realize the necessity of restrictions in becoming healthy" (Goldstein, 1959, p. 10). This has significant consequences for therapy, since, due to the impairments of both the cognitive and emotional functions of the brain injured individual, (1) "a particular part of therapy consists in making the patient understand the problem as much as possible in all of its details. It will help him to take restrictions, particularly if he becomes aware that this situation is in principle not so very different from" normal persons, who continuously through life also must cope with and adjust to losses, restrictions, and diminishing capacities; and furthermore, (2) "we have to decide, for instance, which symptoms can be eliminated and which should remain undisturbed, and shall have to evaluate" (Goldstein, 1959, p. 10) which of the many techniques recommended by the various schools of psychotherapy are suitable for brain-impaired individuals and which are not. Since, "therapy will be successful only if the patient participates in its enterprise adequately" (Goldstein, 1959, p. 11). And the patient's impairments will prevent his or her adequate participation without appropriate modifications in techniques, to fit the patient's capacities.

The NYU Model Program Is the Embodiment of Goldstein's Holistic Concepts

The intensive day program type that was initially piloted in Israel (Ben-Yishay, 1975, 1976; Ben-Yishay *et al.*, 1977) and subsequently at the New York University Medical Center, Rusk Institute in New York (Ben-Yishay, 1977, 1978) is the present-day embodiment of Kurt

Goldstein's notion of an "ordered environment." This type of program is well suited to a particular subset of head-injured patients undergoing postacute rehabilitation (Ben-Yishay & Diller, 1981; Ben-Yishay, 1983; Ben-Yishay *et al.,* 1985). Its added "therapeutic community" features, which were lacking in Goldstein's program in Frankfurt (Goldstein, 1942), complement Goldstein's holistic ideas quite well, as was spelled out in some detail in a recently published article (Ben-Yishay, 1996). This model integrates systematically remedial and therapeutic elements aimed at ameliorating disturbances in the cognitive sphere, the interpersonal and social spheres, and the intrapsychic sphere, or the self, of the individual. In other words, this type of program makes possible the orchestration of the specific cognitive management and psychotherapeutic interventions and the peer group activities, so that each reinforces the effects of the other on the behavior and personality of the rehabilitant.

A Hierarchy of Stages in Clinical Interventions

A basic premise of the therapeutic millieu model is that there ought to be a definite order, with clearly identifiable stages or points of emphasis in the delivery of clinical and remedial interventions aimed at (1) preventing the occurrence of catastrophic responses, (2) overcoming the brain-impaired individual's organismic defensive tendency to avoid engaging in challenging learning situations, (3) assisting the individual in attaining, through compensation, the modified competencies that remain within that individual's potential, (4) becoming productive again, and hence (5) begin to feel "healthy" again.

Extensive clinical experiences have made it possible to identify the clinical "landmarks" and specific process characteristics of successful rehabilitants, as they advance stage by stage toward realizing their ultimate personal rehabilitation potential:

1. *The awareness and understanding stage.* The first of these prioritized phases of intervention is the awareness and understanding phase. In this stage, the successful rehabilitant must achieve awareness and understanding (1) of the nature of his or her core deficits; (2) how these deficits interfere with various aspects of his or her functional life at present, as well as their long-term implications; (3) that the rationale of all the rehabilitation interventions is to attain successful compensations for deficits, rather than achieve genuinely restitutive goals; and (4) the fact that he or she must develop realistic expectations for the future, based on the degree of success in compensating for deficits imposed by the injury.

2. *Malleability to treatment stage.* Malleability to treatments must be actively promoted. Simultaneously with promoting awareness and the understanding of one's disability and its consequences, remedial efforts also must be systematically directed toward rendering the rehabilitant optimally responsive, or malleable, to the guidance and influence of others. Four specific characteristics of optimal malleability must be actively encouraged: (1) an ability to respond empathically to staff and peers; (2) a willingness and ability to actually modify one's behaviors that are defined by trusted others as either dysfunctional or undesirable; (3) complying, in a disciplined and unresentful manner, with instructions of "coaches"; and (4) displaying persistence and diligence as a trainee. Clearly, the process of learning to compensate for one's deficits will not and cannot unfold optimally, nor yield its potential benefits, without awareness, understanding, and optimal malleability.

3. *The compensatory stage.* We seek three specific outcomes during the compensatory stage of the rehabilitation process: (1) making certain that the patient has successfully mastered (and is reliably able to utilize in functional situations) the necessary compensatory props

and metacognitive strategies he or she has been taught; (2) establishing the limits of the patient's ability to learn, retain, and transfer new information, (verbal–ideational as well as practical), hence, to become productively engaged in various types of study and work activities; and (3) determining the patient's capacity to self-correct errors and "troubleshoot" in unexpected situations. For these are the determinants of the patient's future vocational prospects, as well as the ultimate degree of autonomy he or she will prove capable of achieving in managing his or her affairs. The question of compensation touches on many issues concerning the nature, scope, rationale, efficacy, and effectiveness of cognitive remedial interventions following a head injury.

These topics have received considerable attention in numerous publications in recent years and it is not within the scope of this chapter to review these publications, except to reiterate a few points on which all serious students of cognitive rehabilitation agree. The first point is that cognitive remediation is about improving reasoning and problem-solving abilities that have been rendered inefficient by the brain injury. Elsewhere, in a detailed analysis of the objectives, tasks, and conditions of cognitive remediation, Ben-Yishay (1981) has shown that Luria's model of the thinking and problem-solving cycle (Luria, 1973) is an excellent way of defining the tasks of the cognitive remedial endeavor. Accordingly, it is quite obvious that no single training procedure fits all problems. Depending on where along the logical reasoning or problem-solving cycle (to follow Luria's model) the breakdown in functioning has occurred, different types of training procedures are needed. Cognitive exercises designed to improve convergent reasoning functions (e.g., formulating an objective; abstracting the main idea) must be different from exercises designed to improve divergent thinking and mental flexibility (e.g., considering alternative approaches; drawing inferences; synthesizing different ideas). And these types of exercises, in turn, are not suitable to improve executive functions (e.g., organizing, prioritizing, methodically implementing a plan of action, correcting errors, achieving closure).

The second point is that for remedial training to translate into enhanced functional life, (1) the training procedure will have to be sufficiently protracted and intensive to be mastered by the patient; (2) it will have to be rehearsed often enough to become habituated (for only habituation can ensure that the patient could apply it reliably); and (3) the habituated compensatory strategy will have to be applied in the context of concrete functional life activities, and thus (4) become integrated with the person's functional behavior repertoires.

4. *The acceptance stage.* Acceptance is a prerequisite for stable adjustment. Acceptance of one's existential situation is the culmination of success in attaining (1) the minimal criteria of awareness and understanding; (2) malleability to the constructive influences and coaching of other; (3) the realization of the necessity for restrictions on one's future options; (4) success in compensating for the deficits imposed by the brain injury; and (5) the feeling that in spite of achieving less than a full return to one's preinjury abilities after rehabilitation, life is meaningful.

We can recognize that a person has entered the stage of acceptance (1) when he or she ceases to agitate and "mourn" the losses he or she has sustained (e.g., when the person displays the degree of calm and emotional detachment needed to be able to speak about "my head injury" with objectivity); (2) when the person is once again able to enjoy the little pleasures of life, including humor and laughter; (3) when the person is able to view and speak about his or her achievements in rehabilitation as being valuable and meaningful; and (4) when the person speaks and acts in ways that clearly show that he or she has regained a sense of hope, self-worth and self-esteem.

Some Empirical Evidence

The following is a brief summary of some empirical evidence in support of the foregoing assertions: (1) In a 5-year clinical research study (Ben-Yishay *et al.*, 1982), it was found that virtually the same markers of initial baseline competence on a wide spectrum of cognitive measures correlated with both the ability to benefit from systematic cognitive remedial training and from small-group procedures designed to increase malleability and acceptance of disability. (2) In a subsequent analysis (Ezrachi *et al.*, 1983), it was found that a high correlation existed between the cognitive learning index and the small-group assimilation, and that each correlated highly with the vocational outcome index. But when partial correlations were performed, it was found that while the predictive powers of the small group assimilation index remained still high, the predictive powers of the cognitive learning index alone "shrank" considerably. (3) Some years later, in a study involving a large group of patients (Ezrachi, Ben-Yishay, Kay, Diller, & Rattok, 1991), 20 factors were allowed to compete as predictors of vocational success in a multivariate regression analysis. It was found that six factors (of the 20 allowed to compete) have produced a multiple correlation (R) of .81; which means that these six factors were able to account for about 66% of the total variance. When the relative efficiency of each of these six predictor variables was looked at, it was found that duration of coma (an index of the severity of the injury) accounted for only 8% of the variance; (2) the combination of empathic ability displayed by the patients and their ability to regulate their affective behavior in their naturalistic (home) environments and acceptance following intensive rehabilitation accounted for 60% of the variance; and (3) the two cognitive factors—visual information processing and abstract verbal reasoning—accounted for 32% of the variance.

Clearly, acceptance and the ability to regulate one's emotions and to maintain appropriate interpersonal relations proved to have nearly double the predictive powers of the cognitive factors.

Psychotherapeutic Interventions with Brain-Impaired Individuals

Goldstein (1959) explicitly stated that in doing psychotherapeutic work with brain-injured persons, "we have to decide, for instance, which symptoms can be eliminated and which should remain undisturbed" and that we "shall have to evaluate the many procedures which have been recommended in the different schools of psychotherapy" (p. 10) and choose and modify only those that are particularly suited for persons with a head injury. In a previous publication, Ben-Yishay and Lakin (1989) undertook a detailed analysis of the basic assumptions that underlie the various (dynamic types of) insight-producing psychotherapies, and based on that analysis have proposed a parsimonious model for psychotherapeutic intervention with non-brain-injured persons and a model for therapeutic interventions with brain-injured persons.

The scope of this chapter permits merely a summary of the key points: As is commonly assumed, in order to benefit from dynamic, insight-producing psychotherapies, a person (1) must have a minimum degree of awareness and acknowledgment of the fact that he or she needs help; (2) must feel an urgent need to change how he or she feels, acts, or lives; (3) must have the ability to make resolutions to change and then act on this resolution; and finally, (4) that the person must have intact "ego functions." The second point is that, as Hartman (1964) and Bellak (1977) have shown, ego functions are not a unitary entity but rather a construct, which refers to at least seven identifiable capacity levels. Each must reach a certain threshold of adequacy to produce intact ego-functions. The third point is that, since in brain-injured persons a number of the components of ego functions are often impaired, it should be obvious that both the basic assumptions made and the therapeutic techniques that are employed by conventional insight-producing psychotherapies in the case of non-brain-injured (ego-intact) persons are not valid in the case of brain-injured persons. The fourth point is that, based on the foregoing, a specially modified therapeutic methodology—the paradigmatic group exercise—was developed and successfully applied in the context of holistic, therapeutic community types of programs.

The paradigmatic group exercise procedure consists of a number of structural and clinical–didactic features that permit the delivery of standard or individualized exercises in interpersonal communication, in the setting of a "living theater." Built into this flexible procedure (1) are mechanisms capable of ensuring that patients can optimally process and assimilate important "messages," or templates of behavior; (2) is a rehabilitation algorithm (i.e., systematic encouragement coupled with practice to receive help and feedback from others); (3) is the possibility of "calibrating" the level of intellectual complexity of the exercises to suit the capabilities of specific patients; (4) is a public forum (i.e., the peer group) in which the individual repeatedly is encouraged to assert acceptance of his or her situation; and (5) is the possibility of receiving the supports necessary for patients to regain their self-esteem and to reconstitute their ego identity, or sense of self.

Relationships between Acceptance and Ego Identity

Although more empirical studies in neuropsychological rehabilitation are needed to enable us to clearly (i.e., operationally and in a measurable way) elucidate the precise relationships between acceptance and ego identity, extensive clinical experiences in the rehabilitation of brain-injured persons over the past two decades justify (in the opinion of the author) the conclusion that (1) acceptance of one's disability, that is, feeling that life is still worth living despite some changes and reductions in one's living and/or career options, is intimately tied to the persons's ability to reconstitute his or her sense of self, or ego identity; and that (2) successful rehabilitative interventions (especially when carried out in holistic, therapeutic community types of programs) can and do result in both the reconstitution of the person's shattered ego identity as well as acceptance of one's existential situation; but that (3) this can come about only in a particular subset of brain-impaired individuals.

Defining Ego Identity

Of all the ideas that were contributed by Erikson, the most popular is his concept of ego identity (Erikson, 1950, 1958, 1959). The concept has a multiplicity of meanings which are not always easy to follow. Fortunately, Yankelovich and Barrett (1970) have provided a lucid and systematic description of the various meanings of Erikson's thinking on the subject.

The concept of ego identity is seen as evolving aspects of personhood. Ego identify has several distinguishing components, or characteristics: (1) identity as imitation, (2) identity as the persistence of a sense of sameness within oneself, and (3) identity as self-definition. Each component is briefly described:

Identity as imitation. The earliest roots of ego identity are in the psychological mechanism involving imitation. For example, the little girl puts on her mother's shoes and hat and declares: "I am mommy." This earliest version of the imitative process becomes more complex, as the child matures. "The imitation may be of persons, acts, values, roles, attributes, styles, etc. It may be a partial imitation, as when a little girl scolds her doll in the way she herself is scolded, but without adopting her mother's mannerisms" (Yankelovich & Barrett, 1970, p. 123).

A critical phase of the imitative aspects of ego identity takes place during the period of adolescence, at which time, "the synthesizing ego, acting on the sum of all of these partial processes, consolidates them, forges them into a unity, and transforms them to create the unique sense of self known as ego identity" (Yankelovich & Barrett, 1970, p. 124).

But in order to achieve an authentic ego identity these fused and internalized meanings must become a part of the person's inner being.

Identity as the sense of continuity. Ego identity requires "the sense of a persistent sameness within oneself," the subjective sense of coherent memories of one's "self as a stable structure that endures in time" (Yankelovich & Barrett, 1970, p. 127).

Identity as self-definition. Between adolescence and early adulthood, one's ego identity metamorphoses into its two (final) complementary aspects: the self-definition and its corollary, the transcendent aspects. We may find an excellent illustration of what is meant by the term of self-definition in a quote attributed to the Greek philosopher Epictetus, who lived and taught in Ancient Rome nearly 2000 years ago: "You should explicitly identify the kind of person you aspire to become: What are your personal ideas? Whom do you admire? What are their special traits that you would make your own?" (Lebell, 1994, p. 60). As to the transcendent aspect of the fully evolved ego identity, in discussing George Bernard Shaw, Erikson (1959) quotes Shaw's statement to the effect that his identification was with the "mighty dead." Erikson sees this as an illustration of "ego identity as presenting a form of transcendence, a way of reaching beyond one's own self and even beyond the limits of one's own times and culture" (Yankelovich & Barrett, 1970, p. 133).

Thus, ego identity is the culmination of the transformed and crystallized miscellany of all the imitations accumulated throughout one's childhood, adolescence, and early adulthood into a unified sense of selfhood; which, "when in later years, the person's experiences are compatible with this structure of meanings, he feels a sense of fitness, a feeling of oneness with himself, with his environment, and his life" (Yankelovich & Barrett, 1970, p. 132).

The Integrity of Ego Identity Cannot Be Taken for Granted

Erikson, however, cautioned us that this sense of self, or ego identity, though capable of enduring in time, cannot be taken for granted. For, there are a number of situations in life when the sense of continuity can become disrupted, with severe consequences to a persons's life. Thus, in describing his encounters with war veterans who suffered so-called "combat neuroses," Erikson had this to say: "What impressed me most was the loss in these men of a sense of identity. They knew who they were; they had a personal identity. But it was as if subjectively their lives no longer hung together—and never would again" (Erikson, 1950, p. 38). Essentially the same point was made by the British existential psychiatrist Laing (1962) who descried various manifestations of a dissolution of the Eriksonian sense of self as generalized feelings of unreality; a blurred sense of selfhood, only precariously differentiated from the rest of the world; a lack of temporal continuity; and feelings of emptiness.

Summing Up

The central thesis of this chapter is that, as shown by extensive clinical experiences in neuropsychological rehabilitation, that when due to brain impairments brain functions fall short of certain thresholds of intactness, (1) a person's ego identity can become severely disrupted; (2) that this disruption is intimately tied to impairment of aspects of the person's ego functions; and therefore (3) the usual types of dynamic, insight-producing psychotherapeutic interventions are ineffective, indeed even inappropriate in such persons; but that (4) by the systematic application of specially devised therapeutic techniques (adapted to the capabilities of brain-impaired persons) it is possible to reconstitute certain individual's ego identity as well as help these persons achieve true acceptance of their disability; and finally (5) that a holistic program, delivered in the setting of a therapeutic community, is the optimal method of facilitating a stable and enduring postrehabilitative adjustment.

References

Bellak, L. (1977). Psychiatric states in adults with minimal brain dysfunction. *Psychiatric Annals, 7,* 58–76

Ben-Yishay, Y. (1975). An outline of a theoretical frame work for the rehabilitation of persons with severe head trauma. Keynote address. Sixth Annual Rehabilitation Symposium, Chaim Sheba Medical Center, Tel Hashomer, Israel.

Ben-Yishay, Y. (1976). Setting up a therapeutic community for Israeli outpatient war casualties with severe head injuries. Invited panelist. The 13th World Congress of Rehabilitation. Tel Aviv, Israel.

Ben-Yishay, Y. (1977). Innovative treatments for brain damaged persons. Invited lecture. The 1977–78 Scientific Lecture Series on Medical Models in Psychiatry: Toward a New Synthesis. Forest Hospital and Foundation, Des Plaines, IL.

Ben-Yishay, Y. (1978). Organizing a comprehensive rehabilitation program for head trauma patients. Invited lecture. New York University Goldwater Memorial Hospital, Roosevelt Island, New York.

Ben-Yishay, Y (1981). Cognitive remediation: Toward a definition of its objectives, tasks and conditions. In Y. Ben-Yishay (Ed.), New York University Medical Center, Rehabilitation Monograph No. 62, pp. 14–42.

Ben-Yishay, Y. (1983). Cognitive remediation viewed from the perspective of a systematic clinical research program in rehabilitation. *Cognitive Rehabilitation, 1,* 4–6.

Ben-Yishay, Y. (1996). Reflections on the evolution of the therapeutic millieu concept. *Neuropsychological Rehabilitation, 6,* 327–343.

Ben-Yishay, Y., & Diller, L. (1981). Rehabilitation of cognitive and perceptual defects in people with traumatic brain damage. *International Journal of Rehabilitation Research, 4,* 208–210.

Ben-Yishay, Y., & Lakin, P. (1989). Structured group-treatment for brain-injury survivors. In D. W. Ellis & A. L. Christensen (Eds.), *Neuropsychological treatment after brain injury* (pp. 271–295). Boston: Kluwer Academic Publishers.

Ben-Yishay, Y., Ben-Nachum, Z., Cohen, A., Gross, Y., Hoofien, D., Rattok, J., & Diller, L. (1977). Digest of a two-year comprehensive clinical research program for out patient head injured Israeli veterans. In Y. Ben-Yishay (Ed.), NYU Medical Center Rehabilitation Monograph No. 59, pp. 1–61.

Ben-Yishay, Y., Rattok, J., Ross, B., Lakin, P., Ezrachi, O., Silver, S. L., & Diller, L. (1982). Summary of results of the first phase of the study: HEW, RSA, Project RT-1, RT-93, Part of NIHR 16-P-56801/2-19. In Y. Ben-Yishay (Ed.), New York University Medical Center, Rehabilitation Monograph No. 64, pp. 128–176.

Ben-Yishay, Y., Rattok, J., Lakin, P., Piasetsky, E., Ross, B., Silver, S. L., Zide, E., & Ezrachi, O. (1985). Neuropsychological rehabilitation: The quest for a holistic approach. *Seminars in Neurology, 5,* 252–259.

Erikson, E. H., (1950). *Childhood and society.* New York: W. W. Norton.

Erikson, E. H. (1958). *Young man Luther.* New York: W. W. Norton.

Erikson, E. H. (1959). Identity and the life cycle. In *Psychological issues 1* (pp. 102–110). New York: International Universities Press.
Ezrachi, O., Ben-Yishay, Y., Rattok, J., Ross, B., Lakin, P., Silver, S. L., Piasetsky, E., & Diller, L. (1983). Summary of results of the second phase of the study HEN, RSA, Project RT-1, RT-2, NIHR 16-P-56801/2-19. In Y. Ben-Yishay (Ed.), New York University Medical Center, Rehabilitation Monograph No. 66, pp. 53–91.
Ezrachi, O., Ben-Yishay, Y., Kay, T., Diller, L., & Rattok, J. (1991). Predicting employment in traumatic brain injury following neuropsychological rehabilitation. *Journal of Head Trauma Rehabilitation, 6,* 71–84.
Goldstein, K. (1942). *After effects of brain injuries in war: Their evaluation and treatment.* New York: Grune and Straton.
Goldstein, K. (1952). The effects of brain damage on the personality. Presented at the annual meeting of the American Psychoanalytic Association. Atlantic City, NJ.
Goldstein, K. (1959). Notes on the development of my concepts. *Journal of Individual Psychology, 15,* 5–14.
Hartman, H. (1964). *Essays on ego psychology.* New York: International University Press.
Laing, R. O. (1962). *Ontological insecurity in psychoanalysis and existential philosophy.* New York: E. P. Dutton.
Lebell, S. (1994). *A manual for living. Epictetus—A new interpretation.* San Francisco: Harper.
Luria, A. R. (1973). *The working brain: An introduction to neuropsychology.* New York: Basic Books.
Yankelovich, D., & Barrett, W. (1970). *Ego and instinct.* New York: Random House.

9

Empirical Support for Neuropsychological Rehabilitation

LANCE E. TREXLER

The theoretical, clinical, and empirical sophistication of the field of brain injury rehabilitation has evolved exponentially over the last two decades. Traditional physical rehabilitation models did not address the unique needs of the patient with acquired brain injury, particularly the long-term psychosocial and community reentry difficulties experienced by these patients and their families. New models for the rehabilitation of persons with brain damage have of necessity been developed. These new paradigms, particularly in postacute brain injury rehabilitation, transcend physical restoration models to embrace cognitive and neurobehavioral, social, and experiential aspects of recovery and rehabilitation.

The purpose of the present chapter is to provide the brain injury rehabilitation professional with (1) an individualized yet holistic framework for evaluating and conceptualizing the rehabilitation of an individual with acquired brain injury, (2) a description of holistic neuropsychological rehabilitation programs, with particular reference to their structure and characteristics, and (3) a review of the empirical research regarding the efficacy of holistic neuropsychological rehabilitation.

A Clinical and Research Framework for Conceptualizing Brain Injury Rehabilitation

The rehabilitation of the patient with acquired brain injury is a complex task. The variability in clinical presentation of these patients exists across many domains of human functioning, including physical and motor abilities, sensory, perceptual, cognitive, and executive

This chapter is in part based on Trexler, L. E., & Helmke, C. (1966). Efficacy of holistic neuropsychological rehabilitation: Program characteristics and outcome research. In W. Fries (Ed.), *Ambulante und teilstationäre Rehabilitation von Himverletzten* (pp. 25–39).München: W. Zuckschwerdt Verlag.

LANCE E. TREXLER • Center for Neuropsychological Rehabilitation, Indianapolis, Indiana 46260.

International Handbook of Neuropsychological Rehabilitation, edited by Christensen and Uzzell.
Kluwer Academic/ Plenum Publishers, New York, 2000.

functions. Significant individual differences exist in our patients prior to injury that impact on their recovery, psychological reaction to injury and disability, and outcome. Different types of rehabilitation professionals are needed to comprise a brain injury rehabilitation team, but each rehabilitation discipline has a different educational background, different methods of evaluating the patient and monitoring progress, and emphasizes different domains of human functioning. No one rehabilitation discipline has a complete repertoire of brain injury rehabilitation-related knowledge. Nonetheless, brain injury rehabilitation requires a great deal of team integration, communication, and collaboration. Few models exist that provide an organizational template from which brain injury rehabilitation professionals can evaluate and conceptualize the rehabilitation process. Additionally, research in brain injury rehabilitation is similarly methodologically complex, and a need exists for researchers to utilize a common framework for operationalizing and measuring different levels or types of human functioning in a consistent and heuristic manner. A framework developed by the National Center for Medical Rehabilitation Research (NCMRR) (1993) provides a basis for these clinical and research needs and is presented in Table 1. This framework was developed for all types of rehabilitation research, but it can been modified to specifically address the levels of functioning applicable to acquired brain injury rehabilitation and research as presented in Table 2.

As previously noted, the heterogeneity of behavioral and functional consequences characteristic of the patient with acquired brain injury are vast. One of the primary sources of heterogeneity concerns premorbid individual factors. Therefore, the domain of preexisting individual differences was added to the NCMRR model, as noted on Table 2. Studying individual differences in postacute brain injury rehabilitation and research is important not only because they have a significant impact on the rehabilitation process for that individual, but also because they are a source of significant variability in brain injury rehabilitation research. Individual differences can be conceptualized in primarily two domains, including preexisting personological factors and differences in the pathophysiology of the injury, that is, in whose brain did what injury occur? Failure to control for these factors in brain injury rehabilitation research will likely statistically obscure treatment effects. Similarly, failure to study and take into account individual factors in brain injury rehabilitation will likely result in an incomplete or misguided rehabilitation plan and, as a consequence, less than optimal outcome. As a consequence of individual differences among premorbid and pathophysiological factors, individual differences between patients emerge at all other levels of the modified NCMRR model (see Table 2), including resultant impairments, functional limitations, and disability.

Preexisting individual factors that influence recovery from brain injury and response to rehabilitation are potentially numerous, and to address these issues in depth is not the focus of the present work. The reader is referred to Lezak (1995), Trexler and Fordyce (1995), and Trexler and Sullivan (1995) for a more comprehensive review of these factors. Several examples, however, are noteworthy to illustrate the importance of these individual factors. Some patients have a long history of psychosocial adjustment and adaptive coping skills, while others may have few psychological resources with which to manage a new disability. These types of individual differences are likely to influence outcome and need for rehabilitation services, for example, the need for psychotherapy and involvement of the family. Further, in a series of studies by Moore and colleagues (Lubuski, Moore, Stambrook, & Gill, 1994; Moore & Stambrook, 1992; Moore, Stambrook, & Wilson, 1991), it was demonstrated that traumatic brain injury (TBI) patients who had an internal locus of control, meaning that they believed they had control over what happened to them, demonstrated better rates of return to work and

TABLE 1. Domains of Science Relevant to Medical Rehabilitation Research[a]

	Pathophysiology	Impairment	Functional limitation	Disability	Societal limitation
Definition	Interruption of or interference with normal physiological and developmental processes or structures	Loss and/or abnormality of cognitive, emotional, physiological, or anatomical structure or function, including all losses or abnormalities, not just those attributable to the initial pathophysiology	Restriction or lack of ability to perform an action in the manner or within a range consistent with the purpose of an organ or organ system	Inability or limitation in performing tasks, activities and roles to levels expected within physical and social context	Restriction, attributable to social policy or barriers (structural or attitudinal), which limits fulfillment of roles or denies access to services and opportunities that are associated with full participation in society
Level of impact	Cells and tissues Structural or functional	Organs and organ systems Structural or functional	Functions of organs and organ systems Action or activity performance of organ or organ system	Individual Task performance by person in physical and social contexts	Society Societal attributes relevant to individuals with disability
Example	Adult with ruptured cerebral aneurysm	Decreased motor strength; difficulties with problem solving and abstraction; visual impairments	Difficulty with walking, difficulties to organize and plan activities, unable to read	Dependent on others for transportation, needs more time with activities of daily living	No public transportation for wheelchair dependent people

[a] From NCMRR (1993).

psychosocial adjustment, irrespective of severity of injury, as compared to TBI patients who had an external locus of control, meaning that they believed that luck or fate was the primary determinant of what happened to them. Individual differences exist at all levels of the framework presented in Table 2.

Individual differences obviate the need for an individualized assessment and rehabilitation planning. Moreover, significant dissociations are often witnessed clinically in terms of what one might predict a patient's ability to adapt in the real world might be given certain neuropsychological impairments. For example, some patients with relatively mild disturbances of memory may be quite functionally disabled in the real world, perhaps because they are also depressed, which may serve to exacerbate their memory impairments, or because their job requires intricate recall of detailed information. Other patients with severe impairments of memory may have job demands that require only procedural memory and therefore may have relatively little vocational disability. Some patients spontaneously generate compensatory strategies, while others exhibit massive denial. These are just a few examples of individual differences in persons with seemingly similar or identical injuries.

The heterogeneity of clinical presentation, characteristic of acquired brain injury, has necessitated the development of a comprehensive preadmission assessment in postacute brain injury rehabilitation programs. The goals for the assessment are multifaceted and include: (1) determination of the patients impaired and spared brain functions (impairments); (2) the effect these impairments have on everyday behavior (functional limitations and disability); (3) the needed rehabilitation services, with reference to type of postacute program, duration, intensity, and specific therapy interventions; and (4) the goals for rehabilitation (usually set at the level of functional limitation and disability) and the prognosis for reaching these outcome goals. Given these demands, a variety of types of information should be collected. The modified NCMRR framework provides a schematic for the different domains of information which are required.

Information about the patient's premorbid status and individual differences are often obtained through interviews with the patient and family. In the postacute setting, effort must be given to collecting relevant medical records from the acute setting, particularly with relevance to acute and postacute neuroradiological data, duration of unconsciousness, or other factors known to be related to the type, location, and severity of injury. Information about impairments can be obtained through all professionals involved in the evaluation, but in particular through the neuropsychological evaluation and through physical therapy evaluation. Information regarding functional limitations, disability, and societal limitations can be obtained through occupational therapy, social workers, and sometimes including vocational specialists. Moreover, this format can be utilized for individual rehabilitation program goal setting. Most of the time, rehabilitation goals are established at the level of functional limitation (e.g., independence with managing one's own money) or disability (e.g., return to previous job).

The modified NCMRR form is meant to serve only as a guide to organizing rehabilitation-relevant information across all applicable professional disciplines and for conceptualizing individual cases and rehabilitation planning. The intent of utilizing the framework is to obtain a holistic perspective of the patients functioning and the factors that are likely to affect long-term outcome. Of course, it can be modified in structure and function to meet each program's needs. Multidisciplinary assessments integrated through this framework provide the rehabilitation team with much more information than if the evaluations were not organized and shared. This schemata also provides a holistic perspective to predict recovery and outcome and to determine rehabilitation type, duration, and goals.

Holistic Programs of Neuropsyhchological Rehabilitation

No one program can serve the wide constellation of clinical needs that follow acquired brain injury. As a consequence, several different types of postacute brain injury rehabilitation (PABIR) programs have emerged. The different types of PABIR programs that have developed over the last two decades are summarized in Table 3. The different types of programs have evolved not only based on patient characteristics, but also on theoretical and professional differences among providers, as well as economic, demographic, and political factors indigenous to the environment. Consequently, the decision as to what type of rehabilitation each patient receives is driven far less by patient characteristics and empirical studies of efficacy than would be desirable. Hopefully, future outcome research and advances in health care policy will improve these circumstances.

Malec and Basford (1996) completed a comprehensive review of outcome research in different types of PABIR. These authors classified outcome research in PABIR into three types of intervention, including neurobehavioral programs, residential community reintegration programs, and Comprehensive (holistic) day treatment programs. When these authors pooled outcomes for subjects who received PABIR and compared these outcomes to outcomes from studies of TBI subjects who did not receive PABIR, the subjects who received PABIR had significantly better independence in work, training, or homemaking and had significantly lower levels of unemployment. These findings support the efficacy of specialized brain injury rehabilitation programs. Many of the studies included in this analysis were performed in holistic neuropsychological rehabilitation programs.

Characteristics and Structure of Programs of Holistic Neuropsychological Rehabilitation

Of the types of PABIR, the most theoretically and empirically developed is what is most commonly referred to as holistic neuropsychological rehabilitation. The constellation of interventions characteristic of neuropsychological rehabilitation have been defined in several consensus conferences (Bergquist *et al.*, 1994; Trexler *et al.*, 1994). Programs of holistic neuropsychological rehabilitation have been organized to address the difficulties characteristic of most individuals with acquired brain injury, including: (1) neurological impairments of awareness of cognitive deficit; (2) difficulties in psychologically accepting newly acquired cognitive deficits; and (3) impairment of the ability to utilize or generalize learning from clinical environments into real world environments, such as at home, work, or school, all of which often result in functional long-term limitations and disability (Ben-Yishay & Prigatano, 1990; Levin, Benton, & Grossman, 1982; Trexler & Fordyce, 1995; Trexler & Sullivan, 1995). The presence of these neuropsychological disturbances necessitated the development of a different rehabilitation paradigm compared to the organization and structure of rehabilitation services provided for patient populations with intact cognitive abilities. Characteristics of neuropsychological rehabilitation programs are summarized in Table 4. A scale to measure the extent to which a brain injury rehabilitation program falls on a continuum from traditional outpatient rehabilitation therapies to holistic neuropsychological rehabilitation has been developed by Mauer, Glueckauf, Tomusk, Trexler, and Diller (1996), based on the program characteristics described in Table 5. This scale was developed to provide an objective classification and quantification of the type of PABIR program from which research methodologies could compare outcome associated with different types of rehabilitation.

These programs are based on an overall program design that includes group therapies and a therapeutic milieu (Prigatano *et al.*, 1984, 1994; Ben-Yishay & Diller, 1993) to address

Table 2. NCMRR Model Adapted for Brain Injury Rehabilitation

Societal limitation				
	Productivity		Quality of life	
Disability	Competitive work		Intimacy	
	Noncompetitive work		Social-interpersonal integration	
	Student		Family integration	
	Home care and maintenance		Avocational and recreational participation	
	Parenting			
	Mobility	Activities of daily living	Communication	Emotional reactions
Functional Limitation	Transportation	Higher level of financial management	Conversational pragmatics	Loss of identity
	Locomotion	Housekeeping skills	Verbal expression	Attribution for past transgressions
	Architectural barriers	Emergency management	Nonverbal expression	Fear of loss of love and approval
	Wheelchair transfers	Cooking/nutrition	Writing	Feelings of guilt and shame
	Floor mobility	Telephone use	Reading	Depression
	Bed mobility	Medical self-care/medications	Verbal comprehension	Anxiety
	Endurance, speed	Basic money management	Nonverbal comprehension	Catastrophic reaction
		Cooking	Vocabulary/word finding	Spiral of deterioration
		Dressing/undressing	Intelligibility	
		Grooming		
		Toileting		
		Bowel/bladder		
		Showering/bathing		
		Eating/drinking		

	MOTOR-SENSORY FUNCTIONS		EXECUTIVE AND COGNITIVE FUNCTIONS		NEUROBEHAVIORAL FUNCTIONS
IMPAIRMENT	Dexterity	Visual	Anticipation, initiating, planning, organizing, and self-monitoring		Awareness: Intellectual, emergent, anticipatory
	Initiation defect	Tactile	Abstraction		Disinhibition: Verbal, motor, affective
	Coordination/balance	Auditory	Problem solving and hypothesis formation		Confabulation
	Dysarthria	Proprioception	Memory: visual, verbal, motor, episodic and semantic; procedural-declarative; prospective memory		Tangentiality
	Motor programming				Perseveration
	Praxis				
	Limb				
	Verbal				
	Buccofacial		Language functions	Visuoperceptual functions	
	Strength		Language-related functions	Visuoconstructive functions	
	Range of motion		Controlled attention		
	Endurance		Vigilance		
	Speed		Alertness		

	INDIVIDUAL FACTORS	PATHOPHYSIOLOGY		
INDIVIDUAL FACTORS AND PATHOPHYSIOLOGY	Education	Traumatic brain injury	Stroke	Other or complications
	Psychosocial and vocational adjustment	Diffuse axonial injury	Infarction	Encephalopathy
	Preferences	Punctate hemorrhages	Hemorrhage	Metabolic
	Coping skills	Focal cortical contusion	Aneurysm	Infectious
	Substance abuse	Ischemic/hypoxic insult	Embolic	Hypoxic
	Legal problems	Open/closed head injury	Arteriovenous malformation	Seizure disorder
	Psychiatric history	Subdural hematoma		Increased ICP/shunt
	Family support			

TABLE 3. Types of Postacute Brain Injury Rehabilitation

Type	Predominant goals	Patient characteristics	Main program components
Traditional outpatient	Self care and ADL's	Mild to severe	Physical, occupational, and speech therapies
Community reentry	Independent living at home in community, return to work	Mild to moderately injured	Community-based therapies with vocational emphasis
Holistic	Psychosocial adjustment, compensation for cognitive disorders, return to work	Mild to moderately injured, impaired awareness	Therapeutic milieu Neuropsychological orientation Integration of staff
Residential	ADL's and independent living	Moderately to severely injured	Functional skill training provided in residential environment
Behavioral	Behavioral control and stability	Neuropsychiatric and neurobehavioral disorders	Behavioral modification in structured environment
Lifelong living	Quality of life	Moderately to severely injured	Interpersonal and community integration

problems of awareness, acceptance of residual impairments, and compensation in ecologically valid, target environments (e.g., home, workplace). Individual and group psychotherapies have been incorporated into the program to address problems with acceptance and emotional reactions to disability (Prigatano, 1992). The holistic neuropsychological rehabilitation program has typically included functional skills training and discipline-specific therapies, such as speech and language therapy, and occupational and physical therapies as well. These programs are typically structured as day treatment programs, with the average length of treatment ranging from 3 to 6 months, which sometimes includes community-based and vocational trials or training. Some programs utilize a continuous admission and discharge model, while other programs have a fixed cycle where all patients are admitted and discharged at the same time. As presented in Table 4, many programs use a primary therapist model. The role of the primary therapist is to establish a relationship with the patient through which patient awareness can be addressed as well as the patient and family's understanding of the treatment schedule and purpose of the specific therapies. Additionally, the primary therapist will promote the patient's ability to set realistic short-term rehabilitation goals, derive strategies for the accomplishment of those goals, and provide constant feedback as to the effectiveness of the patient's functioning.

Results of Efficacy Research in Holistic Neuropsychological Rehabilitation

A variety of studies have demonstrated improved outcome among brain injury patients who have received holistic neuropsychological rehabilitation (Ben-Yishay, Silver, Piasetsky, & Rattock, 1987; Christensen, Pinner, Moller-Pedersen, Teasdale, & Trexler, 1992; Malec, Smigielski, DePompolo, & Thompson, 1993; Prigatano *et al.*, 1984, 1994). All subjects studied had TBI, except for Christensen *et al.*, where 48% of their sample had TBI. The average sample size for these five studies was 45. The characteristics of the subjects in these five studies are presented in Table 5. The time since injury to time of treatment (chronicity) varied significantly in these studies, but the averages were typically 2 to 4 years postinjury. These studies employed a very similar theoretical orientation to the rehabilitation of brain injury, which was consistent with what has herein been described as holistic neuropsychological rehabilitation.

Detailed information regarding the treatment provided in each of these studies is provided in Table 6. Additionally, these studies compared pretreatment status with discharge and follow-up status, except for the two studies by Prigatano and colleagues who used matched controls. Ben-Yishay *et al.* (1987) and Prigatano *et al.* (1994) followed patients at 6-month intervals for up to 3 years for the former study and for 18 months postdischarge for the latter study. Prigatano *et al.* (1984), Christensen *et al.* (1992), and Malec *et al.* (1993) did follow-up examinations on one occasion either at 1 year postdischarge or all at one time for patients treated in previous years. Measures of outcome were typically status indicators for amount and type of work or productive activity, level of supervision required, and level of independence. Table 7 provides specific information regarding the outcome measures utilized in each study and their results. Christensen also studied amount and type of leisure activities and utilization of health care services. In the case of Prigatano *et al.* (1994), TBI subjects treated with holistic neuropsychological rehabilitation had significantly higher levels of employment than controls. Christensen and co-workers (1992) also demonstrated significant improvements in amount and type of leisure activities and significant decreases in utilization of health care services following holistic neuropsychological rehabilitation for patients on average 2.9 years postinjury.

TABLE 4. Characteristics of Holistic Neuropsychological Rehabilitation Programs

Program characteristic	Description
Individualized goal setting	Patients and families directly involved in deriving short- and long-term rehabilitation goals Outcome goals individualized Type and intensity of specific therapies individualized (e.g., frequency of physical therapy, training compensatory strategies for neglect)
Holistic rehabilitation planning	Primary therapist facilitates patient understanding of the purpose and relevance of program and specific therapies to short- and long-term rehabilitation goals Rehabilitation team staffings and decision making Integrated transdisciplinary progress notes organized around goals Family integrated into rehabilitation process
Neuropsychological orientation	Extent to which impairments of awareness, cognitive deficits, and emotional reactions to injury and disability are directly addressed
Therapeutic milieu	Group therapies for psychotherapy, social pragmatics, and awareness Group sessions for goal setting and review of progress Feedback from others inherent in all aspects of the program regarding awareness, acceptance, use of compensatory strategies, progress toward rehabilitation goals
Outcome-oriented rehabilitation planning	In addition to clinic-based therapies, therapies provided at home, in the community, and in vocationally relevant environments to promote generalization Scheduled follow-up after discharge to monitor maintenance of rehabilitation gains
Intensity of rehabilitation program	Intensity and duration of therapy sufficient to promote learning and generalization
Brain injury rehabilitation expertise	Staff dedicated to brain injury rehabilitation Staff training in brain injury rehabilitation Type and experience of staff

TABLE 5. Subjects in Holistic Neuropsychological Rehabilitation Research

Study	*n*	Age	Edu	M/F (%)	Chronicity	Controls	Diagnoses
Prigatano *et al.* (1984)	18	26.1	12.5	83/17	21.6 months	Yes	Closed head injury
Ben-Yishay *et al.* (1987)	94	27	14	78/22	36.5 months	No	97.0% Acceleration-deceleration concussion 2.0% Anoxic encephalopathy 1.0% Post-infectious sequelae
Christensen *et al.* (1992)	46	30	9.9	60/40	34.8 months	No	47.8% TBI 30.4% Stroke 15.2% Metabolic/toxic/hypoxic 2.2% Tumor 4.3% Gunshot
Malec *et al.* (1993)	29	33.1	13.3	69/31	48.07 months	No	69.0% TBI 13.8% CVA 6.9% Anoxia 6.9% Hydrocephalus 3.4% Postlymphoma
Prigatano *et al.* (1994)	38	29.6	13.5	68/32	43.26	Yes	87.6% Brain contusion or hematoma 7.4% Loss of consciousness only 5.0% Skull fracture

TABLE 6. Treatment Provided in Holistic Neuropsychological Rehabilitation Research

	Treatment		
Study	Duration	Intensity	Type
Prigatano *et al.* (1984)	6 months	6 hr/day 4 days/week	Group and individual Focus on: increasing awareness and acceptance of injury and deficits, development of compensatory strategies, increase understanding of emotional and motivational responses to injury.
Ben-Yishay *et al.* (1987)	4 months	5 hr/day 4 days/week	Three phases: 1. intensive and holistic remedial interventions, 2. individualized, guided occupational trials culminating in actual vocational placement, 3. follow-up.
Christensen *et al.* (1992)	4 months	6 hr/day 4 days/week +F/U: monthly group for 6 months + 2/month neuropsych. visits	Group and individual Focus on: awareness, acceptance and psychosocial adjustments and cognitive remediation.
Malec *et al.* (1993)	28.4 weeks	+/– 4 hr/day 5 days/week	Focus on group therapy: increasing insight into disabilities and compensation, emotional and behavioral self-management; specific group and individual treatment provided as needed; each patient has a team leader
Prigatano *et al.* (1994)	+/– 6 months	4–6 hr/day 4–5 days/week	Group and individual Focus on: increasing awareness and acceptance of injury and deficits, development of compensatory strategies, increase understanding of emotional and motivational responses to injury. 4 months protected work trial for 15–20 hours a week.

These studies have demonstrated that when carefully selected patients are treated with holistic neuropsychological rehabilitation, in most cases quite some time following the usual period of spontaneous recovery, significant improvement in social, interpersonal, and recreational integration, functional independence, and vocational adaptation are obtained at discharge and on follow-up examinations compared to pretreatment status.

Implications for Future Research

The findings of these five studies support the efficacy of holistic neuropsychological rehabilitation, particularly when outcome is measured at the level of functional limitations and disability. There are significant limitations, however, of the aforementioned research.

The extent to which these findings can be generalized to other samples is difficult to determine. In all, only 225 brain-injured subjects were treated with holistic neuropsychological

TABLE 7. Outcome Measures and Results in Holistic Neuropsychological Rehabilitation

Study	Outcome measures	Vocational results	Other results
Prigatano *et al.* (1984)	Neuropsychological testing, Katz adjustment scale, work status	50% of treatment vs. 36% of controls in productive activity at f/u	WAIS, PIQ, Block Design, and WMQ were significantly better for treated as compared to the control patients Positive, but not significant changes in the Katz score for the treated patients
Ben-Yishay *et al.* (1987)	Employability Rating Scale (ERS)	84% of those found to be unemployable previously could engage in productive activities	None
Christensen *et al.* (1992)	Questionnaires for independent living status, help in living situations, utilization of health services, work and leisure activities	Significant from pretreatment to d/c and f/u	Sign. improvement in rates of cohabitation on f/u Sign. decrease in amount of assistance needed in the home between admission and f/u Sign. reduction in general practitioner, outpatient hospital and therapist visits from preadmission to f/u Sign. increases in quantity and quality of leisure activity d/c to f/u preceeded by significant decline preinjury to pre-treatment
Malec *et al.* (1993)	Independent living ratings, work outcome scale, Portland Adaptability Inventory (PAI), Goal Attainment scaling	Significant increases in work status from admission to d/c and f/u	Sign. decrease of supervision required Sign. improvements in PAI scores for functional abilities and physical disabilities sections
Prigatano *et al.* (1994)	Questionnaire regarding school and work status from the Traumatic Coma Data Bank. Ratings of work trial success retrospective ratings of working alliance for patient/family	86.8% of the treated patients were rated as productive at f/u vs. 55.3% of the non-treated ones	None

rehabilitation, and it seems unlikely that these samples were representative of the population of individuals with acquired brain injury. In fact, these programs employ rigorous admission criteria and, as mentioned, perform thorough preadmission evaluations. Second, while many subject variables were included in each of the studies, the studies do not uniformly describe the severity of injury or the severity of functional limitation of the sample that was treated with holistic neuropsychological rehabilitation. Moreover, some programs include persons with a variety of diagnoses, and future studies of necessity will be restricted to a single diagnosis so as to not introduce unwanted sources of variance. Because of the heterogeneity of the population, measurement of severity is complicated and no one measure serves this purpose. Therefore, it is difficult to determine the extent to which these findings can be generalized to persons with acquired brain injury of varying levels of severity of injury and types of injury. Last, because the sample size of the studies tends to be quite small, it is difficult statistically to reliably differentiate individuals who respond favorably from those who do not. Future studies will require larger sample sizes, perhaps gathered through multicenter designs.

There are other methodological limitations of these studies. Obviously, most of these studies are uncontrolled, with the exception of the studies of Prigatano and colleagues. Future studies will of necessity utilize new measures of severity at the level of both pathophysiology and functional limitation. Based on these measures, groups of treated and nontreated (or treated in a different manner) subjects can be matched to ensure that treatment gains are attributable to rehabilitation or a type of rehabilitation. Instruments like the one developed by Mauer *et al.* (1996) allow for an experimental, objective method to classify the type of brain injury rehabilitation program. Second, sampling methodology will of necessity be quasi-experimental. Sufficient evidence exists favoring the efficacy of holistic neuropsychological rehabilitation such that withholding treatment to study outcome is no longer ethical (Brooks, 1991). Nonetheless, a rigorous quasi-experimental methodology can be developed with group matching and sufficient size of sample.

While the methods of rehabilitation used in these studies were heavily neuropsychologically oriented, all outcome measurement strategies focused on measures of real world, functional limitation or level of disability. Christensen and co-workers (1992) also addressed utilization of health care resources pre- and posttreatment. Most of the outcome measures used were status indicators, and new instruments such as the community integration scale (Willer, Rosenthal, Kreutzer, Gordon, & Rembel, 1993) may serve to augment these methodologies.

Many types of postacute brain injury rehabilitation have evolved over the last two decades to address the complex cognitive, behavioral, psychosocial, and vocational challenges faced by the person with acquired brain damage. Of the types of postacute brain injury rehabilitation, holistic neuropsychological rehabilitation has been the most developed theoretically and the most studied. These studies provide very positive but nonetheless tentative support for their efficacy. Future research will need to employ measurement strategies that parallel the framework as provided by the NCMRR model and respond to increasing pressures to also demonstrate cost-effectiveness.

References

Ben-Yishay, Y., & Diller, L. (1993). Cognitive remediation in traumatic brain injury: Update and issues. *Archives of Physical Medicine and Rehabilitation, 74,* 204–213.

Ben-Yishay, Y., & Prigatano, G.P. (1990). Cognitive remediation. In: M. Rosenthal, E.R. Griffith, M.R. Bond, & J.D. Miller (Eds.), *Rehabilitation of the adult and child with traumatic brain injury,* (2nd ed., pp. 393–409). Philadelphia: F. A. Davis.

Ben-Yishay, Y., Silver, S. M., Piasetsky, E., & Rattock, J.(1987). Relationship between employability and vocational outcome after intensive holistic cognitive rehabilitation. Journal of Head Trauma Rehabilitation, 2, 33–43.

Bergquist, T. F., Boll, T. J., Corrigan, J. D., Harley, J. P., Malec, J. F., Millis, S. R., & Schmidt, M. R. (1994). Neuropsychological rehabilitation: Proceedings of a consensus conference. *Brain Injury, 9,* 50–61.

Brooks, N. D. (1991). Editorial. The effectiveness of postacute rehabilitation. *Brain Injury,* 5,103–109.

Christensen, A.-L., Pinner, E. M., Moller-Pedersen, P., Teasdale, T. W., & Trexler, L. E. (1992). Psychosocial outcome following individualized neuropsychological rehabilitation of brain damage. *Acta Neurologica Scandanavia, 85,* 32–38.

Levin, H. S., Benton, A. L., & Grossman, R. G. (1982). *Neurobehavioral consequences of closed head injury.* New York: Oxford University Press.

Lezak, M. D. (1995). *Neuropsychological assessment* (3rd ed.). New York: Oxford University Press.

Lubuski,A. A., Moore, A. D., Stambrook, M., & Gill, D. D. (1994). Cognitive beliefs following severe traumatic brain injury: Association with post injury employment. *Brain Injury,* 8, 65–70.

Malec, J. F., & Basford, J. R. (1996). Postacute brain injury rehabilitation. *Archives of Physical Medicine and Rehabilitation, 77,* 198–207.

Malec, J. F., Smigielski, J. S., DePompolo, R. W., &Thompson, J. M. (1993). Outcome evaluation and prediction in a comprehensive-integrated postacute outpatient brain injury rehabilitation programme. *Brain Injury, 7,* 15– 29.

Mauer, B. A., Glueckauf, R., Tomusk, A., Trexler, L. E., & Diller, L. (1996). Development and initial evaluation of the rehabilitation program styles survey. Paper presented at the proceedings of the American Psychological Association, Toronto.

Moore, A. D., & Stambrook, M. (1992). Coping strategies and locus of control following traumatic brain injury: Relationship to long term outcome. *Brain Injury, 6,* 89–94.

Moore, A. D., Stambrook, M., & Wilson, K. G. (1991). Cognitive moderators in adjustment to chronic illness: Locus of control beliefs following traumatic brain injury. *Neuropsychological Rehabilitation, 1,* 185–198.

National Center for Medical Rehabilitation Research (NCMRR). (1993). *Research plan for the National Center for Medical Rehabilitation Research.* NIH Publication No. 93–3509. Washington, DC: US Department of Health and Human Services, National Institutes of Health.

Prigatano, G. P. (1992). Neuropsychological rehabilitation and the problem of altered self–awareness. In N. von Steinbüchel, D. Y. von Cramon, & E. Poppel (Eds.), *Neuropsychological rehabilitation* (pp. 55–65). Berlin: Springer- Verlag.

Prigatano, G. P., Fordyce, D. J., Zeiner, H. K., Roueche, J. R., Pepping, M., & Wood, B. D. (1984). Neuropsychological rehabilitation after closed head injury in young adults. *Journal of Neurology, Neurosurgery, and Psychiatry, 47,* 505–513.

Prigatano, G. P., Klonoff, P. S., O'Brien, K. P., Altman, I. M., Amin, K., Chiapello, D., Shepard, J., Cunningham, M., & Mora, M. (1994). Productivity after neuropsychologically oriented milieu rehabilitation. *Journal of Head Trauma Rehabilitation, 9,* 91–102.

Trexler, L. E. & Fordyce, D. J. (1995). Psychological perspectives on rehabilitation: Contemporary assessment and intervention strategies. In R. L. Braddom (Ed.), *Physical medicine and rehabilitatio*n (pp. 66–81). Philadelphia: W.B. Saunders.

Trexler, L. E, & Sullivan, C. (1995). Neuropsychological perspectives on traumatic brain injury. In M. Zettin, & R. Rago (Eds.), *Head injury: neuropsychological and behavioral sequalae* (pp. 36–52). Torino, Italy: Bollati-Boringhieri.

Trexler, L. E., Diller, L., Glueckauf, R., Tomusk, A., Anreiter, B., Ben-Yishay, Y., Buckingham, D., Christensen, A-L., Grant, M., Klonoff, P., Malec, J. F., Mauer, B., & Seller, S. (1994). Consensus conference on the development of a multicenter study on the efficacy of neuropsychological rehabilitation. Zionsville, Indiana.

Willer, B., Rosenthal, M., Kreutzer, J. S., Gordon, W. A., & Rembel, R. (1993). Assessment of community integration following rehabilitation for traumatic brain injury. *Journal of Head Trauma Rehabilitation, 8,* 75–87.

10

Neuropsychological Postacute Rehabilitation

ANNE-LISE CHRISTENSEN

Introduction

On the grounds of a lifelong experience with and research into brain injury, its sequelae, and restoration, it is the purpose of this chapter to present theoretical and practical tenets that have given evidence of the validity of neuropsychological rehabilitation.

Originally, the goal of the Center for Rehabilitation of Brain Injury (CRBI),* established in 1985 at the Department of Psychology, University of Copenhagen, was described as follows: "The purpose of the institution is to undertake neuropsychological investigations and treatment in the service of rehabilitating brain-injured persons, and at the same time perform research and teaching within the area." Through experiences and research in the years that followed, gradual changes have occurred. Research and teaching are still main tasks, but the rehabilitative goal has broadened, some aspects have been emphasized, and some additions made.

The goal today is to provide a rehabilitation program that ensures prospects for life after brain injury composed of elements that encourage personal growth, responsibility, attachment to others and to work and enjoyment: to support brain-injured individuals in gaining the ability to live their lives to the fullest and to master the constant changes that are a part of human life. The focus of the chapter will be on the structure and content of a rehabilitation program working for this purpose. Research on outcome and cost-effectiveness are also included.

*The author has been the director of the CRBI from its inception until February 1998. The current director is neuropsychologist Mugge Pinner, a close collaborator during the center's early years.

ANNE-LISE CHRISTENSEN • Center for Rehabilitation of Brain Injury, University of Copenhagen, 2300 Copenhagen S, Denmark.

International Handbook of Neuropsychological Rehabilitation, edited by Christensen and Uzzell.
Kluwer Academic/ Plenum Publishers, New York, 2000.

Theoretical Premises for the CRBI

Rehabilitation after brain injury was originally, and still is in many countries, in the hands of neurological medicine, supported by physical, occupational, and speech therapy. One of the pioneers was Kurt Goldstein, the German neurologist who treated victims of brain injury during and after World War I. In the framework of his organismic theory, Goldstein (1939) stated that rehabilitation after brain injury was a psychological task (Goldstein, 1919). Goldstein's insights into psychoanalysis were derived from the psychoanalytic milieu of Foulkes in Frankfurt where he worked. His knowledge of psychological processes were obtained in his own psychological laboratory, where he collaborated with among others A. Gelb (Goldstein & Gelb, 1918). Both were regarded by Goldstein as necessary additions to the practice of neurology. Goldstein opposed the stressing of the anatomical viewpoint in cerebral localization, stating that a cerebral activity is a total one but with everchanging regional accents, in accordance with the needed and variably activated structures, that is, an ever-changing play of figures and backgrounds (Goldstein, 1959).

According to Goldstein, neurologists observe individuals suffering from disordered functions; the essential characteristics first being disordered behavior, which makes the individual unable to use his or her capacities and come to terms with the demands of the environment, and second, anxiety. For Goldstein, disordered behavior and anxiety were objective and subjective expressions of the situation of danger that the organism experiences when it is no longer able to actualize its essential capacities, that is, to exist (Goldstein, 1952). It is for this "hindrance of self-actualization" that intensive psychotherapy is needed. Goldstein's work (1942) as manifested in *Aftereffects of Brain Injury during War,* shows foresight and is remarkably "modern." His impact on rehabilitation, however, did not occur until his student, Yehuda Ben-Yishay, practiced his model, first in Israel as a result of the Six-Days War, and later at the New York University Medical School with Leonard Diller (Ben-Yishay & Diller, 1993).

Alexandre R. Luria's contribution during and after World War II introduced neuropsychology to brain injury rehabilitation. Luria's work was based on the principles of the historicocultural school, which was developed with L. Vygotsky in the early 1930s (Vygotsky, 1962). This psychology was premised on the assumption of an intimate relationship between culture and mental operations. Furthermore, Luria's medical studies and work at the Bourdenko Neurosurgical University Institute in the late 1930s led to his theory about higher cortical functions and the notion of functional systems. Luria's theories were in detail described in *Traumatic Aphasia* (1970), *Higher Cortical Functions in Man* (1965), and *The Working Brain* (1973). The investigatory method was developed with the main purpose of understanding what happens to the higher cortical functions in the presence of brain lesions. In addition, the method was used to explain which syndrome of disturbed mental activity resulted from the fundamental defect. Syndrome analysis was considered essential in the planning of treatment for the patients.

Luria's investigative method leads to a qualitative analysis of the level of functioning of the patient. The examiner has the task of identifying the disturbed functions. In addition, the examiner is responsible for clarifying how a patient is trying to cope with the problems with which he or she is presented. Proper use of this method further allows for very specific hypotheses about the fundamental defect by selecting different tasks in which the defect is an essential component. The double dissociation principle suggested by Teuber and Weinstein (1958) is in accordance with this method. The distinction between primary and secondary disturbances is important for the planning of the rehabilitation process. In the case of primary disturbances, major reorganization of the cortical processes is a necessity. According to Luria, reorganization can be either intrasystemic or intersystemic. The intrasystemic reorganization can take place in either of two basic ways: in one the same functional system is transferred to a new level of organization, that is, transferred to a level either more automatic or to a higher level, that is, by employing speech to support the performance. In the intersystemic reorganization, different functional systems have to be organized anew. An example is in the case of afferent motor aphasia or apraxic aphasia, where destroyed kinesthetic pathways can be replaced by afferent visual input.

The task analysis performed during the investigation can teach the therapist how to structure a task in order to make the patient use intact functions in the service of reorganization, or in other words, how to compensate in the most effective way. Close collaboration between the patient and the therapist in this process will strengthen the effectiveness of the cognitive training. Four major rules for planning a patient's cognitive rehabilitation have been deducted: (1) Diagnostic qualification is essential and the patient needs to be given exact and complete information at a level that the patient is currently able to integrate. This is accomplished in order to ensure the patient's awareness of the deficits and their implications for functioning. (2) Intact functions should be utilized. (3) Integration of intact automatic functions in the learning process. (4) Systematization and repetition are required (Christensen, 1989).

Luria's theory of brain function has been accepted in the Western world, but his techniques for investigation as yet have not been widely used. Luria's theory defines the processes being examined rather than viewing them as a preconceived classification of "functions" that are in accordance with contemporary psychological ideas, which by no means always reflect the disturbances of mental processes actually resulting from brain lesions. The advantages of a procedure like Luria's neuropsychological investigation (LNI) (Christensen, 1975) has special significance in neurosurgery and neurology due to the comparability of the LNI results with (1) the neurological examination, (2) the objective neuroradiological techniques [regional cerebral blood flow (rCBF), functional magnetic resonance imaging (fMRI), and positron emission tomography (PET)], and (3) the neurosurgical operation techniques. Very early research relating the findings from the LNI with these methods seemed promising (Christensen & Caetano, in press) but has until recently only resulted in limited collaboration (Christensen, Jensen, & Risberg, 1990). However, growing interest and appreciation of the benefits of collaboration between medical and psychological specialities are becoming increasingly accepted. In a recent article on functional systems, Castro-Caldas, Petersson, Reis, Stone-Elander, and Ingvar (1998) presented a brain activation study using PET and statistical parametric mapping confirming behavioral evidence of different phonological processing in illiterate subjects compared to literate. The results indicated that learning to read and write during childhood influences the functional organization of the adult human brain.

The process of investigating and analyzing the psychological functioning of a specific person by using the LNI demands a phenomenological approach where the basic assumptions of the historicocultural school—that the higher psychological processes are social in origin, are structured through the mediation of speech, and function consciously in a self-regulated manner—are incorporated. The approach corresponds well to the phenomenological tradition that through many years has characterized psychology at the University of Copenhagen (Rubin, 1949). The need in rehabilitation to consider the individual differences not only in accordance with the patient's brain injury but also with his or her social situation matches the general approach of Danish psychology. In structuring the CRBI's rehabilitation program, is the notion that complex forms of mediated activity, which arise in society and history and constitute the essential components of complex human mental activity, develop as a result of people's social experiences is incorporated.

Rehabilitation within the above-mentioned theoretical framework expands the premises of cognitive neuropsychology as it has been practiced mainly in the United States and in Britain. It goes beyond psychology into physiology, sociology, linguistics, and even anthropology, into what has in the later years been termed *cultural psychology.* In this context, the ideas presented by Jerome Bruner in his books, *A Study of Thinking* (Bruner, Goodnow, & Austin, 1956) and *Studies in Cognitive Growth* (Bruner, Oliver, & Greenfield, 1966) initially influenced the cognitive retraining at the CRBI. In one of Bruner's (1996) latest books, *The Culture of Education,* the framework for the pedagogical attitude characteristic of a phenomenological, cultural approach is clearly expressed:

> Acquired knowledge is most useful to a learner when it is "discovered" through the learner's own cognitive efforts, for it is then related to and used in reference to what one has known before. Such acts of discovery are enormously facilitated by the structure of knowledge itself, for however complicated any domain of knowledge may be, it can be represented in ways that make it accessible through less complex elaborated processes. (Bruner, 1996, p. XII)

A learning principle particularly suited to purposes of cognitive training in rehabilitation is further expressed by Bruner:

> The object of instruction [is] not coverage but depth: to teach or instantiate general principles that renders self-evident as many particulars as possible. The teacher in this version of pedagogy, is a guide to understanding, someone who helps you discover on your own. (1996, p. XII)

Bruner's approach matches exceedingly well the approach inherent in the LNI. The task of the examiner is to disclose how patients orient themselves in the world and how they try to find meaning in the presence of a brain injury. It is a demand of the LNI that the examiner provide continuous feedback as part of the investigation method. This not only assists the neuropsychologist in dealing with what neuropsychological processes are at work, but also helps the patient become aware of the problems of performance of tasks. This is the basis on which to initiate an individualized program. In order to understand the variations in the problem-solving approaches of different patients, ascertaining their specific social and cultural background becomes particularly relevant. A patient's specific "state of mind" contains his or her specific experiences and background as well as motivational and cognitive characteristics. Recognition of the patient's individuality and the importance of that individuality for the planning of rehabilitation for the specific person in recent years has been generally accepted in most rehabilitation programs. The extent to which rehabilitation can profit from deeper insight into social and cultural factors is a new approach that needs further interest and study. One example regarding the latter is a case study, where specific musical skills supported a remarkable recovery (Christensen, 1998).

The issues described above have been building blocks for the construction of the rehabilitation day program at CRBI. Support for this structure has been found in the research of Donald G. Stein (Stein, Brailowsky, & Will, 1995), whose contributions have influenced and promoted the notion that neurorecovery mechanisms are at work in the service of a positive rehabilitation outcome. Research on the importance of treatment for the central nervous system (CNS) recovery after injury has given evidence of the complexities involved when the CNS is viewed as an integrated and dynamic system. A host of agents including complex proteins, peptides, and hormones are capable of directly stimulating the repair of damaged neurons or blocking some of the degenerative processes caused by the injury cascade. Because the injury–recovery cycle takes place over time, it has been ascertained that individual variables (i.e., such as environmental situations, health status, individual learning, and emotional history) will affect the outcome of any kind of medical or psychological therapy.

In their visions for the future Stein *et al.* (1995) state that we have learned more about neural recovery mechanisms in the last 10 years that in the last 10 centuries. It is no longer questioned that the rate and extent of recovery from traumatic injury can be enhanced by properties inherent in the CNS, but this seems to happen only with "priming." They consider that a combination of therapies or what has been termed a holistic view is necessary for appropriate treatment. The recommendations these three researchers present deal with the following: (1) early treatment, (2) combined pharmacological and psychological intervention, (3) careful attention to the individual's past history, health status, age and experience, (4) a supportive environment, and as a very new and interesting suggestion that is based on gender differences, that (5) particular schedules are advised for men and women.

Treatment at the CRBI

A few comments concerning the transfer from the acute care to postacute rehabilitation are needed. The importance of the treatment in the acute phase after an injury for the course of recovery has become increasingly manifest. The conviction that neuropsychological knowledge should be available and affect treatment in the very first stages after brain injury in the later years has been shared by nurses and doctors in the acute care. There is a growing acceptance that rehabilitation specialists should be available in the neurosurgical department to advise (doctors and nurses) regarding patients' behavioral manifestations and to evaluate baseline functioning. Furthermore, contact with the relatives should be considered not only as a therapeutic means, but also with the aim of obtaining necessary information for the process of the evaluation. In the acute phase of treatment the nursing staff can benefit from collaboration with clinical neuropsychologists for preventing or ameliorating behavioral problems. In addition, interpretation of behavioral patterns, comparisons with neuroradiological findings, and assistance in prognostic evaluations are appropriate tasks for a neuropsychologist. A neuropsychologist on the staff in a neurosurgical department could further evaluate and follow up on the progress of patients and could assist in assessing when the right time for entering a rehabilitation program has come. Close collaboration between hospital staff and rehabilitation center could make the change of environment and the new situation easier for both the brain-injured person and his or her family, and in this way ensure a smooth continuation of the recovery process.

In Denmark, the above-described situation is as yet only taking place at a few hospitals, and thus only for a minority of brain-injured persons. A gap between the acute treatment phase and the starting of a rehabilitation program such as the CRBI is more common. Initially, when a patient was referred to the CRBI, the primary criteria for acceptance was the presence of verified brain injury, with loss of consciousness and objective, neuroradiological findings. This is still the main inclusion criteria. At the start of the program our medical advisors and the paying parties (at that time a group of municipalities in the Copenhagen area) demanded that patients not be accepted until 2 years after an injury because of the expected spontaneous recovery period. However, at the First International Conference held at the CRBI in 1987, an important subject for discussion was the optimal time for the initiation of rehabilitation. Stein (1988) argued

> that various physiological events occurring after injury have a specific time course and may be responsible for the limited "spontaneous recovery" that one often sees. We now know that recovery is not "spontaneous" nor is it time itself that mediates the necessary events. The outcome of brain injury is not a constant. Posttraumatic recovery and/or impairment is rather a

> complex series of environmental events whose outcome depend on the specific context in which the injury occurs. (p. 6).

Stein further argued that these posttraumatic events could be altered by various kinds of therapies most effectively if provided in specific intervals during the time course. Five years later at the Second International Conference at the CRBI, Stein, Glasier, and Hoffman (1994) stated:

> If we have learned anything about treating brain injury over these last years it is that therapy to promote functional recovery must begin as soon as possible after the initial trauma. Delaying the course of treatment to observe how much "spontaneous recovery" is likely to occur, will in most cases result in permanent impairment. For example, inflammatory reactions, edema, production of free radicals, and excess excitatory amino acids must be eliminated before growth promoting and regenerating factors can take effect. (p. 33)

The CRBI criteria for admission were changed, and it was accepted that psychological and social rehabilitation should begin as soon as the patient can tolerate this type of environmental stimulation. A natural limit to very early admission is another criterion, that is, that the person must be self-sufficient, a demand caused by the CRBI's university location. A criterion that is not medically or psychologically defined but determined by public payers is that brain-injured persons accepted to the program should have the potential for work or education. Due to this group of criteria, the CRBI program is tailored to persons with medium to severe brain injury who have recovered enough to be self-sufficient in daily activities. In addition, they must be functioning in the average intellectual range, have had a job or started an education, and want to work or regain the capacity to take care of their own lives. The disturbances they have can be physical or cognitive (including aphasia). Typically, they also have emotional difficulties and show loss of self-esteem, and their social situations are frequently drastically changed. (For a detailed overview of the CRBI selection criteria, see Appendix A Chapter 17, this volume.)

Even within these criteria, the diversity of abilities among the patients is great. The criteria provide a framework that ensures the establishment of a feeling of communality, which is

TABLE 1. Profile of the Students Accepted into the CRBI 1985–1998

Characteristics	Number	Percentage
Injury type		
Cerebrovascular accident	131	42%
Traumatic brain injury	137	44%
Other	41	13%
Total	309	100%
Sex		
Male	184	59%
Female	125	40%
	Years	
Age at injury		
Median	32.7	
Quartile range	22.8–42.8	
Time since injury		
Median	2.5	
Quartile range	1.1–2.7	

necessary for socialization, with reference to the theoretical premises and the goals of the program. In addition to these intake restrictions, further criteria have been developed and proved useful. Up until June 1997, the CRBI has treated 25 day program groups and 10 additional groups where the treatment provided has been less intensive. The allocation to these groups has been decided on the basis of the general conditions of the patients, both physical and psychological. Furthermore, in a number of cases, individual treatment programs have been developed based on the initial evaluations, where these patients did not yet show adequate ability and motivation to take advantage of the intensive day program. Where appropriate, inclusion has taken place at a later stage. For patients with specific and minor problems the possibility for individual treatment exists. The demographic data for the patients accepted to the day program can be seen in Table 1.

Application of Theoretical Premises

The postacute day program at the CRBI has been described in various publications, the latest of which are Christensen and Teasdale (1993), Christensen and Caetano (1999), and Chapter 17, this volume, where the program is illustrated through a case history. In this context, the program elements will be discussed with reference to the theoretical foundations. It is also on the grounds of previously described theories that the goal of the CRBI program has been defined, namely, to promote growth, responsibility, attachment, and enjoyment in life.

Once a person is admitted into the program, he or she will receive a letter of admittance in which the conditions for acceptance are stated. The person is asked to make a commitment to collaborate to the fullest of his or her ability. However, to secure the brain-injured persons interest, motivation, and energy, the first requirement of the program is to ensure a social milieu, where possibilities are available for the person to feel respected as an individual, where trust can be developed, and where anxiety, insecurity, and loss of self-value are met with empathy. The aim is to provide a common working background for the group of 15 brain-injured persons who enter the program at the same time, such that a process of individual growth can occur physically, cognitively, emotionally, and socially. Since it is considered the first and main task of the entire staff to provide this milieu, the rehabilitative work at hand becomes a shared interactive enterprise. The primary task is to support and encourage the brain-injured person's responsibility in the rehabilitative process. The person is no longer a patient in a hospital but a student in an educational situation. Part of the role of the therapist is one of a teacher rather than one of a doctor. Furthermore, as a consequence of the CRBI's location at the university, the program is described as a course that runs for one semester, and the patients taking the course are "students." Taking part in a course requires responsibility, it is socially valued, and it includes the hope that graduation signifies an improved status. At the New York University Medical School, the participants from the start have been termed "trainees," a name with corresponding implications.

After inclusion into the social milieu, the task of developing attachment to the group and its work begins. The goal is to provide content in the daily program activities that captures as much of the complexity of brain injury and its sequelae as possible. To serve this task, the staff at the CRBI is composed of professionals from medicine, psychology, and various therapy areas (physical, speech, voice, educational), working as an interdisciplinary team. To ensure effectivity, the present therapist–student ratio in the program is one to two. Close to half the staff are neuropsychologists–clinical psychologists due to the predominant needs for psychological knowledge and insight. Each student is allocated a psychologist, who serves as the student's primary therapist, who provides overall planning in- and outside the program. The main purpose, however, is the development of a therapeutic relationship, where feedback based on trust is the essential element. The initiation of this trust is most often based on the interaction during the LNI, performed early in the process. The primary therapist is also the student's individual therapist in cognitive training and psychotherapy and he or she also has the primary contact to relatives, friends, and eventually the workplace. An important part of the primary therapist's work is to ensure and promote the student's attachment to the training, but also to the social activities in- and outside the program.

The reason for the introduction of the concept of the primary therapist has been to prevent what Goldstein termed "protective mechanisms," (Goldstein, 1952) and to strengthen motivation and interest, first, through the development of a close relationship, and second, to ensure comprehensive planning, for the specific needs of the individual to be taken care of. Individualizing the daily program content for all students within the common program schedule is of utmost significance and takes place continuously from program start to program completion. In addition, general questions, that is, pedagogical attitude, introduction of new ideas or various suggestions, can be considered and discussed at these meetings. Regarding the development of specific premorbid interests and skills among the students, smaller groups of staff collaborate with the students to create projects to meet these needs. This is done by including as much knowledge about each student as can be obtained by daily observations and interactions and by contact with relatives, friends, and colleagues.

The elements in the program focus interchangeably on working with more general problems and on the losses of specific abilities. This means that some part of the program schedule are the same for everybody, but others vary, as can be seen in the case history (see Appendix B, Chapter 17, this volume). Training in cognition can take place both individually and in groups of various sizes and purposes according to the specific problem or the strategy planned for remediation. Likewise, the psychotherapy is directed toward the psychological changes caused by the brain injury and its consequences. Therapy is viewed within this frame of reference.

A group element containing many different aspects of the theoretical premises directed toward a variety of skills of a general and social character comprises our morning meeting. The 15 students are present with two therapists consistently present, and the primary therapists of individual students occasionally attend according to a student's need for their presence. The meeting has an agenda, including tasks related to everyday life, such as in workplaces or educational contexts. The general purpose is to stimulate activity, interaction, and discussions. Students take turns fulfilling different roles during the meeting. One student is responsible for the agenda and for running the discussion, three for bringing in news, one for leading a light gymnastics program, one for clarifying of a specific problem that previously was raised, and one taking the minutes. The meeting ends with general feedback being provided by all participants. The structure is clear, the sequence of tasks is the same from day to day, and the roles are defined. The meeting is highly accepted by the students and most often fulfills its various purposes; it adds greatly to a feeling of participation and engagement, often leading to new insight for both students and staff. Luria´s four rules of rehabilitation are present in this program element, as well as in the cognitive training in general.

A component of the CRBI's rehabilitation program that most clearly adheres to the motivational aspect is the physiotherapeutic program partly based on Luria's rehabilitation theory as described in Chapter 3 in *The Restoration of Motor Functions after Brain Injury* (Luria, 1963). The development of a physical, neurological examination and a cognitive approach to physical treatment was partly inspired by the American physiatrist, Sheldon Berrol, and his wife, Cynthia Berrol, the dance movement therapist, and partly by the American physical therapist Joan Roush, Mediplex, Philadelphia, who all visited CRBI in its early days for a longer period of time. The main concern in the physical training and education is the improvement of the individual's physical condition and well-being driven by personal interests and ecological values (Rasmussen, 1994). The tasks consist of doing various exercises and training strength and endurance in a social environment, that is, a health center at a nearby hotel. Parts of the training include sports, bicycling (with two or three wheels), sailing, dancing, and other physical activities. The sessions have strong cognitive elements owing to self-monitoring of progress in the exercise series. The main goal is a feeling of well-being through physical activity. The results of the physical training were significant improvement during the 4-month period of the intensive program.

As emphasis is placed on the student's cooperation in treatment, the hopes and wishes he or she may have for the future are the focus of the therapeutic relationship. Weighing reality against hope, but still encouraging hope in the service of energy and effort, is of special importance. Lazarus (1998) stresses that hope more often than not stems from a situation in which we must prepare for the worst while hoping for better. In this sense, hope can be regarded as a form of coping and can be of support in avoiding depression.

The phenomenological approach that governs the process strengthens attempts to understand and guide the systematization and control of the entire rehabilitation. The constant interaction between and within the staff and student groups is indicative of the dynamics in the recovery process and emphasizes the ongoing evaluation of both process and content. The empathy that Prigatano (1997) refers to as "entering the patients′ phenomenological space" is important for knowing the right time for introducing changes that can lead to further development. Shifts in attachment to new endeavors have to be encouraged and followed through both during the course but mainly at the end, where learned patterns can be used in new contexts. Gradual decrease in contact to the program has to be replaced by investment in the social world, through continuing development and maintaining activation. Four months of rehabilitation determined by the practical circumstance of being located at a university may not be the optimal amount of time for everybody, but the sense of group feeling and common experiences strengthen the efforts each individual shows in adapting to the next stage: attachment to ordinary social life. While the fixed time schedule may cause problems, these can be dealt with by the availability of a variable follow-up period, dependent on the individual student's needs.

The need and wish to fulfill the goals of rehabilitation are also supported by the possibility to go back to an education or again find one′s place in the labor market. Discussing these possibilities and working out realistic plans take place in the last part of the program and continues in the follow-up period under the guidance of the primary therapist, collaborating with the workplace (often the original work place) and a social worker from the brain-injured persons municipality. A special research project initiated by the Ministry for Social Affairs, a county (Frederiksborg), and the CRBI has operated for 4 years. The aim is to establish optimal conditions for work reentry by involving a colleague at the workplace, who is interested and willing to spend time in supporting a brain-injured person in relearning and readapting during an introduction period. The workplace is paid for the hours the colleague spends on the project. Both the colleague and the brain-injured person receive advice and guidance from the neuropsychologist in the project (who is the brain-injured person's personal adviser). The department or firm is also provided with information of a more general nature by the neuropsychologist. A cost-benefit analysis is presently being performed by an independent research group and will be published shortly.

Another important aspect of the entire process of rehabilitation is the collaboration with families. The family constitutes the emotional and social universe of the brain-injured person, which is dramatically influenced by the brain injury. The bonds are still there, but the family roles change dynamically in ways that can be difficult to appreciate, accept, and respond to. The entire process of recognizing the impact of the disturbances, understanding the compensatory reactions of the brain-injured person to diminish anxiety, and finding new means to function can be as difficult for family members as for the brain-injured persons. This is mainly because it is looked on from different perspectives, but also because brain injury is a frightening and unknown subject. The role of the therapist as a "knowing mediator" in these relationships is difficult but essential for a positive emotional outcome. At the CRBI, relatives are collaborators invited to participate in a process where the student is the key person, who has to regain his or her place in the family. In support of the relatives, group meetings are available every 2 weeks for groups of spouses, parents, and siblings and close friends, and when needed, children of the brain-injured persons.

The European Brain Injury Questionnaire (EBIQ) (Teasdale *et al.*, 1997; Deloche *et al.*, 1992) is a tool used at the CRBI that clinically serves to eliminate misunderstandings and differences between brain-injured persons and their close relatives. Psychotherapeutic treatment is provided by the primary therapist both individually and occasionally with a close relative (most often the husband or wife).

Research and Outcome

In the first years of the CRBI the demand was to provide results showing the usefulness of rehabilitation. In the first study (Christensen *et al.*, 1992), data from 46 patients were collected concerning the following: living conditions, work situation, and leisure activities. The data showed the four points in time: pretrauma, prerehabilitation, postrehabilitation, and 1 year after graduation from the program. Half the patients were traumatic brain injury, 30% had endured cerebral vascular insults, and the remainder, included tumours, hypoxic and metabolic damages. The results were socially convincing: Living conditions were normalized, dependence reduced (more students lived alone), more than 70% returned to education and work, and leisure activities reached the preinjury level. The general improvement was present at the one year follow-up, a fact that was attributed to the intensive half year follow-up at the CRBI of the brain-injured persons.

The results were supported by a study carried out by an independent research institute sponsored by the Association of Counties and Municipalities in Denmark (Larsen, Mehlbye, & Gørtz, 1991). The time period covered by the study was $3^1/_2$ years and results showed that after treatment the student's quality of life had improved and the public costs were reduced. The distribution of gain (reduced expenditures) differed among public authorities. The conclusion was that the economic indications supported rehabilitation. Later studies within the area of outcome have been performed with larger numbers of patients and a follow-up period of 3 years (Teasdale & Christensen, 1994). Gains confirmed previous results and appeared either in the time following completion of the day program or at the 1-year follow-up. At the 3-year follow-up, gains were substantially sustained.

A later study performed with 96 students who completed the CRBI program during the period 1993 to 1996 was based on a follow-up interview conducted during autumn 1996 through January 1997. Interviews were obtained with 74 students (77%), and the EBIQ was completed. Results were obtained regarding employment and partner relationships. In all, 69%

were engaged in some form of work. Stable partnerships before the inquiry characterized 78%, while 22% had not been cohabiting or otherwise. Among the 78% in stable partnerships, over half (45%) were still in that relationship, 9% had engaged in a new relationship, and 25 % lived alone. Those who were still in a relationship were slightly older at the time of injury. An interesting finding was that a strong association existed in the EBIQ profiles between those not in a stable relationship and those not working.

Conclusion

The goal has been to create a postacute program based on evidence obtained in previous studies combined with new research, but also based on experiences gained in work with brain-injured persons, nationally and internationally. In this context, an editorial on the effectiveness of postacute rehabilitation by Neil Brooks (1991) is illuminating. The point made is that despite a tremendous growth in the field, "figures for late outcome often make a rather gloomy reading" (p. 103). Evaluating change due to rehabilitation is difficult, and Brooks argues that the outcome literature suggests that change should be demonstrated in terms of real life outcome. Four papers in the issue of the journal *Brain Injury* (1991) are referred to as examples of important research in this respect. The papers are written by two groups: two papers by Cope and colleagues in California and two by Johnston and Lewis based in Community Reentry Services, Ann Arbor and Kessler Institute of Rehabilitation in Philadelphia. The studies are well conducted and include population samples, demographic data, and etiologic factors, and severity of initial injury are described, outcome defined, and duration of follow up, treatment effectiveness, and cost effectiveness are described. The overall impression stated by Brooks (1991) is: " The short answer is that rehabilitation works" (p. 106).

The reader, however, is left with only sparse information regarding the theoretical premises of the treatment provided, the content of the programs, the professionals involved, the therapeutic attitude of the staff, the collaboration with families, and how motivation was secured. These issues are addressed with the aim of identifying salient characteristics by Trexler and Helmke (1996), who describe a group of holistic programs in detail, for example, hours of treatment in various therapies, the professionals working in the program, and the kind of therapeutic interventions made.

To become truly convincing and didactic, combining both measurable components of programs and the psychological contents and atmosphere, future research regarding the effectiveness of rehabilitation is necessary. The fact that research becomes more complicated due to measurement difficulties is an aspect that will need close attention, including a humanistic approach.

The value of comprehensive and valid rehabilitation has been difficult to obtain. The old statement, that dead brain cells cannot regenerate, has been long-lived and difficult to defeat. Current neuroscience supports psychologically based rehabilitation, and outcome results from comprehensive programs have proved that economic gains can be achieved. Brain-injured persons should be offered the kind of treatment that corresponds to the complexity of the brain and to our present scientific knowledge. It is time for the treatment offered in Goldstein's rehabilitation center, almost 100 years ago, to be surpassed by the best possible standards of today.

ACKNOWLEDGMENTS The inspiration for the writing of this chapter stems from collaboration with a dedicated and engaged staff and eager and motivated students and families. For this I want to thank everyone. For commenting on the chapter, I want to thank David W.

Ellis, PhD, who worked at the CRBI during the center's first year, and Bjarne Pedersen, PhD, a present collaborator. I especially want to express my gratitude to Tom W. Teasdale, Associate Professor, and Carla Caetano, PhD, for their contribution to the center's research and publications.

References

Ben-Yishay, Y., & Diller, L. (1993). Cognitive remediation in traumatic brain injury: Update and issues. *Archives of Physical Medicine Rehabilitation, 74,* 204–213.

Brooks, N. (1991). Editorial. The effectiveness of post-acute rehabilitation. *Brain Injury, 5,* 103–109.

Bruner, J. S. (1996). *The culture of education.* London: Harvard University Press.

Bruner, J. S., Goodnow, J. J., & Austin, G. A. (1956). *A study of thinking.* London: John Wiley & Sons.

Bruner, J. S., Oliver, R. R., & Greenfield, P. M. (1966). *Studies in cognitive growth.* London: John Wiley & Sons.

Castro-Caldas, A., Petersson, K. M., Reis, A., Stone-Elander, S., & Ingvar, M. (1998). The illiterate brain. *Brain, 121,* 1053–1063.

Christensen, A-L. (1975). *Luria's Neurosychological Investigation. Manual and test materials.* New York: Spectrum.

Christensen, A.-L. (1989). The neuropsychological investigation as a therapeutic and rehabilitative technique. In D. W. Ellis & A-L. Christensen (Eds.), *Neuropsychological treatment after brain injury* (pp. 126–156). Boston: Klüwer Academic Press.

Christensen, A.-L. (1998). 1997 Sheldon Berrol, MD, Senior Lectureship: Sociological and cultural aspects in post-acute neuropsychological rehabilitation. *Journal of Head Trauma Rehabilitation, 13,* 79–86.

Christensen, A.-L., & Caetano, C. (in press). Luria's neuropsychological evaluation in the Nordic countries. *Neuropsychological Review,* special issue.

Christensen, A.-L., & Caetano, C. (1999). Cognitive neurorehabilitation: A comprehensive approach. In D. T. Stuss, G. Winour, & I. H. Robertson (Eds.), *Neuropsychological rehabilitation in the interdisciplinary team: The post-acute stage* (pp. 188–199). Cambridge University Press.

Christensen, A.-L., & Teasdale, T. W. (1993). A comprehensive and intensive program for cognitive and psychosocial rehabilitation. In F. J. Stachowiak (Ed.), *Developments in the assessment and rehabilitation of brain of brain damaged patients* (pp. 465–467). Tübingen, Germany: Gunter Narr Verlag.

Christensen, A.-L., Jensen, L. R., & Risberg, J. (1990). Luria's neuropsychological and neurolinguistic theory. *Journal of Neurolinguistics, 4,* 137–154.

Christensen, A.-L., Pinner, E. M., Pedersen, P. M., Teasdale, T. W., & Trexler, L. E. (1992). Psychosocial outcome following individualized neuropsychological rehabilitation of brain damage. *Acta Neurologica Scandinavica, 85,* 32–38.

Deloche, G., North, P., Dellatolas, G., Christensen, A-L., Cremel, N., Passador, A., Dordain, M., & Hannequin, D. (1996). Le handicap des adultes cérébrolésés: le point de vue des patients et de leur entourage. (Point of view of patients and their close relatives on the handicap of brain damaged adults). *Annales de Réadaptation et de Médicine Physique, 39,* 21–29.

Goldstein, K. (1919). *Die Behandlung, Fürsorge und Begutachtung der Hirnverletzten (zugleich ein Beitrag zur Verwendung psychologischer Methoden in der Klinik).* Leipzig: F. C. W. Vogel.

Goldstein, K. (1939). *The organism. A holistic approach to biology derived from pathological data in man.* New York: American Book Company.

Goldstein, K. (1942). *Aftereffects of brain injury in war.* New York: Grune and Stratton.

Goldstein, K. (1952). The effect of brain damage on the personality. *Psychiatry, 15,* 245–260.

Goldstein, K. (1959). Functional disturbances in brain damage. In S. Arieti (Ed.), *American handbook of psychiatry* (pp. 770–794). New York: Basic Books.

Goldstein, K., & Gelb, A. (1918). Psychologische Analysen hirnpathologischer Fälle auf Grund von Untersuchungen Hirnverletzter. I. Abhandlung: Zur Psychologie des optischen Wahrnehmungs- und Erkennungsvorganges. *Zeitschrift für die gesamte Neurologie und Psychiatrie, 41,* 1–142.

Larsen, A., Mehlbye, J., & Gørtz, M. (1991). *Kan genoptræning betale sig? En analyse af de sociale og økonomiske aspekter ved genoptræning af hjerneskadede.* (Does rehabilitation pay? An analysis of the social and economic aspects of brain injury rehabilitation) Copenhagen: AKF Forlaget.

Lazarus, R. (1998). Coping with age. Individuality as a key to understanding. In I. H. Norhus, G. R. von den Bos, S. Berg, & P. Fromholt (Eds.), *Clinical gerontopsychology* (pp. 109–127). Washington, DC: American Psychological Association.

Luria, A. R. (1963). *Restoration of function after brain injury.* Oxford: Pergamon Press.
Luria, A. R. (1965). *Higher cortical functions in man.* NewYork: Basic Books.
Luria, A. R. (1970). *Traumatic aphasia.* Haag: Mouton.
Luria, A. R. (1973). *The working brain. An introduction to neuropsychology.* Hammondsworth, England: Penguin Books.
Prigatano, G. P. (1997). Learning from our successes and failures: Reflections and comments on "Cognitive rehabilitation: How it is and how it must be." *Journal of International Neuropsychological Society, 3,* 497–499.
Rasmussen, G. (1994). A new approach to physical rehabilitation. In A-L. Christensen & B. P. Uzzell (Eds.), *Brain injury and neuropsychological rehabilitation—International perspectives* (pp. 161–172). Hillsdale, NJ: Lawrence Erlbaum.
Rubin, E. (1949). *Experimenta psychologica.* Copenhagen: Munksgaard.
Stein, D. G. (1988). Contextual factors in recovery from brain damage. In A-L. Christensen & B. P. Uzzell (Eds.), *Neuropsychological rehabilitation* (pp. 1–18). Boston: Klüwer Academic Publishers.
Stein, D. G., Glasier, M. M., & Hoffman, S. W. (1994). Pharmacological treatments for brain-injury repair: Progress and prognosis. In A-L. Christensen & B. P. Uzzell (Eds.), *Brain injury and neuropsychological rehabilitation—International perspectives* (pp. 17–39). Hillsdale, NJ: Lawrence Erlbaum.
Stein, D. G., Brailowsky, S., & Will, B. (1995). *Brain repair.* New York: Oxford University Press.
Teasdale, T. W., & Christensen, A.-L. (1994). Psychosocial outcome in Denmark. In A.-L. Christensen & B. P. Uzzell (Eds.), *Brain injury and neuropsychological rehabilitation—international perspectives* (pp. 235–244). Hillsdale, NJ: Lawrence Erlbaum.
Teasdale, T. W., Christensen, A.-L., Willmes, K., Deloche, G., Braga, L., Stachowiak, F. J., Vendrell, J. M., Castro-Caldas, A., Laaksonen, R. K., & Leclercq, M. (1997). Subjective experience in brain injured patients and their close relatives: A European Brain Injury Questionnaire study. *Brain Injury, 11,* 543–563.
Teuber, H-L., & Weinstein, S. (1958). Equipotentiality versus cortical localization. *Science, 127,* 241–242.
Trexler, L. E., & Helmke, C. (1996). Efficacy of holistic neuropsychological rehabilitation: Program characteristics and outcome research. In W. Fries (Ed.), *Ambulante und teilstationär Rehabilitation von hirnverletzten* (pp. 25–39). (Outpatient rehabilitation for brain injured) München: W. Zuckschwerdt Verlag.
Vygotsky, L. S. (1962). *Thought and language.* Cambridge, MA: MIT Press.

IV

Regional Neuropsychological Rehabilitation Programs

11

Poststroke Rehabilitation Practice Guidelines

LEONARD DILLER

Any consideration of rehabilitation for individuals who have suffered a stroke must take into account two contemporary events: the explosion of knowledge in neuropsychology and rehabilitation and the increase in rehabilitation facilities that treat patients with impairments due to stroke.

The growth in the knowledge base of neuropsychology can be seen in the proliferation in new journals. We can only list some of them: *Journal of Clinical and Experimental Neuropsychology* (1980), *Archives of Clinical Neuropsychology* (1985), *The Clinical Neuropsychologist* (1986), *Journal of Neurological Rehabilitation* (1986), *Neuropsychology* (1986), *Neuropsychological Rehabilitation* (1991), *Applied Neuropsychology* (1994), and *Journal of the International Neuropsychology Society* (1995). This list, which is by no means inclusive, does not include journals focused on interdisciplinary rehabilitation issues or specific conditions, such as stroke. The growth in journals in neuropsychology is paralleled by the growth in journals in other clinical disciplines engaged in rehabilitation. Peer-reviewed journal articles tend to focus on highly specific procedures that may be difficult to translate into practical operations where clinical work may not permit the same degree of focused effort expended in controlled studies.

Growth in stroke rehabilitation is seen in several ways. Stroke patients constituted 29.8% of discharges from hospital-based rehabilitation facilities in 1995 (Fiedler & Granger, 1997). The Commission on Accreditation of Rehabilitation Facilities (CARF) reported a membership of 436 medical rehabilitation facilities in 1986, and a record number of 837 facilities in 1998, of which 678 were level-1, that is, comprehensive medical rehabilitation programs. There is a rise in the other programs that tend to be less intensive and closer to skilled nursing facilities that offer some rehabilitation services. An independent confirmation of the increase comes from the analysis of outcome data from the Uniform Data System, using 26,165 stroke patients

---

LEONARD DILLER • Rusk Institute of Rehabilitation Medicine, New York University Medical Center, New York, New York 10016.

International Handbook of Neuropsychological Rehabilitation, edited by Christensen and Uzzell.
Kluwer Academic/ Plenum Publishers, New York, 2000.

discharged in 1992 from 252 facilities. Data from a 1995 base from 469 facilities used information derived from 55,530 stroke patients (Stineman & Granger, 1998).

The rise of therapeutic services poses a problem in terms of defining the nature and frequency of the services that are most valid and useful. These concerns are driven by costs of health care. Because of the impact on the health care budget, the US government via the Department of Health and Human Services set up the Agency for Health Care Policy and Research to provide guidelines for providers, consumers, and other relevant interested parties. Poststroke rehabilitation was selected as one of the topics for the development of guidelines, because it met criteria for a significant public health problem.

Guidelines reflect a worldwide movement toward evidence-based medical practice. Spearheaded by government interests, every professional group has moved in the direction of developing guidelines for their practices. While it is unclear as to whether guideline recommendations are mandatory or merely suggestive, it is clear that all service providers are affected by guidelines and that future guidelines will be inescapable aspects of professional practice impacting training and research.

This chapter therefore will briefly review basic facts about stroke as a condition but will focus on a discussion of the poststroke rehabilitation guidelines, with a bias toward discussing those recommendations that are of greater interest to clinical neuropsychologists. It may be useful to examine recommendations for clinical practice at this time and the issues behind them, because recommendations in guidelines are evolving statements, subject to change. At this point it is unclear as to whether guidelines actually improve practice.

Stroke and Its Aftermath

Stroke is the leading cause of disability in the United States. Generally accepted data suggest (Gresham *et al.*, 1995) that of the 550,000 individuals who sustain a stroke annually, more than 400,000 survive. Annual costs of stroke in the United States have been estimated to range from $6.5 billion to $12.5 billion (Kaste, Fogelheim, & Rissanen, 1998). Approximately 18% of survivors are referred to rehabilitation programs. This does not include patients who received rehabilitation services during the acute phase. There are more than 3 million stroke survivors in the United States with various degrees of neurological involvement. The epidemiology of stroke is an evolving field. Classic estimates of the incidence of stroke (Gresham *et al.*, 1995) are based on data extrapolated from studies conducted more than a decade ago in Framingham, Massachusetts, and Rochester, Minnesota, small cities with homogeneous Caucasian populations. More recent samples conducted in Cincinnati, Ohio, suggest a figure of 700,000 annually (Broderick, 1998). The latter figure is higher because it included more African Americans, a group with a higher incidence of stroke than Caucasians. It is estimated that the worldwide annual incidence of first-time stroke is 8 million (Sandercock, 1998).

The typical stroke patient experiences a cerebrovascular accident that results in loss of blood supply to the brain, giving rise to acquired brain damage. Whether due to a thrombosis, which occurs in three quarters of the cases, intracerebral hemhorrage, which occurs in approximately 15%, or subarachnoid hemorrhage, which occurs in 4 to 8% of the cases, once the patient has survived 30 days, the etiology is irrelevant for rehabilitation, except for the difference in management of coexisting medical conditions. Survivors of stroke who are referred to rehabilitation generally present hemiparesis as the most frequent problem requiring interventions. However, the hemiparesis, which occurs on the side of the body opposite the damaged hemisphere, is usually accompanied by a one or more of a number of associated neurological deficits, including loss of bowel and bladder control, aphasia, apraxia, dysphagia, visual defects, neglect, apathy, sensory, perceptual, and cognitive problems, and emotional disturbances including depression, anxiety, and irritability. Hemiparesis, the major presenting complaint responsible for functional limitations, poses a burden on caregivers, a threat to productivity, and diminished quality of life. However, the hemiparesis, which presents as a problem in walking and self-care, is often only part of a larger syndromal picture associated with associated neurological deficits.

While stroke can occur at all ages, it is more common in the elderly, with a rising incidence from age 55 onward. With time there appears to be some recovery. Thus, only 12% of individuals are physically independent at 3 months and 47% are independent at 6 months, While 38% are very severely dependent at 3 months and 4% are very severely dependent at 6 months (Wade, 1993). Rehabilitation usually takes place within the first month, so that it is often difficult to tell how much improvement is attributable to natural rcovery and how much is attributable to rehabilitation.

Cognitive Deficits and Rehabilitation

It has long been observed that the side of hemisphere of damage plays a role in the subsequent neurological impairments, so that damage to the dominant hemisphere is associated with aphasia and language-related problems and damage to the nondominant hemisphere is associated with spatial and perceptual problems. In addition to the well-known finding that in right-handed people the left hemisphere subsumes the processing of language and the right hemisphere subsumes the processing of space, other dimensions of cognition are differentially associated with the individual hcmisperes. Thus impairment of the left brain interferes with processing temporal information, which is intrinsically sequential, while damage to the right hemisphere interferes with parallel or simultaneous information processing. Hence, left-brain-damaged people have difficulty in auditory tasks because they require attention to a sequence of stimuli, while right-brain-damaged people may appear normal in auditory sequential tasks but have difficulty with visual tasks, which call for searching for simultaneous information. Furthermore, patients with damage to the frontal system are impaired in executive components of a task. These patterns of impairments, which are useful in differential diagnosis, play prominent roles in naturalistic situations as well as test situations.

Cognitive deficits interfere with learning many activities that are taught in rehabilitation. Dressing becomes a complex task for a learner with impairments. For example, it involves awareness of the relationship between the garment and its location in space relative to the body, correct reaching behavior, proper organization of a sequence of actions, awareness of errors and self-correction of errors, ability to incorporate variations in garments and of presentation of the garment, and ability to recognize when the task is correctly completed. It is clear that such a task requires the assembly of a number of discrete and coordinated skills that must be integrated in a timely fashion. It is therefore not surprising that performance in motoric components of activities of daily living reflect neuropsychological deficits and are correlated with neuropsychological test performance. Individuals with right brain damage and visual neglect will show less improvement and will take more time in mastering the motor skill components of activities of daily living (Warren, 1990). Among activities that are correlated with test performance are academically related tasks (reading, spelling, written arithmetic) and instrumental activities of daily living such as dialing a phone, making change, driving an automobile, reading a menu, grooming (Gordon & Diller, 1983, p. 113–135).

Two people may fail the same task for different kinds of neuropsychological deficits. Both right and left hemiplegics are at risk for having multiple accidents in a rehabilitation program to a much greater degree than other types of patients (Diller & Weinberg, 1970). However the dynamics behind the acccidents may differ, depending on the location of the brain damage. Right-brain-damaged people with visual perceptual problems risk multiple accidents in a rehabilitation setting. Left-brain-damaged patients who process information too slowly risk multiple accidents (Diller & Weinberg, 1970). Thus a visual cancellation test that is sensitive to both errors and to speed of response can be used for differential prediction.

In addition to concurrent correlations between test performance and naturalistic behavior, test scores can predict future behaviors. Motor recovery and functional limitations, 2 years after the onset of stroke, are directly related to indicators of sustained attention capacity assessed at 2 months after a stroke (Robertson, Ridgeway, Greenfield, & Parr, 1997). Right-brain-damaged patients lagged in recovery of motor status and measures of sustained attention in comparison with left-brain-damaged after 2 years post-onset (Robertson *et al.*, 1997). Patients who show evidence of unilateral spatial neglect on tests administered during admission may show no deficits on these tests after 60 days. But when the retest is performed under conditions of distraction, evidence for neglect reappears. Stepping on a force plate during mental testing, for example, creates a dual task condition that maybe sensitive to latent impairments. Activities of daily living performed in nonstandardized environments, once patients leave a program, are subject to conditons of cognitive complexity that reveal the underlying deficits (Suzuki, Chen, & Kondo, 1997). Some argue that any brain damage results in the diminished use of cognitive resources. This is illustrated in a study of errors in performing natural actions in multitask situations such as wrapping gift packages or packing a lunch box (Schwartz *et al.*, 1997, pp. 51–63).

Affective Disturbances and Rehabilitation

Emotional responses of stroke patients have become a source of major investigative concern over the past two decades. A number of critical questions have emerged: (1) What is the incidence of emotional disturbance in stroke patients; (2) what are the risk factors for emotional disturbances; (3) how can depression be properly assessed; and (4) what is the significance of emotional disturbance for rehabilitation, including issues of disability and handicap?

There is widespread disagreement on the incidence of mood disorders, although there appears to be a consensus that the most common problem is depression, followed by anxiety disorder. Follow-up for depression on a prospective basis of consecutive admissions to a regional stroke center yielded estimates of 22% at 3 months and 27% at 12 months (Hermann, Black, Lawrence, Szelely, & Szalai, 1998). These figures are similar to the findings of Sacco, who reported a 30-day follow-up at another regional stroke center (Greshan, Duncan, & Stasson, 1995). Stroke patients in rehabilitation centers show a higher incidence of depression. Thus, in our inpatient program the incidence rate approached 50% (Diller, Goodgold, & Kay, 1989). Kotila, Numminen, Waltimo, Kaste (1998) report an incidence of depression of 41% in patients who have gone through outpatient rehabilitation programs in contrast to an incidence of 51% in patients who have not attended programs when assessed at 3 and 12 months in a follow-up of regional centers in Finland.

The etiology of depression following stroke has generated controversy. The classical and commonsense view is that grief is a natural response to the disruptions and losses incurred by a stroke and that depression in stroke is no more common and of no more specific etiology than among patients with other physical illnesses (Burvill, Johnson, Jamrozik, & Anderson,

1997). Others have proposed biological etiologies. There is some evidence that a small lesion in the prefrontal portion of the dominant hemisphere and a small lesion in the posterior portion of the nondominant hemisphere is associated with depression. In the case of large lesions, edema may confound specific effects of locus. This theory has been modified to apply only to depression in the acute but not the chronic phase of recovery, where depression may be related to social support and disability factors (Morris *et al.*, 1996). It has been noted that in the acute phase, 6% of stroke patients admitted to having suicidal plans; in the chronic phase this figure rose to 11% (Kosier, Robinson, & Kishi,1996a). In the acute phase, suicidal plans are related to premorbid use of alcohol and anterior location of lesion. In the delayed phase, plans are related to social support and posterior lesion.

Gordon and Hibbard (1997) have noted that difficulties in assessing depression after stroke may be a reason for the wide range of estimates (30–65%) on the incidence of depression. For example, accuracy of self-report measures may be subject to cognitive competence, awareness, and aphasia. Reports of anxiety or depression may be related to the hospital stay rather than the stroke. Somatic items as indicators of vegetative dysfunction may not be the result of affective state but of associated conditions. Observer ratings of depression may differ on the basis of who is observing and particular behavioral samples. Another factor might be time since onset. Some have urged a multimodal approach to the diagnosis of depression (Hibbard, Gordon, Stein, Grober, & Silwinski, 1993). Others have argued that somatic symptoms are indeed valid indicators of mood in stroke patients. Furthermore, patients who acknowledge depression tend to have a higher frequency of lesions in the left hemisphere, while those in whom depression was observed but denied by the patient may have different etiologic sources for the depression (Kosier, Robinson, & Kishi, 1996b). Some have pointed to evidence for lack of reliability in reporting mood (Toedter *et al.*, 1995). Others have argued for the use of well-standardized intruments (Gresham *et al.*, 1995). These disparities suggest that clinicians should be cautious in assessing mood disorders. Wherever possible, self-report should be checked against clinical interview as well as observer report.

While affective disturbances are considered as part of mental health, recent studies have examined their implications for rehabilitation more directly. Depressed stroke patients make fewer gains on a rehabilitation program, require longer days of inpatient stays, and improve more slowly (Schubert, Burns, Paras, & Sioson, 1992a). Depression appears to be related to functional limitations (Schubert, Taylor, Lee, Mentari, & Tamiako, 1992b). It has also been observed that negative symptoms, that is, behavioral indicators of underactivity, are related to longer lengths of stay in stroke patients (Galynker *et al.*, 1997)

In assessing affective disturbances a number of standardized assessment instruments have been used. There appear to be no data to support one instrument over another, for example, Beck Depression Inventory, Zung, Center for Epidemiological Depression, Geriatric Depression Scale. The most well known, the Beck Depression Inventory, has been modified (Hibbard *et al,* 1993) to accommodate to the situation of stroke patients. A fuller description of these scales may be found in Gresham *et al.*, (1995).

Because of the difficulties in telescoping the many domains of assessment including the cognitive, affective, and motivational into a single session that can be generated in a brief period of approximately 1 hour, a method for sampling the various domains that combines some test items and interview items has been proposed (Padrone & Langer, 1997). This approach samples orientation, attention, memory, language, and two- and three-dimensional spatial ability, by drawing on test items. It also samples issues of affective, motivation, and denial via interviews. Results and recommendations are translated into scales and transmitted electronically via computer to screens for immediate availability to relevant members of the team. While there has been an increase in the use of psychometric technicians to conduct extensive standard assessments in neuropsychology laboratories, this approach requires a trained clinician who uses assessment to set up and pursue diagnostic pathways in a rapid manner. The virtue of the approach is its brevity, the range of issues it explores while zeroing in on the most essential area relevant to the referral, and the concerns of the rehabiltation treatment team. It permits the psychologist to be in close contact with team management issues as they unfold during the patient's ongoing program. The approach yields satisfactory reliability between two experienced clinicians. Its validity is being tested. With electronic communications in the computor age, it permits accumulation of huge databases in actual clinical settings. The approach was developed at the Rusk Institute of Rehabilitation Medicine, NYU Medical Center, to meet the needs of the rapid turnover of patients. Thus the same number of staff can serve 85% of a population, which has increased from 1400 patients to 2400 patients annually including 350 stroke patients each year.

Time and Recovery

In tracking the course of recovery of cognitive deficits and depression following stroke, it is apparent that time course is more variable and rate of return is slower than in the return of motor factors associated with self-care functions of activities of daily living. While cognitive disturbances are most acute at the time of onset, they may persist for longer periods. Egelko *et al.* (1989) found that hemiparetics evaluated during rehabilitation and again 1 year later continued to show cognitive deficits and lagged behind controls. At 3 months, problems in memory still remain for 29% of a group that returned to the comunity (Wade, Parker, & Langton-Hewer, 1986). Using a functional test of memory, 49% were found to be below the lowest scores of non-brain-damaged persons at 7 months after onset (Lincoln & Tyson, 1989). Hemi-inattention or unilateral neglect is present in 72% of right-brain-damaged (RBD) and 62% left-brain-damaged (LBD) at 3 days after stroke. At 3 months it is still present in 75% of RBDs who originally showed neglect and 33% of LBDs who originally showed neglect (Stone *et al.*, 1991). In theory, in a group of 100 RBDs, 72 would show neglect after 3 days and 54 after 3 months. In LBDs, corresponding figures would be 62 and 21, respectively. Wide variation in estimates occur in part because of the variation in the tests that are used. However, it appears that the more extensive and inclusive the test battery, the higher the reported incidence. As previously noted, deficits in sustained attention in RBDs predict responses of motor recovery 2 years later (Robertson *et al*,. 1997).

Time of assessment also plays a role in depression. Depression is underreported in self-report or medical intake interview (Schubert, Taylor, Lee, Mentari, & Tamiako, 1992c). Depression is likely to decrease during a rehabilitation program (Schubert, Burns, Paras, & Sioson, 1992d). Data are ambiguous with regard to long-term status of depression. It is apparent that some with earlier major depression still remain in this state at 2 years and even longer and that minor depression may get worse (Parikh *et al.*, 1990).

Practice Guidelines

Before considering specific recommendations, the methodology of the guidelines should be noted. Two parallel paths of evidence lead to a recommendation for a given practice or utilization of a given procedure or modality: scientific evidence and clinical consensus. Scientific evidence is graded in terms of three levels based on a literature review. The gold standard for scientific evidence is two or more independent prospective clinical trials with good internal validity that specifically address the question of interest in a sample of patients to which the question applies. A less affirmative level occurs in single random controlled trials, or studies that address the question of interest indirectly or by two or more nonrandomly controlled trials. Weaker evidence is generated by a single nonrandomly controlled trial. The second path of recommendation is based on expert opinion. A strong recommendation is based on a consensus wherein 90% or more of a panel agree. A consensus is considered when 75% of a panel agree. Thus a practice could be recommended with different degrees of weight on either a scientific or a clinical basis or both.

A review of the poststroke guidelines yields some striking observations. Of the 57 recommended practices, 13 refer to rehabilitation practices during the acute hospital phase, 18 to screening procedures for admission to rehabilitation programs, 23 to management practices in the rehabilitation setting, and 4 to community transition. The distribution of recommendations provides comment about where professional investments have been placed in rehabilitation. There are only four recommendations pertaining to community transition, despite evidence for social isolation, depression, and caregiver burdens when formal rehabilitation is completed. Of all recommendations, 12 are based on scientific evidence, that is, controlled trials, while the remaining 45 are based on clinical consensus. Thus only 21% of recommended practices prior to, during, and after rehabilitation are based on scientifically based data. The majority of scientifically based recommendations (8) occur for rehabilitation services during the acute care period. Of even greater interest perhaps is the paucity of evidence for rehabilitation practice. These recommendations present a particular challenge to neuropsychologists (see Table 1).

We focus on those domains of interest to clinical neuropsychologists, but the survey opens many questions about clinical practice. Particularly when it is apparent that following the lead of the Agency for Health Care Policy and Research (AHCPR), professional societies are forging ahead with practice guidelines for each discipline contributing services in rehabilitation. While the regulatory and legal status of guidelines is uncertain, that is, are they recommendations or requirements, it is clear that they will serve as standards for third-party payers in the future. On another level, clinical neuropsychologists can influence rehabilitation practice just as rehabilitation practice influences clinical neuropsychologists. While clinical neuropsychology attempts to understand the relationships between brain dysfunction and behavior by creating a path via testing, rehabilitation presents behavioral challenges in a number of different directions including the organization and management of goals and the influence and modification of sensory and cognitive factors, depression, and family and caregiver burdens.

We consider the recommendations that are directed to practices of psychologists in rehabilitation settings. However, major efforts in rehabilitation of concern to psychologists—team operations and working with families—are noted in general recommendations based on clinical consensus rather than systematic study.

Recommendations for Direct Clinical Practice

There is a clinical consensus that all patients should be screened for signs of psychological problems (Recommendations 26):

> A clinical psychological examination should be performed in patients who show evidence of cognitive or emotional problems on clinical examination or a mental status screening test. Complete neuropsychological testing is required when more precise understanding of deficits will faciliate treatment (Gresham *et al.*, 1995).

TABLE 1. Recommendations for Clinical Practice in Poststroke Rehabilitation

Recommendations	Research Evidence[a]	Expert Opinion[b]
Rehabilitation during acute care		
1. Coordinated services	A	Consensus
2. Clinical evaluation through all phases	NA	Strong
3. Prevent recurrent stroke	A	Strong
4. Preventing venous thromoembolism	A	Strong
5. Managing dysphasia; prevent	C	Strong
6. Skin integrity	C	Strong
7. Preventing falls	C	Strong
8. Managing bladder function	C	Strong
9. Preventing/controlling seizures	NA	Consensus
10. Early mobilization	C	Strong
11. Early self-care	NA	Strong
12. Patient/family education	NA	Consensus
13. Early discharge planning	NA	Strong
Screening for rehabilitation		
14. Screening for admission to rehab	NA	Strong
15. Need program information	NA	Consensus
16. Consensus in decision making	NA	Strong
17. Threshold criteria	NA	Strong
18. Two areas of need; criteria for inpatient	NA	Consensus
19. Medical stablility for rehab	NA	Strong
20. Tolerate 3 hours a day	C	Consensus
21. Mild needs: OPD or home treatment	NA	Strong
22. Limited services for limited impairments	NA	Consensus
23. Baseline assessment in 3 days	NA	Consensus
24. Standardized ADL measure needed	NA	Strong
25. Complete motor evaluation	NA	Strong
26. Psychological exam signs of problems	NA	Consensus
27. Motor speech exam if problems exist		
28. Evaluate family/caregiver support	NA	Consensus
Managing rehabilitation		
29. Set goals: realistic, agreed upon	NA	Strong
30. Develop management plan	NA	Strong
31. Family actively involved	NA	Strong
32. Patient/family education	NA	Strong
33. Monitoring progress	NA	Strong
34. Managing acute illness	NA	Strong
35. Managing nutrition	NA	Strong
36. Managing bladder function	NA	Strong
37. Managing bowel function	NA	Strong
38. Managing sleep disturbances	NA	Strong
39. Remediation of sensorimotor deficits	C	Strong
40. Compenstory methods; motor improvement	NA	Strong
41. Adaptive devices	NA	Strong
42. Wheelchair selection	NA	Strong
43. Fall prevention	NA	Strong
44. Treat/prevent spasticity, contractures	NA	Consensus
45. Painful shoulder	C	Strong
46. Cognitive deficits need treatment plan	NA	Strong
47. Diagnose and treat depression	A	Strong

(continued)

TABLE 1. *(Continued)*

Recommendations	Research Evidence[a]	Expert Opinion[b]
Managing rehabilitation *(continued)*		
48. Symptoms/cause guide depression treatment	C	Consensus
49. Aphasia functional treatment	C	Consensus
50. Discharge on plateau on two reevaluations	NA	Consensus
51. Assessment of factors for discharge	NA	Strong
52. Discharge planning strategies	NA	Strong
Community transition		
53. Promote family/caregiver functioning	B	Strong
54. Continuity/coordination community care	NA	Strong
55. Follow-up visit within 1 month	NA	Strong
56. Monitoring postdischarge	NA	Strong
57. Consider continued rehabilitation	NA	Consensus

[a] Research Evidence A=Supported by two or more randomly controlled trials (RCTs) that have good internal validity and specifically address the question of interest in a population; B=Supported by a single RCT meeting with the criteria given above for level A evidence, by RCTs that only indirectly address the question of interest, or by two or more nonrandomly controlled trials; C=Supported by a single non-RCT meeting the criteria listed above for B level evidence, use of historical controls, or quasi-experimental designs such as pre- and post-treatment comparisons.
[b] Expert Opinion Strong = Agreement among 90 percent or more of panel members and expert reviewers; consensus = agreement among 75–89% of panel members and expert reviewers.

There is strong clinical consensus that cognitive deficits require a treatment plan (Gresham *et al.,* 1995) (Recommendations 46):

> Cognitive deficits that preclude effective learning are contraindication to rehabilitation. Cognitive and perceptual problems not severe enough to preclude rehabilitaion require goal-directed treatment plans.

There is scientific evidence that depression should be diagnosed and treated and that the symptoms and cause of depression should guide treatment (Recommendations 47):

> A high index of suspicion needs to be maintained and appropriate steps should be taken to determine the presence and cause of depression. The diagnosis of depression depends primarily on the clinical examination, supplemented when necessary by the use of selected depression scales.
>
> The choice of treatment for depression will depend on the cause and the severity of symptoms.

Psychological Examination in Rehabilitation

While there are major current disagreements with regard to the nature of neuropsychological test batteries, that is, fixed versus flexible (Russell, 1998), the core clinical management issues requiring assessment are the patient's ability to profit from a program that involves learning, suggestions to facilitate learning, and specific interventions regarding treatment of cognitive and emotional problems. Are comprehensive neuropsychological assessments a cost-effective way to contribute insights into these problems, given the compressed pace of contemporary rehabilitation?

There are few templates to guide answers to these questions to providing rapid, meaningful assessments. Evaluation may be considered as a process framing a diagnostic pathway requiring clinical judgment and sensitivity, rather than mechanical administration of a test battery, particularly if the test battery, is time consuming and has not been devised for the clinical issues in rehabilitation. While formulation in terms of a profile of scores is desirable, the methods for arriving at these scores requires a series of clinically sophisticated judgments.

Our experience in an inpatient setting that averages 300 to 400 admissions of stroke patients as part of 2400 admissions a year indicates that 85% of these patients can be seen using brief assesments. Conventional assessment uses brief standardized cognitive scales. The Neurocognitive Status Examination (Mysiw, Bargin, Gatens, 1989) is a useful modification of the Mini Mental Status for stroke patients because it has verbal as well as nonverbal items and can be administered within a 10- to 20-minute period. Additional quick tests from classical neuropsychological test batteries with demonstrated predictive validity for poststroke rehabilitation are finger tapping (Prigitano & Wong, 1997), motor impersistence (Ben-Yishay, Diller, Gerstman, & Haas, 1968), and cancellation tests, which have been useful in identifying neglect and predicting outcomes (Diller, Ben-Yishay, & Gerstman, 1974; Kinsella, Parker, Olive & Stark, 1995; Stone *et al.,* 1991). One virtue of cancellation tests is their application and sensitivity to treatment. One general caution: Generally, neuropsychological tests are referenced against populations of normal people. They are useful in separating brain-damaged from non-brain-damaged people. But they are not referenced against other stroke patients performing in rehabilitation settings. Useful descriptions of brief tests can be found in Wagner, Nayan, and Fine (1995) and Caplan and Shechter (1995).

One might argue that the task of the evaluator is to provide a data-based judgment on whether the individual is a suitable candidate for the program, what goals should be set, how should a team modify practices to address the needs of a patient, or does the patient require intervention by the psychologist for cognitive deficits and or emotional/motivational reactions. To be able to respond effectively within a time frame that permits only an hour or two for direct contact requires a highly disciplined, yet flexible procedure to flow with particular needs of the patient and the concerns of the team. The evaluator must sample cognitive, affective, and motivational domains. In an ideal world, aside from the classical issues of validity and reliability, methods for assessment should be sensitive, that is, reasonable, relevant, and important testing and reporting formats that are friendly. In one such format, judgments are recorded on electronic information screens rather than hard copy papers. Screens permit immediate transmission of results and recommendations and are available for team meetings and decision making within the same day. Typical screens might include brief surveys of language, attention, memory, spatial ability, awareness, patient-perceived goals, affective state, and relevant premorbid psychiatric factors. In this manner it is possible to convey assessment results quickly and reduce time in team meetings.

A critical domain of assessment in rehabiltation is the congruence between a patient's goals and goals offered by a program. In screening during initial evaluation, the patient may be insufficiently familiar with the details of a rehabiitation program or may be too overwhelmed by the recency of the stroke experience or by the transfer from an acute care setting, so that goal statements must be accepted cautiously. There are no standardized instruments to assess motivation. Motivation involves a goal-directed activity that covers two components: the goal and the drive to execute the goal. Goals may be sampled by direct and indirect questioning. Drive may be inferred from the energy or persistence demonstrated in executing tasks. Deficient drive is usually associated with hypoarousal or depression.

If psychotherapy and/or cognitive rehabilitation are to be recommended, a more intensive workup is necessary. While it is beyond the scope of this chapter to provide details of such a workup, it should address a profile of deficits and assets that could be used to build treatments and to identify associated factors that may affect the treatments. The workup should link behavioral–neuropsychological complaints with test data and link the two to a strategy for interventions yielding clinically meaningful outcomes.

Treatment Plans for Cognitive Deficits

Treatment plans for cognitive deficits should take into account both plans for the team as well as individual remedial–compensatory approaches. There are few reports of the neuropsychologist actually participating in teaching skills in activities of daily living or outlining the ways in which the neuropsychological report can be used by a team in inpatient settings. Hanlon, *et al.* (1992) describes the application of principles of scanning for activites of daily living by a rehabilitation team. Calvanio and Petrone (1997) describe how attention can be kept focused and describe the use of cuing strategies in learning wheelchair transfers in a patient with profound spatial problems. A major problem in applying compensatory strategies is a patient's unawareness, which may range from passive acknowledgment to active resistance to individual sessions that focus directly on cognitive deficits. Patients have difficulty in identifying problems and tend to identify attentional–perceptual problems as memory problems (Diller & Weinberg, 1993).

Interventions that have received the greatest attention from neuropsychology over the past two decades have been strategies for reducing or compensating for the neglect of space; that is, the tendency to minimize responses to stimuli on the side opposite the lesioned hemisphere. Neglect of space appears in right-brain-damaged individuals on the left side of space as part of a syndrome associated with left hemiparesis.

There have been advances in understanding neglect over the past decade, with the publication of a text on the topic (Robertson & Marshall, 1993), an entire journal issue devoted to the topic (Halligan & Marshall, 1994), and a published symposium (Cermak, 1996). The development of techniques to improve management of the problem in rehabilitation has been of equal importance. The rapid growth suggests that specific treatments will be able to be incorporated into practice guidelines.

A major feature of neglect is the individual's unawareness. A number of approaches have been useful in alleviating the condition. In a series of studies based on case reports of Lawson (1962), a set of procedures and principles for training right-brain-damaged patients to overcome neglect was developed (Diller, Ben-Yishay, & Gestman, 1974). This approach featured training in scanning behavior so that individuals were taught to locate a starting point for the scan (anchoring), check their impulsiveness in rushing to complete the task (self-regulation), recite the targets aloud (pacing), respond to demonstration of the correct response (feedback), and practice. Individuals with neglect could be taught to improve reading, arithmetic, and body-image-related tasks. With modifications to accommodate tasks in three-dimensional space, individuals could be taught to avoid accidents while navigating in wheelchairs (Gouvier, Cottam, Webster, Beissel, & Wolford, 1984; Gouvier, Bua, Blanton, & Urey, 1987; Webster, *et al.* 1989), learn transfer behaviors (Calvanio, Levine, & Petrone, 1993). Among the issues raised by these studies are questions of generalization, the role of affect and hypoarousal in modifying response to treatment, and the fact that skills appear to be nested so that improvement in one set of tasks uncovers the presence of another underlying deficit. Some of these considerations are summarized by Gordon & Hibbard (1991, 1992) (see Table 2).

Since the original work on scanning occurred, a number of different behavioral paths have been pursued. These paths might be divided into several categories: (1) Spatial motor cuing, wherein compensation for neglect is facilitated by a motor act on the impaired side of space

TABLE 2. Summary: Interventions for Problems of Neglect

Author	Year	*N*	Design[a]	Results
Scanning approaches				
Lawson	(1962)	2	Cases	Trained to read by scanning
Weinberg *et al.*	(1977)	57	E vs. C	E>C in scanning, reading
Weinberg *et al.*	(1979)	55	E vs. C	E>C body estimation tasks
Weinberg *et al.*	(1982)	35	E vs. C	E>C visual analysis and synthesis
Young	(1983)			E>C
Gordon	(1985)	88	E vs. C	E=C 4 months post; E reads more
Webster *et al.*	(1984)	3	Cases	Scanning reduces wheelchair hits;
Gouvier *et al.*	(1984)			Broad space scan reduces hits
Gouvier *et al.*	(1987)	5	Cases	Broad vs. narrow scan different
Webster *et al.*	(1988)	13	Cases	Scanning reduces direct hits
Pizzamiglio *et al.*	(1992)	13	Cases	Varied scanning improved function
Hanlon	(1992)	1	Case	Team approach to scan aids ADL
Calvanio *et al.*	(1993)	2	Cases	Scan, task analysis = + transfers
Diller and Weinberg	(1993)	35	E vs. C	Breadth vs. depth > control
Antonucci *et al.*	(1995)			Arousal + scan more effective
Stimulus-specific responses				
Seron *et al.*	(1989)	1	S	Turn off buzzer left pocket
Robertson & Cashman	(1991)	1	S	Buzzer under heel improve walking
Lennon	(1991)	1	S	Color-coded edges avoid collisions
Lennon	(1994)	1	S	Verbal regulate steps in transfers
Spatial motor cuing				
Joanette & Brouchon	(1984)	1	S	Left vs. right arm improves pointing
Joanette *et al.*	(1986)	1	S	Left point reduces neglect
Halligan & Marshall	(1989)	1	S	Left arm aids in cancellation
Halligan *et al.*	(1991)	1	S	Left arm adv lost if starts on right
Robertson	(1991)	1	S	Left arm aided by right helps
Robertson & North	(1992a)	3	S	Left arm anchoring reduces neglect
Robertson	(1992b)	1	S	Left finger action reduces neglect
Robertson *et al.*	(1998)	1	S	Limb act improves varied ADLs
Feedback				
Tham & Tegner	(1997)	15	E vs. C	Video feedback helps baking tray
Trunk rotation				
Wiart *et al.*	(1997)	22	E vs. C	Scan + body rotate gains in ADL/FIM
		5	S	Chronic S
Arousal				
Robertson *et al.*	(1995)		S	Arousal reduces neglect

[a] E=Experimental; C=Control-controlled trial; S=Single case design

rather than visual scanning, has been used in a series of single case design studies (Joanette & Brouchon, 1984; Halligan, Manning, & Marshall, 1991; Robertson, 1991a; Joanette, Brouchon, Gauthier, & Samson, 1986); (2) other various behavioral methods have been shown to be effective: for example, some have focused on stimuli that have cuing properties such as buzzers (Seron, Coyette, & Bruyer, 1989; Robertson & Cashman, 1991), color coding schemes (Lennon, 1994), or verbal regulation cues (Lennon, 1994). These approaches have been used to deal with neglect issues that go beyond scanning of two-dimensional space or facilitate compensation in alternate ways. Tham and Tegher (1997) found that video feedback helped individuals. Wiart *et al.*, (1997), drawing on an insight from the original scanning studies (Weinberg *et al.*, 1977, 1979) in which it was shown that body space plays an important part in neglect, found that scanning training combined with trunk rotation facilitated ambulation in stroke. Robertson, I. H., Mattingly, J. B., Rorden, C., & Driver, J. (1998) Phasic alerting of neglect patients overcomes their spatial deficit in visual awareness. *Nature, 395,* 169–172 (1995) showed that arousal can facilitate compensation for neglect.

Management of Depression

Management–treatment of depression requires careful assessment of the presence of depression, its severity, and etiologic factors, including the premorbid history. Psychotherapeutic approaches to the emotional problems are useful. Although, there are few controlled studies of their efficacy, patients can be taught to shift their focus from preoccupation with losses. One helpful method is to have the patient together with the psychologist elaborate the personal losses and then have the therapist point out that the patient is a person beyond the losses. In effect, a boundary is placed after explicating the losses and an attempt is made to enlarge the scope of positive values. Cognitive behavioral treatment of depression has received some empirical support. Lincoln, Flanagan, Sutcliffe, and Rother (1997), using a series of single case designs of 19 patients who were depressed, found that 4 showed consistent benefits, 6 showed some benefit, and 9 showed no benefit. The improvements were not associated with changes in functional status. Grober, Hibbard, Gordon, Stein, and Freeman (1993) have presented 14 principles of cognitive psychotherapy in the treatment of poststroke depression with illustrative cases. While various pharmacological approaches have been found useful, psychotherapy is often helpful not only in its own right, but also because there may be conterindications for pharmacological approaches or patient refusals to comply with pharmacological recommendations.

References

Antonucci, G., Guarglia, C., Judica, A., Magnotti, L., Paolucci, S., Pizzamiglio, L., & Zuccolotti, P. (1995). Effectiveness of neglect rehabilitation in a randomized group study. *Journal of Experimental Clinical Neuropsychology. 9,* 383–389.

Ben-Yishay, Y., Diller, L., Gerstman, L., & Haas, A. (1968). The relationship between impersistence, intellectual function and outcome of rehabilitation in patients with left hemiplegia. *Neurology, 18,* 852–861.

Broderick, J. (1998). The rising number of strokes. February, 7, *NY Times.*

Burvill, P., Johnson, G., Jamrozik, K., & Anderson, C. (1997). Risk factors for poststroke depression. *International Journal Geriatric Psychiatry, 12,* 219–226.

Calvanio, R., Petrone, P. N. (1997). Stroke patients move better when they attend better: Varieties of attentional assistance and their implications. *Archives of Physical Medicine and Rehabilitation, 78,* 913.

Calvanio, R., Levine D., & Petrone, P. N. (1993). Elements of cognitive rehabilitation after right hemisphere stroke. *Neurology Clinics, 3,* 25–57.

Caplan, B. C., & Shechter, J. (1995). The role of nonstandard neuropsychological assessment in rehabilitation: History, rationale, examples. In L. A. Cushman & M. J. Scheerer (Eds.), *Psychological assessment in medical rehabilitation* (pp. 359–392). Washington, DC: American Psychiatric Association.

Cermak, L. S. (1996). Varieties of neglect. *Journal of the International Neuropsychological Society, 2,* 403–406.

Clark, M. S., & Smith, D. S. (1998). The effect of depression and abnormal illness behavior on outcome following rehabilitation from stroke. *Clinical Rehabilitation, 12,* 73–80.

Diller, L., & Weinberg, J. (1970). Evidence for accident prone behavior in hemiplegic patients. *Archives of Physical Medicine and Rehabilitation, 51,* 358–363.

Diller, L., & Weinberg, J. (1971). Differential aspects of attention in the brain damaged. *Perceptual Motor Skills, 1972, 35,* 71–81.
Diller, L., & Weinberg, J. (1933). Styles of response in perceptual retraining. In W. A. Gordon (Ed.), *Advances in stroke rehabilitation,* Boston; Andover Medical Publishers.
Diller, L., Buxbaum, J., & Chiotelis, S. (1972). Relearning motor skills in hemiplegia: Error analysis. *Genetic Psychoogy Monographs, 85,* 249–286.
Diller, L., Ben Yishay, Y. & Gerstman, L. J., (1974) Studies in Cognition & Rehabilitation. Rehabilitation Monograph 50, Department of Rehabilitation Medicine, NYU Medical Center, New York, N.Y.
Diller, L., Goodgold, J., & Kay, T. (1989). Final report. National Institute Disability Rehabilitation Related Research—*Research and Training Center in Stroke and Head Trauma.* New York: NYU Medical Center.
Egelko, S., Simon, D., Riley, E., Gordon, W., Ruckdeschel-Hibbard, M. & Diller, L. (1989). First year after stroke: Tracking cognitive and affective deficits. *Archives of Physical Medicine and Rehabilitation, 70,* 297–302.
Fiedler., R. C., & Granger, C. V. (1997). The Uniform Data System for medical rehabilitation: Report of first admissions for 1995. *American Journal of Physical Medicine and Rehabilitation, 76,* 76–81.
Folstein, M. J., Folstein, S. E., & McHugh, P. R. (1975). "Mini-Mental State": A practical method for grading the cognitive status of patients for the clinian. *Journal of Psychiatric Research,*
Galynker, I., Prikhojan, A., Phillips, E., Focseneau, M., Ieronimo, C., & Rosenthal, R. (1997). Negative symptoms in stroke patients and length of hospital stay. *Journal of Nervous and Mental Disease, 185,* 616–621.
Gordon, W. A. & Diller, L. (1983). Stroke, coping with a cognitive deficit. In T. G. Burish & L. A. Bradley (Eds.) *Coping with chronic disease* (pp. 000). New York: Academic Press.
Gordon, W. A., & Hibbard, M. R. (1991). The theory and practice of cognitive remediation. In Kreutzer, J. S. & Webman, P. H. (Eds.). *Cognitive rehabilitation for persons with traumatic brain injury.* Baltimore: PH Brookes (pp. 13–222).
Gordon, W. A. & Hibbard, M. R. (1992). Critical issues in cognitive remediation. *Neuropsychology, 6,* 361–370.
Gordon, W. A., Hibbard, M. R., Egelko, S., Diller, L., Shaver, M., Lieberman, A., & Ragnaarson, K. (1985). Perceptual remediation in patients with right brain damage: A comprehensive program. *Archives of Physical Medicine & Rehabilitation, 66,* 352–359.
Gordon, W. A., & Hibbard, M. R. (1997). Post-stroke depression: An examination of the literature. *Archives of Physical Medicine and Rehabilitation, 78,* 658–664.
Gordon, W. A., Hibbard, M. R., Egelko, S., Riley, E., Simon, D., Diller, L., Ross, E. D., & Lieberman, A. (1991) Issues in the diagnosis of post-stroke depression. *Rehabilitation Psychology, 36,* 71–88.
Gouvier, W., Cottam, G., Webster, J., Beissel, G., & Wolford, J. (1984). Behavioral interventions with stroke patients for improving wheelchair navigation. *International Journal of Clinical Neuropsychology, 1,* 186–190.
Gouvier, W., Bua, B., Blanton, P., & Urey, J. (1987), Behavioral changes following visual scanning training: Observation of 5 cases. *International Journal of Clinical Neuropsychology, 9,* 74–80.
Gresham, G., Duncan, P. J., Stasson, W., (1995). *Post stroke rehabilitation* (Clinical Practice Guideline No. 16) Rockville, MD: Agency for Health Care Policy and Research, USPHS.
Grober, S., Hibbard, M. R., Gordon, W. A., Stein, P. N., & Freeman, A. (1993). The psychotherapeutic treatment of post-stroke depression with cognitive–behavioral therapy. In W. A. Gordon (Ed.), *Advances in stroke rehabilitation* (pp. 185–211). Boston: Andover Publishers.
Halligan, P. W., & Marshall, J. C. (1989). Laterality of motor responses in visuo-spatial negelect: A case study. *Neuropsychologia, 27,* 1301–1307.
Halligan, P.W., & Marshall, J.C. (1994). Current issues in spatial neglect. *Neuropsychological Rehabilitation, 4,* 101–240.
Halligan, P. W., Manning, L., & Marshall, J. C., (1991). Hemispheric activation vs. spatiomotor cueing in visual neglect: A case study. *Neuropsychologia, 29,* 165–176.
Hanlon, R. E., Dobkin, B. H., Hadler, B., Ramirez, S. & Cheska, Y. (1992). Neurorehabilitation following right cerebral infarct; Effects of cognitive retraining on functional performance. *Journal of Clinical Experimental Neuropsychology, 14,* 433–444.
Hermann, N., Black, S. E., Lawrence, J., Szelely, C., Szalai, J. P. (1998). The Sunnybrook Stroke Study; a propective study of depressive symptoms and functional outcome. *Stroke, 29,* 618–624.
Hibbard, M. R., Gordon, W. A., Stein, P. N., Grober, S.W., & Silwinski, M. A., (1993). In W. A. Gordon (Ed.), *A Multimodal approach to the diagnosis of post-stroke depression. Advances in Stroke Rehabilitation* (pp. 215–241). Andover, MA: Andover Medical Publishers.
Iacoboni, M., Padovani, A., Di Piero, V., & Lenzi, B. L. (1995). Post-stroke depression: Relationships with morphological damage and cognition. *Italian Journal of Neurological Science, 16,* 209–216.
Joanette, Y., & Brouchon, M. (1984). Visual allesthesia in manual pointing: Some evidence for a sensori-motor cerebral organization. *Brain & Cognition, 3,* 152–165.

Joanette, Y., Brouchon, M., Gauthier, L., & Samson, M. (1986). Pointing with the left vs. pointing with the right in left visual field neglect. *Neuropsychologia, 24,* 391–396.

Kase, C. S., Wolf, P. A., Kelly-Hayes, M., Kannel, W. B., Beiser, A., & D'Agostino, R. B. (1998). Intellectual decline after stroke. *Stroke, 29,* 805–812.

Kaste, M., Fogelheim, R., & Rissanen, A. (1998). Economic burden of stroke and the evaluation of new therapies. *Public Health, 112,* 103–112.

Kinsella, G., Parker, S., Oliver, J., & Stark, R. (1995). Continuing issues in the assessment of neglect. *Neuropsychological Rehabilitation, 5,* 239–258.

Kishi, Y., Robinson, R. G., & Kosier, J. T. (1996a) Suicidal plans in patients with stroke: Comparison between acute onset and delayed onset suicidal plans. *International Psychogeriatry, 8,* 623–634.

Kishi, Y., Robinson, R. G., & Kosier, J. T. (1996b). The validity of observed depression as a criteria for mood disorders in patients with acute stroke. *Journal of Affective Disorders, 40,* 53–60.

Kotila, M., Numminen, H., Waltimo, O., & Kaste, M. (1998). Depression after stroke. *Stroke, 29,* 368–372.

Lawson, I. R. (1962). Visual–spatial neglect in lesions of the right cerebral hemisphere. *Neurology, 12,* 23–33.

Lennon, S. (1991). Wheelchair transfer training in stroke patients with neglect: A single case study design. *Physiotherapy Theory and Practice, 7,* 51–55.

Lennon, S. (1994) Behavioural rehabilitation of unilateral neglect In M. J. Riddoch & G. W. Humphreys (Eds.), *Cognitive Neuropsychology and Cognitive Rehabilitation.* Hove, UK: Lawrence Erlbaum.

Lincoln, N. B. & Tyson, D. J. (1989). The relation between subjective and objective memory impairment after stroke. *British Journal of Clinical Psychology, 28,* 61–65.

Lincoln, N. B., Flanagan, T., Sutcliffe, L., & Rother, L. (1997). Evaluation of cognitive behavioral treatment for depression after stroke: A pilot study. *Clinical Rehabilitation, 11,* 114–122.

Morris, P. L., Robimson, R. G., de Carvalho, M. L., Albert, P., Wells, J. C., Samuels, J. F., Eden-Fetzer, D., & Price, T. R. (1996) Lesion characteristics and depressed mood in the stroke data bank study. *Journal Neuropsychiatry Clinical Neuroscience, 8,* 153–159.

Mysiw, W. J., Bargin, J. G., & Gatens, P. E. (1989). Prospective cognitive assessment of stroke patients before inpatient rehabilitation. The relationship of the Neurobehavioral Cognitive Status Examination to functional improvement. *American Journal of Physical Medicine and Rehabilitation, 68,* 168–171.

Osmon, D. C., Smet, I. C., Winegarden, B., & Ghandavadi, B. (1992). Neurobehavioral cognitive status examination: Its use with unilateral stroke patients in a rehabilitation setting. *Archives of Physical Medicine and Rehabilitation, 73,* 414–418.

Padrone, F., & Langer, K. (1997). Adaptation of psychological assessment for inpatient rehabilitation. Presented at symposium. 50th anniversary of the Rusk Institute: Developments in Psychological rehabilitation: *105th annual meeting American Psychological Association* Chicago, IL.

Panisset, M., Roudier, M., Saxtion, J., & Boller, F., (1994). Severe Impairment Battery. A neuropsychological test for severely demented patients. *Archives of Neurology, 51,* 41–45.

Parikh, R. M., Robinson, R. G., LIpsey, J. R., Starkstein, S. E., Fedroff, J. P., & Price, T. E. (1990). The imapct of poststroke depression on recovery of activities of daily living over a two year follow-up. *Archives of Neurology, 47,* 785–790.

Pizzamiglio, L., Antonnucci, G., Judaica, A., Montenero, P., Razzano, C., & Zoccolotti, P. (1992). Cognitive rehabilitation of patients with the hemineglect disorder in chronic patients with unilateral right brain damage. *Journal of Experimental and Clinical Neuropsychology, 14,* 901–923.

Prigatano, G. P. & Wong, J. L. (1997). Speed of finger tapping and goal attainment after unilateral cerebral accident. *Archives of Physical Medicine and Rehabilitation. 78,* 847–852.

Robertson, I. H., (1991). Use of left hand vs. right hand in responding to lateralized stimulation in unilateral neglect. *Neuropsychologia, 29,* 1129–1135.

Robertson, I. A., & Cashman, E. (1991). Auditory feedback for walking difficulties in a case of unilateral neglect: A pilot study. *Neuropsychological Rehabilitation 1,* 175–183.

Robertson, I. H., & Marshall, J. C. (Eds.) (1993). *Unilateral spatial neglect.* Hove, UK: Lawrence Erlbaum.

Robertson, I. H. & North, N. (1992a). Spatial motor cuing in unilateral neglect. The role of hemisphere, hand and motor activation *Neuropsychologia, 30,* 553–563.

Robertson, I. A. & North, N., (1992b). Spatial motor cuing in unilateral neglect; The role of right hemispace, hand motor activation. *Neuropsychologia, 30,* 553–559.

Robertson, I. A., North, N., & Geggie (1992). Spatiomotor cuing in unilateral neglect: Three single case studies of its therapeutic effects. *Journal of Neurology, Neurosurgery, and Psychiatry, 55,* 799–805.

Robertson, I. H., Tegner, R., Tham, K., Lo, A., & Nimmo-Smith, I. (1995). Sustained attention training for unilateral neglect: Theoretical and rehabilitation implications. *Journal of Clinical and Experimental Neuropsychology, 17,* 416–430.

Robertson I. H., Ridgeway, V., Greenfield, E., & Parr, A. (1997). Motor recovery after stroke depends on intact sustained attention; A 2-year follow-up study. *Neuropsychology, 11,* 290–295.

Robertson, I. H., Hogg, K., & McMillan, T. M. (1998). Rehabilitation after unilateral neglect. Improving function by contralateral limb activation. *Neuropsychological Rehabilitation, 8,* 19–30.

Robertson, I. A., Mattingly, J. K., Rorden, C. & Driver, J. (1998). Phasic alerting of neglect; Patients overcome the spatial defect in visual awareness. *Nature, 395,* 169–171.

Russel, E. W. (1998). In defense of the Halstead Reitan Battery: A critique of Lezak's review. *Archives of Clinical Neuropsychology, 13,* 365–384.

Sandercock, P. (1998). What questions can large and simple trials answer? *Cerebrovascular Disease, 8* (Suppl. 2), 30–36.

Schubert, D. S., Burns, R., Paras, W., & Sioson, (1992a). Increase of medical hospital length of stay by depression in stroke and amputee patients: A pilot study. *Psychotherapeutics and Psychosomatics, 33,* 61–66.

Schubert, D. S., Taylor, C., Lee, S., Mentari, A., & Tamiako, W. (1992b). Physical consequences of depression in the stroke patient. *General Hospital Psychiatry, 14,* 69–76.

Schubert, D. S., Taylor, C., Lee, S., Mentari, A., & Tamaiko, W. (1992c). Detection of depression in the stroke patient. *Psychosomatics, 33,* 290–294.

Schubert, D. S., Burns, R., Paras, W., & Sioson, (1992d). Decrease of depression during stroke and amputee rehabilitation. *General Hospital Psychiatry, 14,* 135–141.

Schwartz, M. F., Buxbaum, L. J., Montgomery, M. W., Fitzpatrick-Desalme, E., Hart, T., Ferraro, M., Lee, S. S., & Coslett, H. B. (1997). Naturalistic action production following right hemisphere stroke. *Neuropsychologia, 37,* 51–66.

Seron, X., Coyette, F., & Bruyer, R. (1989). Ipsilateral influences on contralateral processing in neglect patients. *Cognitive Neuropsychology, 6,* 475–498.

Soderback, I., Bengsston, I., Ginsburg, E., & Ekholm, J., (1992). Video feedback in occupational therapy: Its effect in patients with the neglect syndrome. *Archives of Physical Medicine and Rehabilitation, 73,* 1140–1146.

Stineman, M., & Granger, C. V., (1998). Outcome, efficiency, and time trend pattern analysis for stroke rehabilitation. *American Journal of Physical Medicine and Rehabilitation, 77,* 193–202.

Stone, S. P., Wilson, B., Wroot, A., Halligan, P. W., Lange, S. L., Marshal, J. C., & Greenwood, R. J. (1991). The assessment of visual spatial neglect after acute stroke. *Journal of Neurology, Neurosurgery, and Psychiatry, 54,* 345–350.

Suzuki, E., Chen, W., & Kondo, T. (1997). Measuring unilateral stepping behavior during stepping. *Archives of Physical Medicine and Rehabilitation, 78,* 173–179.

Tham, K., & Tegner, R. (1997). Video feedback in the rehabilitation of patients with unilateral neglect. *Archives of Physical Medicine and Rehabilitation, 78,* 410–415.

Thompson, S. C., (1991). The search for meaning following stroke. *Basic and Applied Social Psychology, 12,* 81–86.

Toedter, L. J., Schall, R., Reese, C. A., Hyland, D. T., Berk, S. N., & Dunn, D. S., (1995). Psychological assessment in stroke. *Archives of Physical Medicine and Rehabilitation, 76,* 719–725.

Wade, D. T. (1994). Health care needs assessment. In A. Stevens & J. Raferty (Eds.) *The epidemiology based needs assessment review Vol. 1* (pp. 111–255). Oxford: Radcliffe Medical Press.

Wade, D. T., Parker, V., & Langton-Hewer, R. L. (1986). Memory losses after stroke: Frequency and associated losses. *International Rehabilitation Medicine, 8,* 68–74.

Wagner, M. T., Nayan, M., & Fine, C. (1995). Bedside screening of neurocognitive function. In L. A. Cushman & M. J. Scheerer (Eds.), *Psychological assessment in medical rehabilitation* (pp. 145–198). Washington DC: American Psychological Association.

Warren, M. (1990). Identification of visual scanning deficits in adults after cerebrvascular accidents. *American Journal of Occupational Therapy, 44,* 391–399.

Webster, J. S., Cottam, G., Gouvier, W. D., Blanton, P., Bussel, G. F., Woford, J., (1989). Wheelchair obstacle course performance in right cerebrovascular victims. *Journal Clinical Experimental Neuropsychology, 11,* 295–311.

Webster, J., Jones, S., Blanton, P., Gross, R., Beisel, G., & Wofford, L. (1984). Visual scanning training with stroke patients. *Behavior Therapy, 15,* 129–143.

Weinberg, J., & Diller, L. (1968). On reading newspapers by hemiplegics. Denial of visual disability. *Proceedings of the 76th Annual Convention* (pp. 655–656) Washington, DC: American Psychological Association.

Weinberg, J., Diller, L., Gordon, W. A., Gerstman, L., Lieberman, A., Lakin, P., Hodges, G., & Ezrachi, O. (1977). Visual scanning training effect on reading-related tasks in acquired right brain damage. *Archives of Physical Medicine and Rehabilitation, 58,* 479–486.

Weinberg, J., Diller, L., Gordon, W. A., Gerstman, L., Lieberman, A., Lakin, P., Hodges, G., & Ezrachi, O. (1979). Training sensory awareness and spatial organization in people with right brain damage. *Archives of Physical Medicine and Rehabilitation, 60,* 491–496.

Weinberg, J., Piasetsky, E., Diller, L., & Gordon, W. A. (1982). Treating perceptual organization deficits in non neglecting RBD stroke patients. *Journal of Clinical Neuropsychology, 4,* 59–75.

Wiart, L., Saint Come, A. B., Debelleix, X., Petit, H., Joseph, P. A., Mazaux, J. M., & Barat, M. (1997). Unilateral neglect syndrome rehabilitation by trunk rotation scanning training. *Archives of Physical Medicine and Rehabilitation, 78,* 424–436.

12

Therapeutic Milieu Day Program

ELLEN DANIELS-ZIDE AND YEHUDA BEN-YISHAY

Introduction

The holistic, therapeutic milieu approach provides a conceptual as well as practical setting for meeting the complex and multifaceted remedial and therapeutic challenges encountered in postacute neuropsychological rehabilitation of the brain-injured adult. The conceptual underpinnings of the approach have been articulated by Ben-Yishay in a companion chapter in this volume (see Chapter 8). It is the aim of this chapter to describe the practical implementation of the holistic approach, as represented by the New York University Medical Center, Rusk Institute Brain Injury Day Treatment Program. It explains how the structural, programmatic, and specialized cognitive–psychotherapeutic elements, combine and reinforce one another to foster the levels of awareness, malleability, compensation, appropriateness of interpersonal behaviors, and acceptance of the consequences of the brain injury, which are essential for achieving optimal rehabilitation outcomes.

Brief History

The New York University Medical Center, Rusk Institute Brain Injury Day Treatment Program (formerly called the Head Trauma Program) was established in 1978 as a federally funded 5-year clinical research and demonstration program. The program was based on the results of a pilot study of the efficacy of holistic neuropsychological rehabilitation, which was conducted in Israel, between 1974 and 1976, with a group of head-injured Israeli war veterans (Ben-Yishay, 1975, 1976, Ben-Yishay & Diller, 1976; Ben-Yishay *et al.,* 1977). Based on the successful outcome of this 5-year research study, the program has been operating, since 1983, as an outpatient clinical service of Rusk Institute. While initially the program accepted almost exclusively persons who sustained traumatic brain injuries in motor vehicle accidents, it currently accepts persons with other types of brain injuries, as well. However, the program's

ELLEN DANIELS-ZIDE AND YEHUDA BEN-YISHAY • Brain Injury Day Treatment Program, New York University Medical Center, New York, New York 10016.

International Handbook of Neuropsychological Rehabilitation, edited by Christensen and Uzzell. Kluwer Academic/ Plenum Publishers, New York, 2000.

structural elements and its methods of remedial and psychotherapeutic intervention have remained essentially unchanged since the program's inception.

Over the years, there have been numerous publications outlining the conceptual foundations of the program (Ben-Yishay *et al.*, 1985; Ben-Yishay & Diller, 1993), its structural and programmatic elements (Ben-Yishay & Prigatano, 1989; Ben-Yishay & Lakin, 1989), and an illustration of the utilization of the therapeutic milieu to achieve individual clinical objectives (Ben-Yishay & Gold, 1990). Succinctly summarized, the therapeutic milieu program setting possesses three mutually reinforcing features: (1) the program's multilayered interventions are carefully prioritized, time-sequenced, and coordinated, to ensure an optimal integration of the unfolding remedial interventions; (2) the therapeutic community provides (a) the individual patient with a supportive peer group and a (psychologically)safe environment in which to practice newly acquired modifications of cognitive and interpersonal skills, as well as (b) the "therapeutic leverages," that is, the inspirational and persuasive influences of peers, needed to induce compliance and motivation to alter maladaptive behaviors and to adopt realistic expectations from rehabilitation; and, (3) the therapeutic milieu setting makes possible the orderly transition from remedial experiences, within the program, to the application of these lessons in the home environment, in other words, from the intensive remedial (preparatory) phase to the functional application phase, including the explorations of the person's work potential. In the following sections, each of the program features is briefly described.

A Program in Three Phases

The New York University program delivers its rehabilitation interventions in three phases: the intensive remedial phase, the guided work trials phase, and the follow-up and maintenance phase. The treatment sequence unfolds gradually, over a long enough period (typically 1 full year), to permit the realization of multiple clinical objectives.

Phase One

The first phase is devoted to the initial intensive remedial interventions and the preparation of the patient (or "trainee" in the parlance of the program) for the two stages that follow. During the first phase, the focus is on: fully engaging the trainees and "enrolling" them as members of a therapeutic community; helping them gain self-awareness and understanding of the consequences of the brain injury; fostering optimum malleability to the remedial interventions of the program staff and their peers; systematically training them to master and habituate compensatory strategies and props; and, helping the trainees attain self-acceptance and a readiness to pursue realistic and achievable functional goals.

The rehabilitative interventions during the intensive remedial phase take place in "cycles." This makes possible the orderly delivery of carefully prioritized cognitive remedial training modules, which, in tandem with individualized interpersonal therapeutic "exercises," gradually and incrementally promote the attainment of the foregoing clinical objectives. Each cycle consists of 20 consecutive weeks. Treatments are delivered 4 days a week, 5 hours per day, for a minimum of 400 treatment hours per cycle.

The orderly implementation of a carefully formulated "master plan" is made possible through a combination of two structural features of the program: (1) a peer group of 10–12 trainees (the appellation "patient" or "client" is frowned on in this therapeutic community), who commence their treatment together and remain together for the duration of a cycle; and,

(2) the complementary nature of the various program components. Since all the members of the peer group begin and end the cycle together, it is possible to pursue common objectives. Nevertheless, while pursuing these common clinical objectives, the application of the remedial and therapeutic interventions must be personalized to accommodate the particular needs and capabilities of each of the trainees comprising the peer group. A detailed illustration of the manner in which this is accomplished within the setting of the therapeutic community was provided elsewhere by Ben-Yishay and Gold (1990).

Based on the experience of the past decade, nearly two thirds of the individuals who have attended the NYU program required two cycles of intensive remedial training, before they were prepared to advance to the next stage of their rehabilitation.

Patient Selection

During the years immediately following its inception, the NYU program accepted, almost exclusively, persons who sustained traumatic brain injuries (in work-related or motor vehicle accidents, falls, or assaults). For the past 10 years, it has served persons with diverse, acquired brain injuries. These include persons with: open and closed head, acceleration–deceleration brain injuries; strokes; aneurysms; anoxia; postinfectious cerebral encephalopathies; and, post-surgical and/or radiation sequelae. These persons have been discharged from conventional in- and/or outpatient rehabilitation programs and have been unable to resume productive lives, despite (often extensive) previous rehabilitation efforts. Typically, these persons sustained their brain injuries about 2 years prior to entering the NYU program. However, in a significant number of instances, the injuries have been more recent or have occurred 7 or more years prior to a person's entering the NYU program.

Qualifying For Entry

To qualify for entry into the NYU program, a person must: (1) be between 18 and 60 years of age; (2) have an intellectual aptitude within the "educable" range; (3) possess reliable, two-way communication skills (e.g., if aphasia and/or dysarthria are present, these should not preclude participation in interpersonal group activities); (4) be capable of residing within the community (either independently or with supervision from a significant other); (5) be manageable without physical restraints (e.g., socially unacceptable behaviors must be amenable to control by verbal persuasion); (6) be willing to agree to participate voluntarily in the program (e.g., a candidate may need urging, but cannot be compelled to attend by family or the courts); (7) refrain from abusing drugs and/or alcohol while attending; (8) be free of major disabling psychiatric conditions (e.g., psychosis); (9) be willing to submit to a period of intensive assessment before commencing treatment; (10) be willing to commit to a full 20-week treatment cycle, without interruption; and, (11) be willing to have significant others participate in the rehabilitation process.

Initial Comprehensive Assessment Procedures

The assessment process includes: clinical interviews; naturalistic behavioral observations; a broad spectrum of standardized neuropsychological tests, as well as special measures developed within the program setting to assess specific cognitive abilities, motivational factors, awareness, malleability, and acceptance of the injury; and, remedial training probes designed to assess cognitive learning potential, as well as motivation and capacity to respond to the group therapeutic interventions. This evaluation procedure thus aims to: (1) provide a comprehensive picture of the candidate's current intellectual functioning; (2) assess his or her current interpersonal skill repertoires; (3) gauge the candidate's malleability, that is, ability to respond to individually administered and small-group rehabilitative interventions; and, (4) explore his or her potential to benefit from systematic cognitive remedial training methods, by obtaining learning samples that demonstrate the feasibility of retraining.

The evaluation is conducted over a period of 1 to 2 weeks (25–35 hours). Typically, a candidate undergoes the evaluation process, while in direct contact with trainees whose treatment is already in progress. This affords the staff an opportunity to assess a prospective candidate's rehabilitation potential and interpersonal skill repertoires, by means of direct observation within the therapeutic setting. It also provides the candidate, as well as his or her significant others, an opportunity to experience what it would entail to participate in an intensive day program. Those individuals who are found to be qualified for the program are placed on a waiting list until the next treatment cycle begins. Candidates from this waiting list are accepted for the intensive phase of their remedial treatment two times a year (in September or March), in groups of 10 to 12 trainees per cycle.

Unfolding of a Treatment Cycle

On the appointed date, the 10–12 trainees who have been previously assessed and found to be suitable program candidates present for treatment. Trainees are typically accompanied by significant others. These 10–12 trainees, with their respective significant others, are inducted into the program through a carefully "staged" and choreographed orientation procedure.

Of the 10–12 trainees who now comprise the membership of the therapeutic community, typically 50 to 60% are "veterans," that is, trainees who have already completed one cycle of treatment and are now returning for a second, follow-up cycle of intensive treatments. These veterans and the new trainees participate, sometimes together and at times separately, in the various program activities. The mixing of new trainees with veteran trainees is calculated to facilitate the realization of the program's overall clinical objectives, as well as the specific clinical objectives of each individual trainee.

Within the first 2 weeks of a treatment cycle, each trainee is assigned to one member of the staff for personal counseling. This staff member provides personal counseling for the duration of the treatment cycle. Since the ratio of staff to trainees is 1:2, the individualized, small-group, "community," and personal counseling treatments are intensive.

Daily Program Features

10–10:30 AM: Orientation. Each program day begins with the assembly of the entire group of trainees, the significant others present on that day, and the clinical staff for the orientation session. This is a small-group procedure designed to: establish continuity; teach the trainees how to set realistic remedial goals (for a day, for a week, for a weekend, and for longer periods); promote the use of compensatory props and compensatory strategies; and, foster willingness on the part of the trainees to assess their progress and difficulties in the presence of peers, staff, and significant others. At the beginning of each cycle, based on the results of the initial assessment, the clinical team prepares a poster for each trainee. This poster identifies for the trainee the first core cognitive or neurobehavioral problem that, in the opinion of the staff, must be ameliorated by the trainee, so that meaningful progress will become possible in the remedial process. Outlined on this poster are the problem (e.g., "Dysinhibiton, manifested as impulsivity"); the solution sought (e.g., "Become a deliberate preplanner and thoughtful responder"); and a four- to five-step operational action sequence, or "strategy," describing how the trainee can ameliorate the problem.

These posters are presented to one trainee at a time, each morning, in the presence of the entire community. The presentation and the dialogue with the trainee receiving the poster are videotaped. Once the logic underlying the staff's selection of the particular problem area and the method for ameliorating it are explained to the trainee, he or she is asked to restate the message on the poster, in his or her own words. The trainee is then asked to endorse the staff's recommendation and to work on this deficit area. The poster is then hung on the wall, in full view of the community, and remains there throughout the treatment cycle. This procedure is repeated until each trainee's personal poster is presented. Thus, all trainees and significant others can appreciate, at a glance, the particular problem that each trainee must learn to compensate for, as a first clinical priority.

10:40 AM–12:00 Noon:Interpersonal Group Exercises. This individualized daily exercise is conducted in the presence of the therapeutic community. It is designed to improve interpersonal communication skills, malleability, and self-acceptance. The exercises consist of a series of rehabilitation-relevant themes that serve as the vehicles for the attainment of various clinical psychotherapeutic goals. Trainees gradually learn how to acknowledge and speak about their losses in the cognitive, social, and vocational domains, while also regaining their sense of self-worth and dignity. The level of difficulty of the themes, from both a cognitive and an emotional point of view, is gradually increased over the course of the cycle. Each day, one trainee is asked to take the "hot seat" and make a presentation on the given theme in the presence of peers, staff, and significant others. The performance is videotaped and forms part of the videotape library that the trainee is encouraged to view with significant others and staff.

Each trainee on the hot seat is coached by a staff member. At the end of the exercise, the trainee receives organized feedback from the entire community about how effectively ideas were formulated and presented, the adequacy of the interpersonal communication style, and the manner in which guidance ("coaching") was accepted. The trainees who observe and give feedback to the person on the hot seat at the conclusion of the exercise are also coached on how to adequately analyze a peer's presentation and how to provide constructive criticism, in an appropriate manner. No one is permitted to decline participation, either in presenting or offering feedback.

This group exercise procedure was described by Ben-Yishay and Lakin (1989). It is the paradigm for therapeutic intervention with brain-injured survivors. The trainee is systematically induced to do as he or she is asked or is shown, do it of his/her free will and make these behaviors part of his/her habit system. The result is that when the trainee has incorporated these "templates" into his/her behavioral repertoire, both the trainee's mental outlook and lifestyle will have improved.

Trainees who are returning for an additional intensive remedial cycle receive "graduate-level" group exercises. These exercises are tailor designed to systematically address remaining problems in awareness, malleability, acceptance, or style of interpersonal communications. In the more advanced versions of the paradigmatic group exercises, typically two trainees are paired and helped by staff coaches to interview each other according to predetermined themes and procedures. Through such carefully orchestrated dialogues, which are calibrated according to the specific trainees' intellectual and emotional capabilities, they are guided by the staff to encourage, gently challenge, and support each other in the difficult process of coming to terms with their existential situation.

12:00–1:00 PM Peer Lunch. Trainees are encouraged to take their lunch hour with peers and those significant others who are present. This informal interpersonal hour provides trainees with an opportunity to practice communication and socialization skills in a naturalistic setting. Trainees are encouraged to invite prospective candidates, who are undergoing assessment, to take lunch with them. Members of the staff are not, as a rule, included in these peer lunches.

1:00–2:30 PM Individualized Cognitive Remedial Training. Individualized cognitive remedial training exercises are carried out in accordance with a preset curriculum and tailored to each trainee's unique constellation of deficits. Thus, trainees are clinically matched, each day, with one or two of their peers to perform (according to their respective treatment plans and under the guidance of a staff coach) cognitive exercises designed to ameliorate difficulties in: initiating purposeful activities or ideas; controlling impulsive behaviors; focusing attention (due to difficulties in "screening out" internal or external distractions) and/or sustaining concentration for required durations; effectively processing visual–perceptual and spatial–motor information; and, higher-level (convergent, divergent, and executive) reasoning functions.

The individualized cognitive remedial training sessions are conducted in a manner that integrates three cardinal principles: (1) The cognitive training is executed hierarchically, focusing initially on the amelioration of basic attentional functions and ending with the remediation of higher-level logical reasoning deficits. (2) The training is conducted according to the principle of "saturation cuing," whereby the trainee is initially provided with maximum cues (or receives demonstrations of how to perform tasks in the most optimal fashion) and, gradually, receives fewer cues, until he or she achieves mastery of the training task. Successful mastery of a training procedure is demonstrated when the trainee can perform that procedure adequately, unaided by others, any time after mastery has taken place. Included in the principle of saturation cuing is the notion of "habituation," that is, that a newly acquired compensatory skill must be practiced until it becomes a semiautomatic behavioral procedure. (3) The third principle is that a newly mastered compensatory skill must be applied in as many real-life situations as possible for it to become part of the trainee's functional repertoire. In other words, it is not realistic to expect true generalization of learned compensations. Rather, the practical goal is to achieve a transfer of learning, which can be attained only through repeated applications, in a variety of functional contexts.

2:30–3:00 PM Community Hour. This daily group exercise is conducted with the participation of the full community. It is designed to: (1) foster a sense of "citizenship" and group belonging; (2) improve social appropriateness of behavior; (3) enhance the trainee's willingness and ability to comply with socially acceptable rules of conduct; and, (4) promote a sense of competence and a reconstituted sense of self. Elsewhere, Ross *et al.* (1982) have provided a detailed discussion of the specific functions that are served by the daily "community hour," in the overall context of the program. With the entire community seated in a large circle, each day, one of the trainees volunteers or is selected to chair the session. Typically, one question, which has been prepared in advance of the daily community hour, is raised. The question is written down by the trainees who proceed to prepare, in writing, a concise and well-targeted response to that question. Then, each trainee in turn is called on by the chair to articulate, in front of the community, his or her response. Others (e.g., staff, significant others, and visitors) are then called on by the chair to comment. The sources of these questions vary. Often they are raised by one member of the staff, with the foreknowledge and agreement of the others. At other times, a particular trainee will ask a question that the trainee discussed and rehearsed with his or her personal counselor. Occasionally, a significant other or visitor will pose a question.

While the sources of these questions vary, they are designed to provide the trainees with repeated experiences in articulating their ideas in front of their peers and hearing what others have to say on the same topic. The topics discussed during the "community" hour deal with issues such as the need to accept one's disability with "calm dignity," the rationale for rehabilitative training, and the possibility of finding meaning in life following rehabilitation, despite the restrictions imposed by the brain injury. The frequent presence of visiting professionals from different countries provides an opportunity for trainees to "think on their feet" and "teach" the visitors about a particular facet of the program or the rehabilitation process. Thus, the cumulative effect of chairing the sessions and responding effectively to challenging questions bolsters the trainees' self-esteem and confidence. As they advance in the treatment cycle(s), trainees are helped to formulate and pose challenging and controversial rehabilitation-relevant questions to their peers, thereby increasing their ability to deal with the "give and take" of real-life social situations.

Periodic Program Features

Weekly Personal Counseling Sessions. Two hours per week, the trainee meets with his or her personal counselor. These sessions are designed to: help the trainee understand the overall program objectives, in terms that have relevance to his or her individual needs; develop the necessary rapport with the counselor, so that the counselor may serve as the trainee's "ombudsperson"; coach the trainee on how to optimally implement compensatory strategies and techniques; foster, in the more reticent and/or socially isolated trainee, a sufficient degree of confidence to bring relevant personal concerns to the therapeutic community; and, help the trainee to transfer gains made in the program to the home environment. Personal counseling is viewed as an adjunct to the broader behavior-shaping activities and psychotherapeutic influences engendered by other program activities.

Family–Significant Other Counseling. The personal counselor assigned to each trainee meets 1 to 2 hours per week with the trainee's family and/or significant others, either individually or jointly, as clinically indicated. The therapeutic approach with family or significant others is principally psychoeducational in nature. It is designed to provide the significant others with the necessary understanding of the purposes and possibilities of rehabilitation, as well as the skills and emotional supports they will require to be able to cope effectively with their respective trainees and the changed family and/or social roles that were caused by the injury.

Weekly, Multiple Significant Others Group Session. The significant others and family members of all the trainees meet once each week, for a $1\frac{1}{2}$ hour multiple family, group session. These sessions are not attended by the trainees. The meetings (a combination of lectures, presentations, and group discussions) are focused around a core curriculum that parallels the educational process of the trainees. These include: topics concerning awareness and understanding of the nature of the brain injury; issues relating to malleability and coaching; questions about how best to help their loved ones implement compensations they are being taught in the program and how to facilitate their transfer to the home environment; and, finally, questions concerning acceptance of the permanence of the brain injury and its future personal, social, and vocational implications. Significant others are provided with guidelines for managing (in the parlance of the program, "coaching") the trainee at home. They are also helped to develop an in-depth understanding of the purpose, techniques, and outcomes that can be realistically expected from the rehabilitation process.

These sessions are attended by significant others whose trainees are in various phases of the remedial process (e.g., first or second intensive remedial cycle, guided work trials, or undergoing follow-up/maintenance therapy). The levels of insight and sophistication of the more experienced significant others is particularly helpful to those in the early stages of the process. Significant others and family members are urged to attend the program during the intensive remedial phase, as frequently as possible, even on a daily basis. This constant exposure to the rehabilitation process, within a community setting that is composed of persons with different types of problems and capabilities, accelerates the educational process and fosters the objectivity that is required for significant others to become effective "frontline" coaches.

Ad Hoc Crisis Interventions and/or Clinical Management Sessions. During any treatment phase, a trainee and his or her significant others may meet with the clinical team for special "poster" sessions. These poster sessions are designed to provide optimal clinical "leverage," to make possible the desired modifications in the trainee's attitude and/or behavior, and to form a therapeutic alliance between the trainee's significant others and the staff. These sessions are called "poster" sessions because the staff employs large colorful posters on which the problem and suggested solutions are outlined. Each poster session is videotaped to provide an audiovisual record for the trainee and significant others to review at home.

Mid-Cycle and Graduation Parties. Twice during each intensive remedial cycle (at weeks 10 and 20), the trainees prepare a carefully written and well-rehearsed formal presentation to an audience consisting of families, friends, and invited others (including former trainees and their families). Although the audience is "friendly" and a number of its constituent members are often familiar to the trainees, it nevertheless represents the "outside world" to them. The presentations are videotaped and subsequently are used in individual counseling or small-group sessions to enhance the trainees' awareness and acceptance. Participation in the preparation and delivery of the presentations is compulsory, as is the need for each trainee to accept the clinical inputs and editorial suggestions provided by the staff during the preparation of the speeches.

During the mid-cycle presentation, each trainee is required to deliver a well-written and carefully edited didactic speech describing a particular facet of the program, such as its philosophy, the purpose of the interpersonal groups exercises, the role of cognitive remediation, and the benefits of significant other participation. Following the didactic presentations, trainees deliver a personal statement as well. These statements describe their deficits, as they have come to understand them, as well as the progress they are making in rehabilitation. For many, the mid-cycle party is the first public admission that they have sustained a brain injury, which has produced intellectual and/or behavioral limitations, and that these problems necessitate intensive remedial training, as well as the need to "gracefully" accept assistance from others. This "owning up" prepares the way for further progress in awareness and malleability. The fact that the personal speeches are well-rehearsed "plays," much appreciated by the audience, ensures that the trainees experience their public disclosures as ego-enhancing. The applause and the respect paid by the audience also enhance the trainees' self-confidence and self-acceptance.

Phase Two: Guided Work Trials

Upon completion of the intensive remedial phase, once the team has determined that the trainee has achieved the minimum requirements in each of the five clinical "landmarks" (see Chapter 8, this volume), the trainee is deemed ready to advance to the second phase of the program. This phase entails a series of tailor-designed, prework and/or actual work explorations under the supervision of the program's vocational counselor. The second phase of the program typically lasts 3 months but may be extended. Each trainee is assigned to a series of supervised *in vivo* work experiences based on the individual's current capabilities. The work assignments are selected to assess the individual's generic work skills and behaviors (e.g., attendance, punctuality, receptivity to supervision, self-monitoring of one's performance, interpersonal skills with co-workers, reliable application of compensatory strategies). Each trainee begins at the most basic level of work assignment. Gradually, as task efficiency is established, the trainee is advanced to more complex work experiences. The trainee has an on-site work supervisor, who consults with the program's vocational counselor on a daily basis.

In addition to the on-site supervision, the trainee receives 1 to 2 hours per week of individual counseling from the vocational counselor and 1 hour of small-group counseling, with peers who are also participating in the guided work trials. The vocational counselor also provides guidance in the areas of independent living and self-management of one's affairs. The vocational counselor is an integral member of the program staff and attends all clinical team meetings, while the trainee is still undergoing treatment during the intensive remedial phase. Likewise, the progress of each trainee during the guided work trials phase continues to be monitored by the entire clinical team, at triweekly staff meetings.

Once the trainee's work potential has been established, he or she receives a final "employability" rating. This consists of a report documenting the level of work competence achieved by the trainee, the types of jobs for which he or she would qualify, and whether he or she would be capable of engaging in full- or part-time competitive work (or, if this proves untenable, whether the trainee could engage in some unpaid volunteer experience). Then, the program assists the trainee in finding work commensurate with his or her current capabilities, which includes helping the individual to become integrated into the new work setting.

The Follow-up/Maintenance Phase

The program provides follow-up vocational and maintenance therapeutic support on a fee-for-service basis, for indefinite periods after discharge. For those trainees who do not reside within the New York metropolitan area, the program staff helps in the search for appropriate assistance within their respective communities.

Integration of the Complementary Program Elements

The orchestration of the different program elements so that they are maximally complementary and, therefore, more readily integrated by the brain-injured trainee is achieved only when the individual staff members function as a clinical council. The team members of the program spend a minimum of 15 hours per week (from 9:00 AM to 10:00 AM each program day before the treatments begin, two clinical meetings per week at the close of the program day and all day Friday, when the trainees are not present) in an ongoing planning process. This process begins with the joint formulation of individualized treatment plans, continues with the daily assessment of each trainees's progress, with respect to his or her rehabilitation objectives, and culminates with the staff's final recommendations.

The fact that all team members interact with each other and with all the trainees on a continuous basis enables them to respond to the various individual trainees in a complementary manner and with a "single voice." Although each staff person is assigned two trainees whose individual and family counseling he or she will oversee, all team members are interchangeable within the context of the therapeutic setting. Since each staff member works daily with all of the trainees for some portion of the one-on-one or small-group remedial activities, it is possible for the interventions to be clinically well-coordinated and systematically applied. This, in turn, helps maintain the necessary consistency that brain-injured trainees require for optimal assimilation of newly learned compensatory practices in their functional life.

Creating an Atmosphere of Empowerment

A central feature of the therapeutic community approach is the deliberate creation of a special atmosphere in which trainees can feel secure, respected, productive, and hopeful. From the moment the trainees commence the intensive remedial phase, they are informed that they are no longer "patients." Rather, they ought to consider themselves "trainees," who, together with the staff and their significant others, are equal partners in the recovery process. All members of the community are referred to by their first name and the trainees quickly learn that all community members are expected to follow the same rules of conduct (e.g., raising a hand to be recognized to speak, punctuality) and share the same responsibilities as "citizens" (e.g., tidying up, collecting work materials, setting up tables, showing courtesy to one's peers).

Persuasion, Articulation, Inspiration

As was previously argued by Ben-Yishay and Diller (1983), brain-injured individuals learn best when instructions or therapeutic messages are maximally articulated, so that the cause–effect relationships or the merits of a given course of action are made explicit for them. In addition, frank persuasion and the use of exhortative techniques are utilized to motivate trainees to exert themselves optimally.

Summary

The Brain Injury Day Treatment Program is the present-day embodiment of Kurt Goldstein's concept of an "ordered environment." In combination with the features of a therapeutic milieu, this model provides a framework for systematically ameliorating disturbances in the cognitive, interpersonal, and intrapsychic spheres of the brain-injured adult. This type of program permits the systematic remediation of problems in awareness, malleability, compensation, and acceptance of the disability, and thus, facilitates a stable personal, social, and vocational adjustment following brain injury.

References

Ben-Yishay, Y. (1975). An outline of a comprehensive theoretical framework for the rehabilitation of persons with severe head trauma. Keynote Address, Sixth Annual Rehabilitation Symposium, Sheba Medical Center, TelHashomer, Israel.

Ben-Yishay, Y. (1976). Setting up a therapeutic community for the rehabilitation of Israeli out-patient war casualties with severe head injuries: Structure and remedial systems. Invited expert panelist, the 13th World Congress of Rehabilitation, Tel-Aviv, Israel.

Ben-Yishay, Y. (1996). Reflections on the evolution of the therapeutic millieu concept. *Neuropsychological Rehabilitation, 6,* 327–343.

Ben-Yishay, Y., & Diller, L. (1976). A multi-impact clinical experiment in rehabilitation of problematic brain injured war veterans. Presented at the 13th World Congress of Rehabilitation, Tel-Aviv, Israel.

Ben-Yishay, Y., & Diller, L. (1983). Cognitive remediation. In M. Rosenthal, E. R. Griffith, M. R. Bond, & J. D. Miller (Eds.), *Rehabilitation of the head injured adult* (pp. 367–380). Philadelphia: F.A. Davis.

Ben-Yishay, Y., & Diller, L. (1993). Cognitive remediation in traumatic brain injury: Update and issues. *Archives of Physical Medicine and Rehabilitation, 74,* 204–213.

Ben-Yishay, Y., & Gold, J. (1990). Therapeutic millieu approach to neuropsychological rehabilitation. In R. L. Wood (Ed.), *Neurobehavioral sequelae of traumatic brain injury* (pp. 194–215). London: Taylor and Francis.

Ben-Yishay, Y., & Lakin, P. (1989). Structured group treatment for brain-injury survivors. In D. W. Ellis & A. L. Christensen (Eds.), *Neuropsychological treatment after brain injury* (pp. 271–295). Boston: Kluver Academic Publishers.

Ben-Yishay, Y., & Prigatano, G. (1990). Cognitive remediation. In M. Rosenthal, E. R. Griffith, M. R. Bond, J. D. Miller (Eds.), *Rehabilitation of the adult and child with traumatic brain injury* (2nd ed., pp. 393–408). Philadelphia: F. A. Davis.

Ben-Yishay, Ben-Nachum, Z., Cohen, A., Gross, Y., Hoofien, D., Rattok, J., & Diller, L. (1978). Digest of a two-year comprehensive clinical research program for out-patient head injured Israeli veterans. In Y. Ben-Yishay (Ed.) *New York University Medical Center Rehabilitation Monograph No. 59* (pp. 1–61).

Ben-Yishay, Y., Rattok, J., Lakin, P., Piasetsky, E., Ross, B., Silver S. L., Zide, E., & Ezrachi, O. (1985). Neuropsychological rehabilitation: The quest for a holistic approach. *Seminars in Neurology, 5,* 252–259.

Ross, B., Ben-Yishay, Y., Lakin, P., Rattok, J., Silver, S. L., Thomas, J. L., & Diller (1982). Using a "therapeutic community" to modify the behavior of head trauma patients in rehabilitation. In Y. Ben-Yishay (Ed.), *New York University Medical Center, Rehabilitation Monograph No. 64* (pp. 57–91).

13

Milieu-Based Neurorehabilitation at the Adult Day Hospital for Neurological Rehabilitation

PAMELA S. KLONOFF, DAVID G. LAMB,
STEVEN W. HENDERSON, MARIE V. REICHERT,
AND SUSAN L. TULLY

History

The Adult Day Hospital for Neurological Rehabilitation (ADHNR) has been providing a milieu-based rehabilitation program for persons with acquired brain injury at the Barrow Neurological Institute in Phoenix, Arizona, since January 1986. The ADHNR program was initially implemented by George P. Prigatano, PhD and Pamela S. Klonoff, PhD, based on a similar program at Presbyterian Hospital in Oklahoma City that Dr. Prigatano directed from 1980 to 1985. The Neuropsychological Rehabilitation Program at Presbyterian Hospital in Oklahoma City was a milieu-based program that assisted patients in becoming aware and acceptant of the neuropsychological consequences of their injuries, improving their personal reactions to their injury, and obtaining employment commensurate with their abilities (Prigatano *et al.,* 1986). Morning hours were devoted to the remediation of and compensation for changes in cognitive, personality, and physical functioning. As time passed, the program was modified to include a structured work experience in order to enhance the effects of therapy within a work setting. The program emphasized developing a good working alliance, not only with patients, but also with family members.

Much of the conceptual framework of both programs was derived from the work of Luria (1963, 1974) and Ben-Yishay (for reviews see Ben-Yishay & Diller, 1993; Ben-Yishay &

PAMELA S. KLONOFF, DAVID G. LAMB, STEVEN W. HENDERSON, MARIE V. REICHERT, AND SUSAN L. TULLY • Adult Day Hospital for Neurological Rehabilitation, St. Joseph's Hospital and Medical Center/Barrow Neurological Institute, Phoenix, Arizona 85013-4496.

International Handbook of Neuropsychological Rehabilitation, edited by Christensen and Uzzell.
Kluwer Academic/ Plenum Publishers, New York, 2000.

Prigatano, 1990). Luria's theory of restoration of higher brain functions has been applied to both diagnostic and cognitive remediation techniques. Ben-Yishay developed the holistic approach to neurorehabilitation, which incorporated cognitive remediation into a therapeutic community. According to his theory, the patient progresses through a hierarchy of six stages, including engagement, awareness, mastery, control, acceptance, and identity, after which the patient should have become successfully reintegrated into the community and attained the highest level of productivity.

Program Philosophy and Description: An Overview

The current program at the ADHNR incorporates all the concepts and philosophy described above. Although for several years Dr. Prigatano has not been involved in administration or direct treatment efforts at ADHNR, the program still relies on the critical theoretical underpinnings he helped to create. For example, there is still an active emphasis on developing a positive working alliance with patients and families (Prigatano *et al.,* 1986) and helping patients improve their levels of awareness, acceptance, and realism about the effects of their injury (Klonoff, 1997). Awareness has been defined as the patients' level of understanding of their areas of strength and difficulty. As part of the process of improving awareness, the patient often experiences a strong emotional reaction (e.g., anger, frustration) when he or she perceives that failure on a task is due to the effects of the brain injury. When such emotional reactions occur, each patient is helped to understand the concept of "catastrophic reactions" (Goldstein, 1952) in order to better recognize and manage their particular form of the catastrophic reaction (Klonoff, Lage, & Chiapello, 1993). Many of the individual and group therapies that directly address cognitive, communication, and physical deficits are also designed to assist patients in improving their awareness of the effects of their injuries.

The second major facet of the rehabilitation process is improving the patients' acceptance of the functional impact of their injury. Patients are given therapeutic suggestions for coping and adapting to their injuries. Individual and group psychotherapy, as well as family support and education, are important vehicles for increasing acceptance levels in both the patients and their families.

Finally, patients are assisted in developing the skills necessary to make good decisions about their future. Such judgments are relevant to independent functioning in the home and community, as well as a return to work or school. Patients and families are taught the value of pursuing attainable goals, which in turn helps restore productivity and meaning in their lives. This frequently requires substantial modification of preinjury goals and aspirations. Participation in structured work and school experiences as part of the rehabilitation process greatly assists patients in becoming realistic about the effects of their injury. Independent feedback from "real-world" evaluators is quite valuable, since it typically provides external validation of the observations and strategies provided in the rehabilitation process.

While the philosophy of the program remains relatively unchanged, the structure and scope of the program have broadened substantially. The current ADHNR program incorporates two programs: Home Independence and Work/School Reentry.

The current treatment team consists of three neuropsychologists, one speech and language pathologist, one occupational therapist, one physical therapist, one recreational therapist, and one neurorehabilitation aide. The team consults on a regular basis with the program medical director or the referring neurologist to review the patient's progress and medical needs. A consultant psychiatrist is also available to help address patients' emotional status. The team functions as an interdisciplinary team, with a strong emphasis on intercommunication and continuity of care. This is accomplished via four 1-hour staff meetings from Monday through Thursday. Aside from providing treatment associated with their particular discipline, the staff performs multiple other roles, including conducting cognitive retraining, co-leading treatment groups, facilitating home and community independence, and establishing and monitoring work trials.

Home Independence Program

The Home Independence program is designed to meet the needs of acutely brain-injured patients, most of whom enter the program directly from an inpatient rehabilitation setting. These patients are actively reintegrating into their home environments and reestablishing meaningful roles within their families. Most patients begin the Home Independence program requiring 24-hour supervision and some level of assistance with activities of daily living. The goals of the Home Independence program are to assist these patients in becoming progressively more independent at home and in the community and to function as productive members of their families.

Patients in the Home Independence program generally attend the program 5 days per week, from 8:15 AM to 2:30 PM. Criteria for admission include:

1. Continence of bowel and bladder.
2. Sufficient cognitive and personality skills to allow participation in six to seven therapy sessions per day (including small group interactions) within 4 to 6 weeks of entering the program.
3. No major psychiatric disturbance that would interfere with the patient's ability to function in the program.
4. The capacity to progress to staying unsupervised in the home for a minimum of 4 hours per day.
5. Family members who are willing to attend weekly individual family meetings and/or Relatives' Group.

The occupational therapist takes the lead role within the treatment team to evaluate and address issues related to home independence. Upon admission into the Home Independence program, the occupational therapist evaluates each patient to determine his or her current and premorbid levels of functioning in activities of daily living. This evaluation necessarily includes an interview not only with patients but also with their available family members, since the acuteness of cognitive deficits oftentimes leads to patients' overestimation of their current level of independence. The evaluation process also includes a home evaluation, wherein the occupational therapist observes the patient in his or her home environment to determine whether any barriers exist to mobility or performance. Recommendations for adaptive equipment or compensatory strategies can be made at this time and supplemented with continued training and education in future treatment sessions.

Next, the occupational therapist meets with both the patient and family members to develop a Home Independence checklist. This checklist is a list of tasks that the patient and his or her family agree represent premorbid levels of functioning. The checklist is updated by the occupational therapist on a weekly basis so that it gradually increases the expectations relative to independence in self-care and home management activities of daily living. Each patient is encouraged to actively use the checklist, that is, initiating, completing, and checking off tasks independently. They are also required to turn the checklist in to the occupational therapist on a weekly basis. At that time, the percentage of completed items is calculated. The checklist serves several purposes. In part, it represents an agreement between the patient, family members, and therapy staff that the patient will make an effort to accomplish the tasks on the list and that the family members will support that effort. It is, therefore, very important that the patient have a key role in contributing to the development of the first and subsequent checklists to avoid feeling as though the checklist is merely a list of assigned "chores." Additionally, the checklist serves as a memory aid for some patients, cuing them to the activities they must complete on a daily or weekly basis. The occupational therapist raises patient progress in Milieu (to be described below) on a regular basis by reporting the percentage of completed items to the community. This provides an opportunity either to recognize patients for good effort or to problem solve and discuss issues that seem to be preventing adequate performance. Overall patient progress in the Home Independence program is assessed and updated on a month-to-month basis.

In order to successfully complete the Home Independence program, patients must demonstrate their ability to function independently for no less than 2 weeks, as defined and agreed to by the patient, family members, and therapists. Typically, discharge criteria also include the demonstration of adequate initiation, judgment, and safety awareness during regular periods of unsupervised time. Such levels of unsupervised activity in the home range from 4 to 24 hours.

Work/School Reentry Program

The Work Reentry program is designed to help patients become productive, whether through gainful employment or volunteer work. For some patients this goal means returning to their former job. For others, it may mean working in a job with less pay or status than preinjury. This may be with their former employer or if necessary in a new work environment. The staff attempts to help patients find a permanent job by the time of program discharge. At times, a vocational assessment is conducted by a program consultant in order to assist the patient with career changes.

The School Reentry program focuses on facilitating the patient's return to school, whether at a high school, community college, or university level. Often high school students will begin with homebound course work on the unit before progressing back to the school environment. On average, 12.5% of our program admissions over the past 5 years have participated in the School Reentry program. Therapists work actively with school personnel to identify and address whatever special needs the patient will have on returning to the classroom. This includes dialogue and meetings with teachers (including input in developing Individual Education Plans), observing students in the classroom, and helping patients access resources for students with special needs on campus. Patients in the School Reentry program eventually transition back to the school environment while they are still receiving program therapies. Usually the speech and language pathologist and/or a neuropsychologist act as liaisons to the school environment.

Criteria for the Work/School Reentry programs are similar to those of the Home Independence program. However, patients must also be able to participate in some form of productive work or school activity within 4 to 8 weeks of program admission. Also, as part of the criteria for program admission, the patients' preinjury work status (e.g., basic job skills, job stability) is evaluated. Such basic work abilities may be further assessed by way of a volunteer work trial within the hospital setting. Many patients progress from completing the Home

Independence program into the Work/School Reentry program. Over the past 5 years, 17% of patients have participated only in the Home Independence program, 47% of patients attended both programs, and 36% participated only in the Work/School Reentry program.

The patients in the Work/School Reentry program generally attend therapies from 8:15 AM until noon, 4 days per week (Monday through Thursday), since they typically spend afternoons and Fridays at work. Whenever possible, program therapists work directly with employers to facilitate the return to work process. At least one therapist supervises the patient at the work site, acting as a liaison between the work environment and the treatment team. Patients who have demonstrated a minimum of 6 to 8 weeks of successful participation, either in a work or school environment, are discharged from the Work/School Reentry program.

Program Therapies

Individual Therapies

ADHNR therapies are divided into group-based sessions and individual sessions. Individual sessions address the specific discipline-related needs of the patient within the context of improving home independence and addressing return to work/school. The patients' treatment programs are individualized (i.e., they receive as much individual therapy as necessary), and patients are often seen several times a week for treatment by individual therapists. Individual therapies are in part directed by feedback from other therapists in daily staff meetings and group therapies. Importantly, many program activities are transdisciplinary in nature, and thus these activities are performed by multiple program therapists in individual sessions. For example, although there is a specific Datebook Group (described below), all program therapists will assign and track memory assignments.

Group Therapies

Milieu

The Milieu session is 15 minutes in length and takes place at the end of the morning. All patients and staff participate. As with all groups, the purpose is reviewed, which in this case is to "discuss the business, progress, and concerns of the day in a community fashion." Patients are given the opportunity to lead the group and are responsible for calling on those individuals who wish to raise issues. This session is also used to monitor the smooth operation of the program, for example, the status of completion of weekly checklists, and how work and school trials are proceeding. Every Monday, the designated leader of the Community Outing reviews relevant assignments and goals with each participant during Milieu. This type of activity holds patients accountable to their treatment goals in a therapeutic manner.

Milieu is also utilized to review and recognize individual patient's progress, for example, accomplishments during Cognitive Retraining, progress with physical therapy goals, and so on. Patient's birthdays and graduation from the program are recognized and celebrated with a cake. Alternatively, if a problem is interfering with a patient's progress, this is discussed in the group, and input and suggestions are requested from staff and other patients.

On a monthly basis, input from all patients is requested regarding their impressions of all individual and group therapies. This information is discussed in staff and is utilized in program development. In many ways the Milieu session is a pivotal illustration of the milieu treatment process at work.

Cognitive Retraining

The various cognitive retraining tasks used at the ADHNR offer an opportunity to work on a broad range of cognitive skills, including attention and concentration, memory and learning, language, visuospatial abilities, executive functions (i.e., impulse control, planning, and organization), abstract thinking, and mental flexibility. Although it certainly seems reasonable to assume that exercising these abilities may facilitate neurological recovery, a detailed description of the theoretical and practical issues involved in cognitive retraining is beyond the scope of this chapter. The interested reader is directed to Klonoff *et al.* (1996) for a presentation of such topics. In essence, the ADHNR approach to cognitive retraining is one of enhancing functionality. Toward this end, efforts have been made to arrange the sessions so as to extract as much practical information as possible, to teach useful compensations, and to apply the experience to the work or school setting. These factors will be briefly described below.

Cognitive Retraining is the first formal therapy session of the day, which mirrors the expectation that one must be productive from the beginning of the work day, as is usually the case for most jobs. It is conducted at several tables arranged within a large room in relative proximity to each other. This arrangement produces a background ambient noise that approximates many work environments. Also, each staff member typically works with two patients during Cognitive Retraining sessions, producing a smaller social unit which requires the patient to interact with those in both a supervisor and co-worker role. Finally, Cognitive Retraining places the patient in a situation where they must strive to meet certain expectations relative to performance levels and work behaviors, while under close observation by a "supervisor."

Because of the above efforts to simulate a real-world environment, Cognitive Retraining provides an excellent opportunity for treatment staff to observe how patients behave in such a setting. Such *in vivo* data are essential in guiding treatment decisions about whether and when to return a patient to the workplace. It has been a consistent clinical observation that problems that occur in Cognitive Retraining are those that will be seen at work, only in a more severe form. For example, normal activities at nearby tables provide ample opportunities for the emergence of impulsivity, distractibility, and social disinhibition. In addition, difficulties with turn taking, intolerance of others' deficits, and procedural rigidity will become evident within the smaller work group interactions. In general, Cognitive Retraining allows therapists to quickly evaluate each patient's ability to follow directions, overall social skills, level of awareness of deficits, and extent of defensiveness and the form it may take (see Klonoff, O'Brien, Prigatano, Chiapello, & Cunningham, 1989). All this information is valuable in directing treatment efforts and determining the appropriate time for a patient to return to work.

Once problem areas have been identified, the next task is to help patients develop effective compensations. Cognitive Retraining assists this process in a number of ways. There are numerous opportunities to discuss each patient's cognitive strengths and difficulties, which facilitates the development of appropriate compensations for work. Daily sessions allow for repeated practice in utilizing compensations. Also, because of the highly quantifiable nature of the tasks, the effectiveness of a proposed compensation is immediately apparent. Weekly graphing of task performance provides an opportunity for observation and discussion of changes in performance based on effective use of compensations, neurological recovery, the benefits of practice, and so forth. Finally, therapists use information shared in staff meetings to coordinate treatment interventions and tie Cognitive Retraining compensations into those used in other program therapies (e.g., procedural checklists for computer-based tasks).

Cognitive Group

In keeping with the overriding goal of enhancing the development of a therapeutic milieu, Cognitive Group provides a common foundation for all patients by presenting information relevant to brain injury across a wide spectrum of etiologies. More specifically, it is anticipated that such knowledge increases meaningful patient interaction about the recovery process and promotes group cohesion. Information is transmitted via the use of lectures, review of handouts, viewing of videotapes, and participant exercises. Sessions are typically conducted by two staff members: a neuropsychologist and a speech and language pathologist.

Cognitive Group modules cover a variety of topics, including "Neuroanatomy," "the Wall Chart," "Strengths and Difficulties Lists," and "Memory." Each module offers considerable opportunity to increase the patient's level of awareness, as discussed below. Depending upon the topic, size of the group, and amount of discussion, modules can continue from 3 to 8 weeks.

The longest and most intensive module covered is Neuroanatomy. Information is provided about the different parts and functions of the brain, as well as different ways in which the brain can be injured. Toward the end of this module, patients view and discuss the available scans of their own brain, and the discussion is then related to the material learned in Neuroanatomy and to their own injury. The Wall Chart module examines the typical course of a neurological patient's treatment, from injury through post-ADHNR discharge. This "roadmap of recovery" covers the process of brain injury, recovery, and rehabilitation, with each patient placing themselves in the process and assessing the progress of their efforts.

Because recall of information is an almost universal deficit of brain injury, an entire separate module is dedicated to memory. This Memory module looks at the complex process of memory in detail and provides numerous methods to deal with memory loss as well as extensive opportunities to practice such compensations. Finally, the Strengths and Difficulties Lists module requires each patient to generate a list of their own areas of strength and deficit since the injury. In order to enhance awareness, each patient receives feedback both from therapists and other patients regarding the accuracy of their list.

As can be seen from the above descriptions, Cognitive Group closely simulates a classroom environment. Patients are expected to take notes and three of the four modules have tests that are given at the end of material presentation. After attempting to answer the questions from memory, patients then use their handouts to go over the test again and answer the items with a different colored pen. Although Cognitive Group is particularly relevant to patients attempting a return to formal education, it provides all patients with a basis for comparison to earlier academic performances, which again promotes increased awareness of the nature and extent of their injury related deficits.

Current Events Group

This group meets once a week and is generally led by the speech and language pathologist. It provides patients with the opportunity to become refamiliarized with local and world news events, a process that is usually interrupted during the early phases of recovery. It also offers another chance for patients to address a variety of cognitive and language deficits, including oral and written formulation, reading comprehension, memory, and abstract reasoning.

This group also lends itself well to addressing pragmatic issues such as problems with hyperverbality, concrete thinking, and tangentiality. As with other group therapies, patients identify and review on a weekly basis their main area of focus for the group. Each patient is expected to read a newspaper article and summarize it. During the session, each patient presents their article and then a discussion is held regarding other group members' opinion of the issues raised. Each week a patient is selected to lead the overall discussion and another is chosen to review the previous week's articles. Patients returning to higher-level administrative or professional positions are given the opportunity to oversee the smooth operation of the session, for example, time management of all segments.

Group Psychotherapy

The structure and purpose of this session have been reviewed in detail elsewhere (Klonoff, 1997). This group meets four times per week at the end of the morning, thus enabling patients the opportunity to discuss relevant issues that may have occurred earlier in the treatment day. The group is open entry–open exit and is composed of patients from both the Home Independence and Work Reentry programs. The decision of when to begin patients in this group depends on a number of factors, including their ability to follow group discussion, sufficient impulse and temper control to tolerate discussion of sensitive issues, and a willingness to discuss personal issues. Additionally, most of the group discussion focuses on helping patients become more acceptant of and realistic about the effects of their injuries; therefore, most patients must have at least some beginning awareness of their injury-related deficits before starting the group.

Note taking is utilized to help recall prior discussions. At times, handouts are developed that summarize important topics that may cover several sessions (e.g., the cause and management of depression). This group is much less structured than other groups in that patients are encouraged to bring up any topic of relevance to their recovery that is of a "feeling" nature. Often, patients use this session to elicit opinions or feedback from other patients who may have experienced similar challenges. Other media are incorporated into Group Psychotherapy, including art therapy and music. At times "guest speakers" (usually prior patients) talk with current patients about their postprogram progress and how their experiences have affected their impressions as they reflect on their own rehabilitation process. Such talks for current participants are usually quite inspirational and helpful, as they let the current patients know there is "life after rehabilitation."

Datebook Group

Datebook Group meets twice weekly to assist patients in using datebooks to compensate for memory difficulties, to plan and organize their daily schedules, and to become more independent in keeping track of appointments, events, and important information. Real-world examples of the importance of organization and follow-through at work and school help underscore the need to consistently use a datebook as a compensation.

Patients are given multiple memory assignments by program therapists as a way of practicing a number of skills. For example, the patient must:

1. Listen effectively to the assignment to ensure staff expectations are fully understood and important details have not been missed, asking for clarification if necessary.

2. Develop the habit of carrying the datebook at all times, to prevent the pitfall of jotting an assignment on a scrap of paper, which could then be misplaced, forgotten, or lost in the disorganized clutter of a purse or wallet.
3. Write a relevant note in the correct location in the datebook. The note must be concise but contain enough detail so that the full assignment can be recalled and understood at a later time.
4. Establish a routine for regularly checking the datebook both in the program and at home in order to be cued by his or her note to fulfill the assignment.
5. Not wait for the therapist to ask for the assignment to be completed (thereby cuing the patient), but rather take the initiative to complete the assignment by the due date.

A memory assignment tracking sheet is kept for each patient in a central location in the unit to which all therapists have access. The staff records the date an assignment was given, the nature of the assignment, the date it is due, and whether it was successfully completed. Each patient's progress in using the datebook is then measured on a weekly basis by calculating the percentage of assignments completed accurately. The goal is for patients to improve their datebook skills to the point of successfully following through on at least 95% of their memory assignments.

Community Outings

Following an initial evaluation period, a general opinion is formed by the recreational therapist and other team members as to whether or not a patient would be appropriate to participate in a group activity within the community. Community outings take place on Monday afternoons from 12 PM to 2:30 PM. Outings usually encompass both a meal at a restaurant and a visit to a local recreational resource (e.g., museum, shopping mall, park, etc.). The recreational therapist and neurorehabilitation aide oversee the organization and implementation of the outings. Depending on patient needs, other therapists frequently attend outings, including the occupational therapist, speech and language pathologist, or physical therapist. This allows the recreational therapist and other team members to further assess a patient's skill level and the impact physical, language, and/or cognitive deficits have on community functioning. Most important, any behavioral or interpersonal problems a patient may demonstrate can be addressed in a supportive, yet therapeutic manner both within the community and later during individual sessions. Patients are also encouraged to generalize strategies learned in therapy to the outing. For example, the focus of outing strategies is often directed at consistent use of a datebook system to compensate for memory difficulties.

Two weekly outing planning sessions are used to first plan and then review each outing. Using a structured worksheet, the recreational therapist determines with the patient whether each task was completed independently, with cuing, or with assistance by a therapist. This worksheet also allows patients to independently chart their own progress, which highlights areas of concern in a manner similar to the Home Independence checklists or Cognitive Retraining graphs. Generally, before successfully "graduating" from community outings, patients are expected to take on the role of "leader," where they plan and implement the outing.

Relatives' Group

As stated above, the weekly Relatives' Group is an integral part of the rehabilitation process. It not only provides an opportunity for the staff and family to discuss the patients' progress or problems, it also facilitates dialogue among family members, who are all attempting to cope and adapt to the injury of their loved one. It is interesting and rewarding to watch more "senior" family members who have been affiliated with the program for a longer time instruct and encourage new members. Understandably, relatives sometimes benefit more from discussion among themselves than from input from the therapists.

The structure and intent of this group have been reviewed elsewhere (Klonoff, 1997). Briefly, the session begins with the purpose of the group being reviewed and any new members being introduced. Next, the patient's progress and relevant treatment issues are discussed in a round-robin format. As many staff members as possible are scheduled to attend the group, providing feedback from the perspective of multiple disciplines. At times, general topics are also discussed in a didactic format, including the use of handouts and research articles. Examples of such topics include a description of the rehabilitation process via the Wall Chart, review of basic neuroanatomy, overview of different types of memory disorders and their compensations, and definition and management of the catastrophic reaction.

Case Study: AB

The above has described many of the philosophical and structural elements currently present in the ADHNR milieu program. The following case study will illustrate how these are integrated into the overall rehabilitation of a patient who attended the Work Reentry program.

Case History

AB was in her 40s when admitted to the ADHNR. Since suffering a traumatic brain injury (TBI) as an adolescent, she had experienced complex partial seizures. She had taken numerous medications, none of which completely controlled seizures. Three years prior to admission to the program she underwent a left anteromesial temporal lobectomy. Prior to surgery, AB had completed a neuropsychological evaluation, the results of which indicated mild-to-moderate verbal memory deficits. Follow-up testing was conducted more than 3 years postsurgery as part of the admission to the ADHNR. Although the results of that assessment revealed multiple areas of adequate cognitive functioning, mild restrictions in confrontation naming and complex visual sequencing abilities were observed. Also, mild-to-moderate restrictions were found in rote verbal learning and memory functions. These data are consistent with sequelae associated with dominant temporal lobe insult.

AB's psychosocial history is significant for severe intermittent depression since the onset of her seizures. Several years after the onset of her seizures, she attempted suicide. She was married for many years to an alcoholic and physically abusive husband, during which time she gave birth to a child. She reported ongoing problems with depression during this period, often not getting dressed or leaving her home for days at a time. She then divorced her husband and went to live with her parents. Her level of functioning improved, and she began to attend community college courses and worked for 2 years as a secretary/receptionist. Unfortunately, her teenaged child was killed as a passenger in a motor vehicle accident. AB became severely depressed. Although she attempted to continue community college and work, she was fired from two jobs within a 1-year period. AB was referred to ADHNR by State Vocational Rehabilitation Services to help her develop compensations for her memory difficulties and find some form of productive gainful employment.

AB is like many of our early program referrals in that she was referred for services after multiple job failures. She had a poor understanding of her neuropsychological difficulties. In her case, she also had multiple prior psychosocial stressors, which contributed significantly to her adjustment difficulties.

Treatment

The milieu program was very helpful in further identifying both AB's assets for and barriers to gainful employment. AB's scores on Cognitive Retraining exercises revealed many strengths: she showed good speed of information processing, a positive learning curve, and good procedural memory. In individual speech and language therapy, her performance on tasks of word retrieval, vocabulary, abstract reasoning, and reading comprehension reflected improvement and appeared functional for secretarial work. She had no significant physical deficits and was independently exercising at a local health club. Because of these many strengths and the length of time postsurgery, 2 weeks after program admission it was decided to have her begin a structured volunteer placement in the afternoons after therapy. Three weeks later she began a second volunteer job due to an insufficient workload at the first work trial. In total, she worked five afternoons per week, approximately 3–4 hours per day. Because of her apparent talent and interest in secretarial/computer work, the two volunteer jobs focused on these areas. She also worked with one of the staff neuropsychologists to become better versed with various computer software systems.

Despite her initial progress in the program, a variety of problematic cognitive, interpersonal, and behavioral problems were observed within the milieu environment that ordinarily would be difficult to detect in traditional treatment programs. For example, it became evident in both structured (e.g., therapy) and unstructured (e.g., lunchtime and community outings) situations that AB was hyperverbal, suspicious, and defensive. Related to her left temporal lobe deficits, she often misperceived and misinterpreted conversations in a negative light. At times the situation escalated to where AB would become verbally attacking and paranoid. A number of episodes arose not only within the treatment environment, but also at her volunteer job in the hospital, though it took several weeks for the seriousness of these difficulties to emerge.

AB was initially highly resistant to feedback regarding these difficulties. Instead, she tended to deflect the cause of the problems to external sources (e.g., other people) and generally became "defensive about being defensive." Many individual psychotherapy sessions were spent developing the working alliance, as attempts were made to help her recognize and monitor the social impact of these symptoms. Eventually over the course of 6 to 8 weeks, progress was made, and AB began to better self-monitor and take more responsibility for her interaction style. These interpersonal and behavioral problems were addressed across a variety of program sessions. The speech and language pathologist addressed some of the specific pragmatic difficulties (e.g., hyperverbality), using role playing as a tool. Pragmatic difficulties were also closely monitored in group settings, often using a hand signal in Group Psychotherapy, Milieu, and Cognitive Group to cue her regarding turn taking and verbal expansiveness. Her parents were a strong asset to the rehabilitation process. They were unfailing in their attendance of the weekly Relatives' Group. Several additional individual family meetings were held with AB, her parents, and the treating neuropsychologist to help confront and discuss these issues. In these meetings AB's parents were highly supportive of the treatment team's perceptions. They were also helpful in providing additional personal examples from home in a manner that AB could hear and to which she would agree.

Lastly, AB was closely supervised by treatment staff at her volunteer work placements, with daily visits for the first several weeks. Both oral and written feedback regarding AB's work performance and interpersonal style were obtained from on-site supervisors and co-workers. Not surprisingly, at one of the volunteer jobs AB received confirmatory feedback suggesting she was hyperverbal and distracting to other employees. She also had difficulty perceiving subtle nonverbal cues from others that they wanted to disengage from a discussion. In the other job environment, AB worked essentially alone and interacted only intermittently with a supportive and patient supervisor. It became clear that this latter type of work setting would be most ideal for AB.

The other major area addressed as part of AB's program involvement was the use of her datebook. Although AB could keep track of two to three assignments per week without using an external compensation, the extent of the memory difficulties grew more apparent as the number and complexity of her responsibilities grew via outside responsibilities and two work settings. AB was inconsistent in remembering to make entries into the datebook and was generally forgetting to check the datebook regularly. Therefore, AB participated in Datebook Group and was trained by the occupational therapist and recreational therapist to make entries consistently and check the datebook regularly throughout the day.

Outcome

After $3^1/_2$ months of therapy, AB obtained a new paid position. Although the actual job placement was facilitated by a state agency, program therapists helped her to practice interview skills and fill out applications. AB works as a secretary for a local health care agency. She works primarily alone, which limits opportunities for problems with hyperverbality and distracting others. Her supervisor is highly understanding and supportive of AB. Two staff neuropsychologists continued to provide treatment to AB for several months after starting this job. One went to the job site for the first 3 months once or twice each week and closely monitored AB's interpersonal style and demeanor. The other neuropsychologist saw AB at the program in weekly individual psychotherapy sessions. Her parents also continued to attend the weekly Relatives' Group until AB completed her 3-month probationary employment period. AB continued with individual psychotherapy for the next several months, three to four times per month, in order to monitor her work status and address any interpersonal difficulties that arose. A good working alliance was maintained with both AB and her family. Because she was able to develop a sense of trust in the treatment team, for the first time in her adult life she was able to successfully maintain competitive gainful employment.

Evolutionary Changes

When examining the demographic and clinical data of recent ADHNR patients in comparison to patients at its inception, a number of changes are revealed. Changes reflect a number of factors, including maturation of the staff's clinical decision-making abilities, generally improved patient treatment over the years, and the impact of managed health care in the United States.

Injury–Admission Interval and Length of Stay

Table 1 provides a comparison of the first 50 ADHNR patients to the most recent 50 patients. Because of skewed distributions of data, median values are reported and nonparametric statistical analyses were used to compare these two groups. Statistical analysis reveals that while age and education have remained the same, the typical patient now seen at ADHNR has a more acute brain injury and stays in the program for a shorter period of time.

TABLE 1. Comparison of Selected Variables of First 50 to Most Recent 50 ADHNR Patients

Demographic variable	First 50 ADHNR patients	Most recent 50 ADHNR patients
Age (years)		
Median (*range*)	33.9 (*14–60*)	38.0 (*15–65*)
Education (years)		
Median (*range*)	12.5 (*10–19*)	12.5 (*8–19*)
Chronicity (months since injury)		
Median (*range*)	5.5 (*1.4–72*)	1.9 (*0.6–318*)[a]
Length of stay (months)		
Median (*range*)	6.5 (*1.9–22.0*)	4.1 (*1.3–8.2*)[a]
Etiology		
TBI	36	27
CVA	4	4
Aneurysm/AVM	4	5
Anoxia	2	0
Infection	1	3
Hydrocephalus	0	1
Tumor	2	6
Epilepsy Surgery	0	3
Other	1	1

ªP< .05 as determined by Mann-Whitney U test.

Because of the increased acuteness of injury of its patients, the ADHNR treatment approaches have been modified. Many patients are transitioned directly from an inpatient environment and have had little or no opportunity to try to function in their home or community since their injury. As a result, the staff has needed to modify the pace of insight-oriented therapy so as not to unduly alienate the patient or family. This means substantially more time is spent helping patients recognize that they have in fact suffered a brain injury resulting in functional problems that will impact their future. Therefore, many of the individual and group oriented therapies focus on awareness training, particularly during the first several weeks postadmission.

Also, as seen in Table 1, the length of stay at ADHNR is now significantly shorter than it was for the first ADHNR patients. Although one might argue that over time the team has become more efficient in helping patients achieve rehabilitation goals, it is our clinical impression that staff, patients, and families often feel "rushed" by third-party payers to accomplish goals and discharge the patient. As a consequence, the clinical director spends a substantial amount of time communicating with third-party payers on behalf of the patient, not only to obtain funding for services, but to extend funding so that treatment goals can be accomplished. The unfortunate reality of the current health care system is that at times the program has had to limit its scope of treatment to only certain goals, in order to accomplish them within the externally imposed time limit.

Patient Populations

As seen at the bottom of Table 1, the current patient population of ADHNR differs from the original 50 patients in terms of brain injury etiology. While the first 50 patients were predominantly people who had sustained traumatic brain injuries (almost three quarters of this group), the most recent 50 patients have a wider range of etiologies, with 54% being post-TBI, 8% poststroke, 10% postaneurysmal or arteriovenous malformation rupture, and 6% post-surgery for epilepsy treatment. While the reasons for this shift in etiologies are unclear, it may be a function of the community's growing familiarity with the services provided by the ADHNR and a greater willingness to refer a variety of neurological diagnoses to the program, as physicians obtain evidence of success with patients of different types.

Also, very recently the ADHNR has begun to treat patients with brain tumors of high malignancy who are in the early phases of their illness and are still relatively healthy. The overall purpose of treatment for these patients is to improve quality of life and help them find some form of productive volunteer activity, even if it is time limited. The milieu of patients, staff, and other family members provides invaluable support to the patient and his or her family, as most often they have been displaced from their work and community support network. Individual and group psychotherapy services and the Relatives' Group are important sources of emotional support and education to both the patient and family. The staff works closely with community resources to facilitate a smooth transition to hospice services when the patient is no longer able to attend the program. Overall, the patient is helped to come to terms with the prognosis of their illness and participate in a supportive, therapeutic environment as long as possible.

Modified Programs

Occasionally, patients are admitted who do not require full-time program involvement. Such cases are discussed extensively in staff meetings to ensure that important treatment goals are not overlooked and that alterations to the standard program are a better course of action than referral to a different, less structured outpatient rehabilitation setting. These program modifications can be due to a number of factors. First, a language barrier can reduce the number of therapies available for a patient who has limited English-speaking abilities. However, since several staff members are fluent in Spanish, the program can be modified to focus on the specific job skills necessary for primarily Spanish-speaking patients to return to gainful employment. Also, some patients have had very negative experiences in school and are therefore resistant to the "academic" nature of some of the tasks and groups. The program is then geared toward more hands-on tasks that are more easily seen as relevant to their actual work. Additionally, a modified program (with limited therapies and an accelerated return to work via a supervised work trial) may be considered appropriate for patients with mild or very circumscribed deficits. Finally, when a patient is suffering from a severe case of unawareness and is threatening to leave the program precipitously, an earlier return to work will be allowed despite strong staff misgivings. This is done in the belief that it is better for the patient to be involved at work with some staff involvement than to return independently without support. As a result, staff members can then assist with developing compensations at work and can provide a buffer with the employer in the event of difficulties. Also, in such cases the patient remains in the program, if only on a part-time basis, to continue to work on improving awareness of deficits. Finally, it is important to maintain ties to the program in the event of job failure, since the patient will then be in even greater need of assistance than before.

Role of Psychiatric Consultation

As the ADHNR has evolved, a consultant psychiatrist also has become progressively more involved in patient care. Although only a single psychiatrist has worked with the program over the past 10 years, his role has expanded over time. Over the last several years, the psychiatrist has begun attending staff meetings on a monthly basis to discuss patients' psychiatric status and assist the staff with their empathic understanding and treatment of the patients. Given the complex interplay between preexisting psychiatric disturbance, neuropsychological deficits, and patients' emotional reactions to their injuries, the psychiatrist's invaluable input has improved the staff's understanding of the patients' overall emotional status. He prescribes psychotropic medications when appropriate for patients experiencing significant depression and temper control problems. The psychiatrist has assisted in helping all the staff to be more alert to issues of suicidality (Klonoff & Lage, 1995). At times when patients have become dangerous to themselves or others, he has helped find more appropriate treatment environments (e.g., inpatient psychiatric hospitalization). The psychiatrist also facilitates discussion within the staff meetings on how the staff is reacting to and coping with the demands of their work. This has become particularly valuable as the treatment milieu has expanded to include terminally ill brain tumor patients.

Additionally, the psychiatrist is available on a consultant basis to meet with the neuropsychologists to review important psychological constructs and treatment approaches. As a direct result, psychotherapy services have benefitted from his insights into narcissistic injury (Klonoff & Lage, 1991), depression, and suicide.

Documentation

The documentation process for patients at the ADHNR reflects the overall philosophy of the program. An initial program summary is compiled by program staff after the patient has completed a 2-week evaluation. This report is generally reviewed in detail with the patient and family members. Often this is the first opportunity the patient and family have had to see injury-related deficits in writing. The process is approached therapeutically in that an attempt is made to begin to increase the patient's and family's level of awareness, but not to overwhelm or discourage them from continuing the rehabilitation process. Usually the treating neuropsychologist is involved in the presentation of the initial program summary, so that any emotional reactions can be addressed quickly. Follow-up reports are prepared on a monthly basis and again a draft of the report is reviewed with the patient and family.

As the program has evolved, there have been some modifications and additions to the documentation process. First, we added a section in 1992 for Working Alliance ratings. For each report, ratings are reported that reflect the staff's rating of the working alliance with the patient and family. We also obtain and report the patient's and family's ratings. (For an explanation of how ratings are derived, see the "Research" section below). Reporting the working alliance from the points of view of the staff, patient, and family enables ongoing dialogue about how the rehabilitation process is unfolding and holds all parties accountable for their level of communication and engagement. Additionally, patients and families have an opportunity with each report to document their impressions of the rehabilitation process and their feedback about the report.

Very recently, we have modified the report review process for selected patients. Some patients have significant cognitive or language deficits and are in the very acute phase of their recovery at the time of program admission. If it is the team consensus (usually with input from the consultant psychiatrist) that full review of the reports would be counterproductive, we review the summary section of the report only, which focuses primarily on the intended therapies and goals. This recommendation is discussed with the patient and they are aware that a summary of the report is being presented to them. With their permission, and if appropriate, the full report is reviewed with the family. It is not uncommon for the report to be reviewed in more detail with the patient as the rehabilitation and recovery process unfolds.

After Care Programs

Within the last 5 years, there have been increasing requests from former patients for some type of assistance after formal discharge from ADHNR. This postprogram treatment is provided in several ways. First, a number of patients continue with individual psychotherapy services, often for several months. At times, it is not until months or even years after discharge that patients begin such individual or family therapy sessions. Additionally, an After Care Support Group for patients who had completed the program was initiated in September 1994. This group consisted of a core of five to eight individuals who attended the twice-monthly meetings on a regular basis. Meetings were held after work hours in the late afternoon, since many of the members were involved in gainful or volunteer positions. The sessions were facilitated by the two senior staff neuropsychologists and usually divided into two parts. The first portion of the session was spent with each group member providing an update about events in his or her life during the previous 2 weeks and the remaining time was used to discuss topics of common interest. These topics were either generated by the members in relation to issues they were dealing with at the time, or if there was no particular need among the members, one of the neuropsychologists would provide a topic for discussion. Examples of topics include depression after traumatic brain injury, relationships with family, whether and how to discuss their brain injury with others, avoiding burnout of supervisors and/or spouses. To help with recall and facilitate behavioral change, the minutes of each meeting were summarized (using members' initials to protect confidentiality) and provided at the following meeting.

This initial group lasted just over 2 years, ending in October 1996. This occurred when several of the core group decided they were functioning well enough to continue without the additional support of the group. Of interest, a majority of this initial core group returned when the After Care Support Group was resumed approximately 1 year later. Again, this was due to a demand for such a service by former patients. The structure of these sessions is basically unchanged from the earlier group, except there is a greater emphasis on members developing a specific plan of action to address the particular concern at issue for them at the time. Also, for the first time there was sufficient interest so that an After Care Support Group for the relatives of patients has been created. This group meets monthly and generally consists of spouses of former patients, although parents and friends have also attended. The fact that a substantial portion of patients continue with individual psychotherapy and/or the After Care Support Group for patients and families clearly points to the need to address long-term adjustment concerns of people with brain injuries.

ADHNR Research

Comprehensive, integrated outpatient day treatment programs such as the ADHNR are not only an intensive, demanding process for the staff and patients involved, but they represent a considerably greater expense than traditional outpatient approaches. While this can be justified to some extent by examining the overall costs of acquired brain injury to society as a whole (Klonoff, Shepherd, & Lamb, 1994), it must first be demonstrated that such programs are actually effective in improving the productivity of participating patients. Empirical evidence is necessary in establishing the need for such multidisciplinary day treatment programs in the continuum of care for neurological patients. The following section will outline: (1) the first major outcome study at the ADHNR, (2) a recently published extended replication examining other etiological groups, as well as the effects of injury severity, and (3) a current long-term follow-up study designed to evaluate program efficacy in improving and maintaining productivity status of patients 3 months to 11 years postprogram discharge.

Productivity, Working Alliance, and Work Trials in TBI Patients

In an effort to produce more methodologically sound research in the neurorehabilitation arena, Prigatano *et al.* (1994) used a historical control group within their outcome study of milieu-based rehabilitation. This was accomplished by comparing the productivity status of 38 patients who had completed the ADHNR program with 38 patients who were provided services in the same hospital prior to the initiation of the ADHNR. Only TBI patients were included in the design, first because they comprised the majority of rehabilitation patients at the ADHNR, and second to minimize variance due to etiologic differences.

In addition to predicting a higher incidence of productivity in patients who completed rehabilitation, the authors also examined the effect of working alliance and completion of a supervised work trial on outcome. More specifically, they hypothesized that productivity rates would be greater among ADHNR Work Reentry participants who had (1) either "excellent" or "good" working alliance ratings (as opposed to "fair" and "poor"), (2) family working alliance ratings of "excellent" or "good," and (3) successfully completed a supported work trial experience.

Treated patients were matched with control patients for gender, age at injury, and Glasgow Coma Scale score. Although years of education and chronicity of injury between the groups were not equivalent, these variables were taken into consideration during analysis of the results. When asked "What best describes what the patient was doing most of the last week," 62.9% of the treated patients were gainfully employed on a full- or part-time basis, as contrasted with 47.2% of the control patients. If school is classified as productive, the difference in the combined totals (86.8% vs. 55.3%) was statistically significant. Of particular interest was the finding that while only one treated patient (2.9%) was considered by the respondent to be unable to work, 36.1% of the historical controls fell in this category.

This study also demonstrated the clinical utility of staff working alliance ratings. When grouping treated patients with "excellent" or "good" working alliance ratings versus those rated as "fair" and "poor," there was a significantly greater number of productive patients with positive ratings. Likewise, a similar comparison based on working alliance ratings of family members proved statistically significant, with better ratings being associated with a productive outcome. The final hypothesis approached significance ($P < .07$), providing some support for the idea that successful completion of a protected work trial contributes to better outcome relative to productivity status.

Outcome Adjusted for Injury Severity in Patients of Mixed Etiology

A second research study involving ADHNR patients incorporated functional impairment ratings at program admission into measures of rehabilitation outcome (Klonoff, Lamb, Henderson, and Shepherd, 1998). This study examined consecutive ADHNR admissions from March 1992 to May 1996, and included 64 patients with heterogeneous brain injury etiologies. A unique feature of this study was the utilization of an Adjusted Outcome score, which was defined as level of discharge productivity adjusted by staff ratings of functional severity of injury at program admission. The intent of the Adjusted Outcome measure was to provide an indication of the patients' outcome *relative to* their level of functional severity at program admission. Thus, if a patient exceeded outcome expectation based on the functional severity of his or her injury, a positive Adjusted Outcome score would be seen. At discharge, 89.5% of patients showed a fair or good Adjusted Outcome, with 62% being gainfully employed or full-time students and 15.6% having resumed preinjury job status. When full- or part-time volunteer work is included, 82.8% of the patients in this sample were productive at discharge.

This study also examined the relationship of "process variables" to rehabilitation outcomes. Such process variables included a Work Readiness rating, which was defined as the patients' ability to return to preinjury level of work/school (without modification) or, if they were not working at the time of their injury, to hold a minimum wage job. A second process variable was a Work Eagerness scale, which dealt more with patients' attitude and attempted to define patients' level of motivation for returning to work or school. Each staff member independently rated each patient on the Work Readiness and Work Eagerness scales and mean data were utilized for data analyses. Finally, ratings of the working alliance between staff and patients were again examined as they related to patient outcomes.

Results of this study found that staff ratings of the patients' work eagerness related to level of outcome at the time of program discharge, with lower motivation associated with less productivity at the time of discharge. Also, reduced motivation to work was more often found in those patients actively seeking compensation. This finding suggests that staff members' clinical impression of the quality of the patients' motivation to work is an important factor in patients' level of benefit from milieu-oriented rehabilitation and ultimate level of work–school attainment. Additionally, as seen in the previous study, a better working alliance between patient and staff predicted better adjusted outcome. These data suggest that therapists who do not incorporate a "holistic" approach to patient treatment may overlook important attitudinal variables, which may predispose patients to an unsuccessful outcome regarding work and school reentry.

Long-Term Productivity Status

Currently, information is being collected from former ADHNR patients at varying postdischarge intervals. Research staff attempts to call patients within 2 weeks of the postdischarge intervals of 3 months, 1 year, and then every 2 years after that time (e.g., 3 years, 5 years, etc.) up until 11 years postdischarge. The purpose of this study is to determine the long-term productivity of patients who have undergone treatment at the ADHNR. Specifically, the study aims to determine how many patients are still working long-term after discharge and how former patients are functioning in their everyday life. This is accomplished by way of a survey that takes approximately 5 minutes to complete. The survey asks questions regarding work or volunteer activities since discharge, modifications to the job from preinjury status if it is the same job as preinjury, ratings of difficulties in areas of work/everyday life since injury (e.g., interpersonal, emotional, or job task difficulties), involvement in additional rehabilitative therapies since discharge, and additional questions about activities of daily living and current use of compensations. Attempts are made to obtain similar information from family members in an effort to provide data about the accuracy and validity of the former patients' responses. Currently, data have been collected for 164 patients representing approximately 74% of total eligible past Work Reentry program patients. Of this total sample, 83.5% were productive in some capacity up to 11 years post-discharge; 67% were in paid employment or school, and 12.2% were volunteers (Klonoff, Lamb & Henderson, 1998).

Future Directions

The ADHNR has now been in operation for 13 years (1986–1999). The staff continues to build on available clinical and research knowledge in an effort to refine the holistic approach to treatment of neurological insult. We are convinced the milieu approach facilitates the patients' level of awareness and acceptance of their injury and assists with their reintegration into the home, community, work, and school environments. We will continue to maintain a strong commitment to the research component of the program, with an emphasis on demonstrating efficacy of services. Research endeavors will not only track long-term outcomes, but will continue to identify and measure important "process" variables reflecting the underlying constructs of therapy, such as working alliance and motivation to work.

References

Ben-Yishay, Y., & Diller, L. (1993). Cognitive remediation in traumatic brain injury: Update and issues. *Archives of Physical Medicine and Rehabilitation, 74,* 204–213.

Ben-Yishay, Y., & Prigatano, G. P. (1990). Cognitive remediation. In M. Rosenthal, E. R. Griffith, M. R. Bond, & J. D. Miller (Eds.), *Rehabilitation of the adult and child with traumatic brain injury* (2nd ed., pp. 393–409). Philadelphia: F.A. Davis Press.

Goldstein, K. (1952). The effect of brain damage on the personality. *Psychiatry, 15,* 245–260.

Klonoff, P. S. (1997). Individual and group psychotherapy in milieu oriented rehabilitation. *Applied Neuropsychology, 4,* 107–118.

Klonoff, P. S., & Lage, G. A. (1991). Narcissistic injury after traumatic brain injury. *Journal of Head Trauma Rehabilitation, 6,* 11–21.

Klonoff, P. S., & Lage, G. A. (1995). Suicide in traumatic brain-injured patients: Risk and prevention. *Journal of Head Trauma Rehabilitation, 10,* 16–24.

Klonoff, P. S., O'Brien, K. P., Prigatano, G. P., Chiapello, D. A., & Cunningham, M. (1989). Cognitive retraining after traumatic brain injury and its role in facilitating awareness. *Journal of Head Trauma Rehabilitation, 4,* 37–45.

Klonoff, P. S., Lage, G. A., & Chiapello, D. A. (1993). Varieties of the catastrophic reaction to brain injury: A self-psychology perspective. *Bulletin of the Menninger Clinic, 57,* 227–241.

Klonoff, P. S., Shepherd, J., & Lamb, D. G. (1994). Management of patients with traumatic brain injury. In C. N. Simkins (Ed.), *Analysis, understanding, presentation of cases involving traumatic brain injury* (pp. 107–124). Washington, DC: National Head Injury Foundation.

Klonoff, P. S., Lamb, D. G., Chiapello, D. A., Kime, S. K., Shepherd, J., & Cunningham, M. (1996). Cognitive retraining in a milieu-oriented rehabilitation program. In M. E. Maruish & J. A. Moses (Eds.), *Theoretical foundations of clinical neuropsychology for clinical practitioners* (pp. 219–236). Mahwah, NJ: Lawrence Erlbaum.

Klonoff, P. S., Lamb, D. G., & Henderson, S. W. (1998). Productivity of patients with brain injuries up to 11 years post-discharge from milieu-based rehabilitation [Abstract]. *Archives of Clinical Neuropsychology, 14,* 151–152.

Klonoff, P. S., Lamb, D. G., Henderson, S., & Shepherd, J. (1998). New considerations for assessing outcome after milieu-oriented rehabilitation. *Archives of Physical Medicine and Rehabilitation, 79,* 684–690.

Luria, A. R. (1963). *Restoration of function after brain injury.* NewYork: MacMillan.

Luria, A. R. (1974). *The working brain.* London: Penguin Press.

Prigatano, G. P., Klonoff, P. S., O'Brien, K. P., Altman, I. M., Amin, K., Chiapello, D., Shepherd, J., Cunningham, M., & Mora, M. (1994). Productivity after neuropsychologically oriented milieu rehabilitation. *Journal of Head Trauma Rehabilitation, 9,* 91–102.

Prigatano, G. P., Fordyce, D. J., Zeiner, H. K., Rouche, J. R., Pepping, M., & Wood, B. C. (1986). *Neuropsychological rehabilitation after traumatic brain injury.* Baltimore: Johns Hopkins University Press.

14

Models and Programs of the Center for Neuropsychological Rehabilitation

Fifteen Years Experience

LANCE E. TREXLER, REBECCA EBERLE, AND GIUSEPPE ZAPPALÁ

Introduction

The Center for Neuropsychological Rehabilitation (CNR) is a department of Community Hospitals Indianapolis. It was founded in 1983, and has enjoyed a leadership role in the field of postacute brain injury rehabilitation. It was developed at a time when patients with acquired brain injury received inpatient rehabilitation for sometimes 6 to 12 months, but thereafter were left without resources to facilitate reintegration into their relationships, communities, or place of employment. The program was developed with many of the program structures and characteristics of a holistic neuropsychological rehabilitation program described in Chapter 9, this volume. Several developmental concepts were central to our program and merit further elaboration.

The Primary Therapist Model

CNR was one of the first postacute brain injury rehabilitation programs to employ the concept of the primary therapist within the context of a multidisciplinary team. The relationship between the patient and the primary therapist was conceived as the patient's main alliance with the program. In brief, the main priorities of this relationship are to address: (1) the patient's awareness of their impairments and the impact of the these impairments on functional

LANCE E. TREXLER AND REBECCA EBERLE • Center for Neuropsychological Rehabilitation, Indianapolis, Indiana 46260. GIUSEPPE ZAPPALÁ • Division of Neurology, Garibaldi Hospital, Catania, Italy

International Handbook of Neuropsychological Rehabilitation, edited by Christensen and Uzzell. Kluwer Academic/ Plenum Publishers, New York, 2000.

adaptation and rehabilitation goal setting; (2) the cognitive and executive impairments characteristic of acquired cerebral lesions; (3) the psychological aspects of the patient's experience of the rehabilitation process; and (4) change in the treatment schedule, the focus, and the strategies of rehabilitation on a day-to-day basis. The purpose is to ensure that the services are individualized and responsive to the dynamic changes characteristic of recovery of function.

Impairments of awareness are unique to patients with acquired cerebral lesions, particularly for lesions involving heteromodal association cortex (Mesulam, 1985). For this very fundamental reason, brain injury rehabilitation necessitates unique and specialized neuropsychological interventions not required in rehabilitation for persons with other diagnoses. Unawareness following brain injury is a multifaceted construct (Prigatano & Schacter,1991), composed of psychological and neurological factors, that has a significant impact on the patient's motivation to participate in rehabilitation therapies, as well as to set and participate in rehabilitation goals. Patients who are unaware of their acquired impairments are reluctant to utilize compensatory strategies, and therefore often do not generalize these strategies outside of the clinical rehabilitation environment. First, in the programmatic design of CNR, we thought it essential to provide a therapeutic relationship to consistently address unawareness syndromes that follow acquired cerebral lesions.

The second major factor that was considered in deriving the primary therapist model was the nature of cognitive and executive deficits, which are also unique to brain injury rehabilitation. As mentioned, cognitive (attention, memory, language, and spatial) and executive (initiating, planning, sequencing and organizing, monitoring goal attainment) impairments that follow acquired brain injury impede the patient's utilization and generalization of rehabilitation strategies to target real-world environments. In the design of CNR, we wanted to provide a means to consistently provide rehabilitation strategies to promote generalization for cognitive and executive impairments that by nature were highly specific and unique to each patient. It was thought that these strategies should be developed in individual therapy with the patient, but also provided in group therapies and in interventions outside of the clinic. Therefore, the role of the primary therapist is to facilitate the patient's utilization of these strategies in different settings as well as to communicate the applicability of these strategies to other staff interacting with the patient.

The third factor taken into account in development of the primary therapist model was the psychological aspects of learning and the rehabilitation environment. Rehabilitation is a learning environment, and one must have the cognitive strategies to learn and generalize this learning to applicable, target environments. The patient also must be motivated, which is dependent on an awareness of one's impairments and the relevance of those impairments to one's functional goals. Last, the patient needs the therapeutic alliance with the therapist not only to bring meaning to the rehabilitative tasks, but also to obtain a sense of self-efficacy over his or her rehabilitation gains. In this context, a group of investigators have demonstrated that those patients who perceive themselves as having some control over their own functioning and their response to rehabilitation have better outcomes than those patients who feel that the doctors or therapists are responsible for their recovery (Lubusko, Moore, Stambrook, & Gill, 1994; Moore & Stambrook, 1992, 1995; Moore, Stambrook, & Wilson, 1991). This issue of locus of control, ranging from internal to external, represents usually long-standing beliefs about the extent to which one has control over one's behavior and one's own life. These findings have very important implications for the rehabilitation process. If patients feel that the therapists and doctors are setting goals for them, this encourages an external locus of control. Rather, it is the role of the primary therapist to facilitate the patient's awareness of their impairments and resources and the relevance of those impairments and resources for reaching rehabilitation goals. However, the role of the primary therapist is not to dictate rehabilitation goals, but to facilitate the patient's setting of their own goals. In a study done in part at CNR, Webb and Glueckauf (1994) found that brain-injured patients who were more involved in their own goal setting maintained their rehabilitation gains much longer than patients who were not actively involved in their own goal setting. Similarly, Bergquist and Jacket (1993) differentiate goal *imposition* as compared to goal *development*. They described goal development as involving facilitation, encouragement, and questioning by the therapist, with directive advice kept to a minimum. The role of the primary therapist at CNR provides a relationship through which awareness, self-efficacy, locus of control, and goal setting can be addressed in an individualized and dynamic manner.

The therapeutic alliance between the primary therapist and the patient is concerned not only with goal-setting process and awareness, but it also emphasizes a kind of meaningfulness and relevance to which the patient can relate. Meltzer (1983), who was a psychologist with hypoxic encephalopathy, wrote an article that was very influential on our thinking as we developed the primary therapist concept. In his article, Meltzer describes his experiences in rehabilitation following hypoxic encephalopathy and at the end of the article makes recommendations as a patient to therapists. One of the more interesting recommendations to therapists is as follows: *"Realize that the patient may feel alone and incompetent, and more important than the rehabilitation techniques used is the relationship with you—somebody who is interested and cares" (p. 9).*

The issue of the therapeutic alliance is not unique to rehabilitation, and there is a long history of research in psychotherapy with respect to this issue. In brief, irrespective of the specific type of psychotherapy utilized, many researchers have found that the quality of the therapeutic alliance predicted more improvement (Raue, Goldfried, & Barkham, 1997). A therapeutic alliance was conceived as agreement between the patient and therapist on the task of therapy, the goals of therapy, and the development of a therapeutic bond. Additionally, ratings of the therapeutic alliance provided by the patient are stronger predictors of treatment outcome than the ratings provided by therapists (Hovarth, 1994; Hovarth & Symonds, 1991). While this type of research has not been conducted in rehabilitation, the importance of therapeutic alliance has been emphasized by at least Meltzer (1983) and Bergquist and Jacket (1993). It should be reemphasized, however, that the quality of the therapeutic relationship between patient and primary therapist largely determines the extent to which the patient can find meaning in the rehabilitation interventions.

The Therapeutic Milieu

The impairments of awareness characteristic of brain injury and the emotional reactions that ultimately evolve cannot be addressed only through the interventions of the primary therapist. We thought it important to place the therapeutic alliance in context of a therapeutic milieu designed for the patient with an acquired brain injury. We were also quite influenced by the work of Ben-Yishay (1996; see also Chapter 8, this volume) with respect to the need and structure of the therapeutic milieu. As discussed by Ben-Yishay (1996), a holistic neuropsychological rehabilitation program is not just the sum of program components: remedial interventions for cognitive disorders, psychotherapy, physical therapy, or training for functional skills. Consequently, it is imperative that the staff and patients appreciate the dynamic interaction among these aspects of human functioning. The emotional, cognitive, and interpersonal aspects of adaptation interact and fluctuate on a minute-by-minute and day-by-day basis, and the therapist's task is to capture and understand the very individual dynamics of these interactions as a basis from which to intervene. The concept of the "spiral of deterioration" (also referred to by Wrightson, 1989), was in part based on Kurt Goldstein's (1948) concept of the "catastrophic reaction," characterized by the panic and anxiety associated with the realization that one's own functioning is impaired and the attendant threat to the ego that accompanies this awareness. The spiral of deterioration is presented in Fig. 1. The evolutionary dynamics of the interaction among these factors in large part determines the individual's long-term adaptation following brain injury. Individuals who learn to compensate for their cognitive impairments and who manage to find self-worth, self-efficacy, and value in their ability to function and contribute to the lives of others are able to meaningfully integrate with others, in the context of their families, friends, and perhaps co-workers. On the other hand, brain injury and the associated confrontation of one's own impairments can precipitate a spiral of deterioration characterized by the catastrophic reaction, depression, feelings of inadequacy and shame, and social withdrawal, all serving to ultimately exacerbate neurological-based cognitive impairments. At a minimum, holistic neuropsychological rehabilitation should serve to provide an optimum environment in which the benefits of physiological recovery can manifest. More ideally, holistic neuropsychological rehabilitation enables the brain-injured individual a conscious utilization of spared neurological and psychological resources with which to adapt and find purpose and meaning in their life. With three main components, the therapeutic milieu at CNR was designed to benefit staff and patients.

First and most important, the therapeutic milieu incorporates a culture of shared values and attitudes that promote coping, growth, and openness to feedback. When it functions at its optimum, the therapeutic milieu at CNR provides patients with interpersonal and social support and promotes knowledge that people and their experiences are valued, regardless of their level of functioning or the struggles they may experience in adapting to their environments. For the patients of CNR and their families, it is intended to promote a nondefensive acceptance of acquired impairments and a sense of worth and dignity.

A therapeutic milieu does not exist just for the patients but for the staff as well. The intellectual, professional, and emotional challenges of brain injury rehabilitation necessitate a milieu where staff feel accepted and supported. For example, staff need to feel professionally respected and accepted when they ask questions about brain functions or rehabilitation strate-

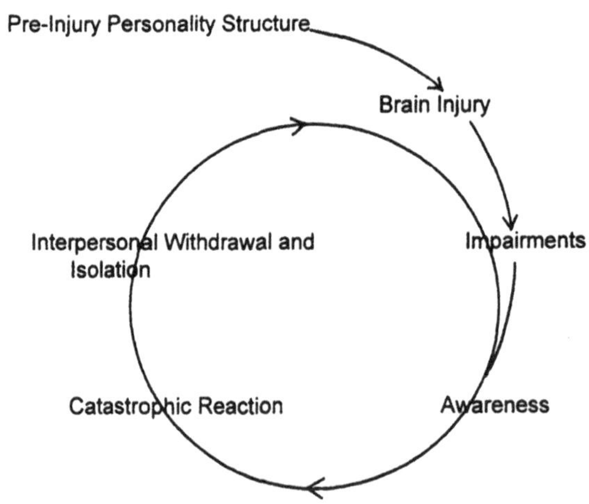

FIGURE 1. Spiral of deterioration.

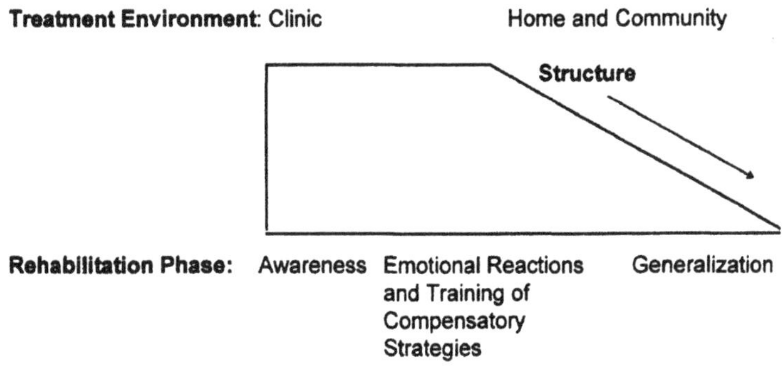

FIGURE 2. Relationship between treatment phases and rehabilitation environment.

gies, reflecting interest and curiosity rather than anxiety about how others may perceive them for not knowing. Additionally, staff need ongoing consultation and feedback regarding the relationship with their patients, their understanding of the rehabilitation process, and their emotional reactions to their patients and the struggles they encounter. Brain injury rehabilitation is a very complex endeavor and no one rehabilitation professional can possess a repertoire sufficient to address the many dimensions characteristic of our patients. The therapeutic milieu provides a social and cultural basis for sharing of knowledge and support that can be received in a nondefensive, open, and stimulating manner.

The second component of the therapeutic milieu at CNR involves group interaction and process. For the patients, this includes the use of a variety of group therapies that are designed to address neurobehavioral and cognitive impairments characteristic of acquired brain injury These impairments sometimes do not manifest in a structured one-on-one context, as in a traditional rehabilitation therapy session. Rather, social and interpersonal situations that are inherently less structured and involve interdependence of multiple people for completion of tasks are particularly disrupted by cognitive and neurobehavioral disorders following brain injury. Obviously, much of our lives are spent in interaction and in cooperation with others, and group therapies for cognitive and neurobehavioral disorders provide a naturalistic context in which to promote adaptation and social integration. For staff, working in a therapeutic milieu means that decisions about each patient's rehabilitation program and the overall rehabilitation program functioning are made as a group, transcending the priorities and biases of each rehabilitation discipline, with a focus on the individual needs of the patient.

The third component of the therapeutic milieu concerns the process of extending the psychological and interpersonal benefits of the therapeutic milieu into the family and into community-based settings. Toward these ends, families are involved from the beginning of holistic neuropsychological rehabilitation, through family education and family therapy. Second, as patients are learning new strategies to compensate for cognitive impairments and are more confident in their ability to manage less-structured situations, individual and group interventions are provided in their homes and in the community. Figure 2 provides an overall model for the stages of rehabilitation and the environmental characteristics in which it is provided. Similar to Ben-Yishay (Chapter 8, this volume), we conceptualized the first stage of rehabilitation as addressing impairments of awareness and establishing rehabilitation goals. The second stage provides psychotherapeutic interventions for the inevitable emotional reactions that follow the emergence of awareness and training of compensatory strategies for cognitive and neurobehavioral impairments. Generalization and integration of compensatory strategies into less structured, target community-based environments are conceptualized as the third phase of the rehabilitation process. In practice, these phases are of course overlapping and continuous, varying as a function of the individual's recovery and progress. CNR has three major programs: the neurobehavioral diagnostic clinics, the day treatment program, and the community employment services.

The Neurobehavioral Diagnostic Clinics

The neurobehavioral diagnostic clinics (NDC) is a 2- to 3-day multidisciplinary evaluation designed to provide a holistic perspective of factors, which determine a person's potential for recovery and response to rehabilitation. These factors include the person's premorbid emotional, educational, and vocational stability, severity of injury, results of neuroimaging studies, neuropsychological and physical status, emotional reactions to the injury, and family structure and support. The NDC includes neuropsychological consultation and testing, evaluation of the family, physical therapy evaluation, occupational therapy evaluation, speech and language therapy evaluation, and, when indicated, vocational evaluation. The findings of the NDC are conceptualized and organized according to the structure of the modified National Center for Medical Rehabilitation and Research (NCMRR, 1993) model (as presented in Table 2 in Chapter 9, this volume) to facilitate communications among rehabilitation team members and establish an individualized diagnosis-based rehabilitation plan. All staff involved in the NDC evaluation meet to integrate findings in an NDC staffing, led by the neuropsychologist. The neuropsychologist then holds a conference with the patient and family to present and discuss the information gathered during the NDC and subsequent recommendations.

The goals of the NDC vary from patient to patient so as to address various referral questions and individual differences in the clinical presentation of the patient. However, several categories of goals of the NDC can be discussed.

Neuropsychological Diagnosis

There are three levels of neuropsychological diagnosis provided through the NDC. The first level concerns the etiology of the impairments. For example, a decline in memory functioning may be caused by a neurological injury, but may also be attributable to depression, medications, or environmental factors. Obviously, a differential diagnosis is crucial for intervention and rehabilitation planning.

The second level of neuropsychological diagnosis concerns not the etiology of abnormalities in behavior, but rather the analysis of cerebral functions, such as memory, executive functions, or language. Significant individual differences follow from neurological disorders in terms of the presenting behavioral, cognitive, or motor sequelae, and neuropsychological diagnosis is required to determine what functions have been impaired or preserved. Each patient presents with a unique syndrome that must be described quantitatively (i.e., the severity of impairment and the extent of preserved functions) and qualitatively (e.g., the types of strategies that enhance the patient's functioning, the environmental conditions that maximize the impairment, and the types of errors that the patient exhibits) for rehabilitation planning. This second level of neuropsychological diagnosis should provide for each patient a description of the unique constellation of impaired and preserved cerebral functions and some indication of the organismic and environmental dynamics that positively and negatively affect his or her functioning.

The third level of diagnosis concerns the identification of variables that may affect the expression of neuropsychological impairments, either positively or negatively. Certainly, psychological factors and certain medications can have a deleterious influence on underlying neurologically based cognitive impairments. Additionally, spontaneous compensatory strategies generated by the patient utilizing spared functions or preexisting strengths can minimize the effects of neurologically based cognitive impairments. Rehabilitation interventions need to eliminate or reduce those factors that negatively impact on the behavioral expression of a lesion and utilize either internal psychological resources or medications that minimize lesion-induced impairments.

Integrating Neuropsychological Diagnosis with Functional Limitations and Disability

The goals of holistic neuropsychological rehabilitation include not only improvements in awareness and psychosocial adaptation, but invariably optimal daily living skills, return to work, and participation in recreational activities or other functions or roles that are important and meaningful to the patient and family. Moreover, neuropsychological diagnosis does not necessarily predict the patient's ability to function at the level of functional limitations or disability. It was therefore thought important to integrate neuropsychological diagnosis with the evaluations of other rehabilitation professionals, specifically physical, occupational, and speech and language therapy. These latter evaluations provide information about the patient's functioning at the level of functional limitations and disability, particularly mobility, activities of daily living, and communication. Evaluations by neuropsychology, vocational specialists, and social workers also provide information regarding family stability and resources, vocational goals and opportunities, the patient's recreational interests, and emotional adjustment. The NDC is a unique process through which data derived from varying levels of human functioning are integrated and conceptualized so as to derive a holistic perspective of each individual. This holistic perspective permits the formulation of a neuropsychological diagnosis and the associations or dissociations with functional limitations and disability. For example, the holistic and integrated assessment provides for determining the extent to which hemispatial neglect affects reading, mobility, self-care, and relevant behaviors required to return to work, as well as the patient's awareness of and emotional reaction to the impairment. Moreover, this perspective provides the basis for determining an overall prognosis for: (1) recovery of functions impaired by the lesion, (2) the extent to which intact functions can be utilized for compensation and adaptation, and (3) what areas of functioning are most likely to respond to rehabilitation efforts. An individualized plan of rehabilitation and appropriate rehabilitation goals can then be established.

Derivation of Individualized Plan of Rehabilitation

The NDC provides a basis for determining an estimated or anticipated plan of rehabilitation to obtain outcome goals usually defined at the level of functional limitations and disability. The plan of rehabilitation is individualized for each patient. The first component of this plan concerns the role of the primary therapist, with specific reference to the intervention strategies for (1) impairments of awareness, (2) impairments of cognitive and executive functions that will effect generalization of learning, and (3) the psychological and personological variables to be considered in establishing a therapeutic alliance. Second, the rehabilitation plan includes a determination of the configuration or mix of required therapies, which includes the different types of individual and group therapies, the intensity of therapy, and an estimate of the duration of rehabilitation therapies. Third, the rehabilitation plan includes some indication of the location in which different interventions may be provided, such as in the home or in a variety of community-based sites. Last, the rehabilitation plan includes an identification of how the patient's family will be involved in the rehabilitation process. This plan is of course tentative and the constellation of rehabilitation interventions changes dynamically according to the course and evolution of the patient's recovery and response to rehabilitation. Nonetheless, the NDC provides a holistic and individualized framework from which to initiate neuropsychologically oriented rehabilitation through a multidisciplinary team of rehabilitation professionals conceptualized and communicated through the modified NCMRR model.

Day Treatment Program

The day treatment program at CNR was designed primarily to promote optimal long-term reintegration within the family and community at large for patients with acquired cerebral injuries, particularly those who present with impairments of awareness or other neurobehavioral disorders and a multiplicity of impairments of cognitive and executive functions. Patients who present with more circumscribed and specific neuropsychological, physical, or sensory impairments who present with intact awareness may not require admission to the day treatment program, and are therefore referred to more traditional outpatient therapies.

Overall Program Structure

The day treatment program offers services up to 5 days a week and operates from 9:00 AM until 3:45 PM each day, except for Wednesdays when clinical services stop at 12:30 to allow for clinical staffings and meetings on Wednesday afternoons. Patients participate in clinical services at varying intensities, ranging in general for 3 days a week to 5 days a week, according to the findings of the NDC.

Approximately 19 professionals comprise the clinical staff of CNR, including four neuropsychologists, three physical therapists, five occupational therapists, three speech therapists, two neuropsychology technicians, one social worker, and one rehabilitation nurse. There are six administrative and support staff at CNR as well. The staff of CNR treat 15–25 patients at any one time, depending on the intensity required and staff schedules. Individual differences at all levels of functioning necessitates that each person's rehabilitation goals and processes be individually derived. For these reasons, we decided not to employ a fixed duration of treatment with all patients starting and stopping treatment at the same time. Patients within this model do not likely experience the same degree of collegiality as patients in a fixed program, but the intensity, duration, and types of individual and group therapies can be provided according to individual needs. The average length of treatment at CNR is approximately 4 months, ranging from 2 to 9 months. Patients with a variety of acquired cerebral lesions are admitted, including traumatic brain injury, stroke, tumor, as well as a variety of diffuse encephalopathies. Chronicity of injury varies widely, ranging from 2 weeks but more commonly from 3 to 6 months; however, some patients come to CNR many years after injury as well. The age of our patients in general ranges from 18 to 65.

Role of the Primary Therapist

The primary therapist at CNR can be any of the rehabilitation professionals working within the day treatment program. The primary therapist will see the patient three to five times a week, depending on the intensity of service the patient is receiving. The conceptual framework for the role of the primary therapist has been previously described, but this role is guided and assisted by the entire rehabilitation team throughout the patient's course of rehabilitation. In addition to providing individual therapies consistent with the role previously described, the primary therapist serves to communicate with the other members of the rehabilitation team who may be treating the patient regarding appropriate rehabilitation strategies to be utilized in the other individual or group therapies, changes in treatment schedule, and day-to-day variations in the patient's functioning according to a variety of environmental, medical, and psychological variables. Additionally, the primary therapist serves as a central point of communication between the program and the family to allow for an exchange of information to promote family integration and generalization of rehabilitation interventions. Finally, the primary therapist is responsible, in concert with the neuropsychologist who leads the NDC through which the patient was admitted, for monitoring progress and goal attainment throughout the course of rehabilitation and facilitates team interaction to modify the treatment schedule as needed.

The determination of which staff member will serve as primary therapist is a multifaceted decision, based on the specific needs of the patient and the particular expertise of individual staff. Consequently, an aphasic patient will likely be assigned a speech and language pathologist as a primary therapist, for example. Additionally, the primary therapist chosen for a particular patient also depends on the overall rehabilitation goal(s) for the patient, such as return to work or school or independence in the home and community. Last, individual preferences and personalities of the primary therapists are considered when assigning a primary therapist to maximize the probability of a meaningful therapeutic alliance forming between the patient and primary therapist.

Group Therapy

Group therapy is an integral dimension of the therapeutic milieu at CNR. Group therapy offers many advantages, including the opportunity (1) to address the effects of cognitive, executive, and neurobehavioral impairments on social interaction and cooperative performance of group activities, particularly in a less structured, more diverse and naturalistic context than individual therapy; (2) to provide modeling, rehearsal, and feedback regarding specific rehabilitation strategies; and (3) to facilitate social and interpersonal support among group members.

CNR maintains a schedule of group therapies offered at any one time in the program. The group schedule is, however, dynamic as a function of the needs of the patient's receiving therapies at any one time and is updated every 3 to 4 months. The program schedule of group therapies includes "core" groups, which are considered necessary and integral components of the program to provide rehabilitation services targeting issues of awareness and the effects of cognitive and executive disorders on psychosocial and interpersonal integration and maintain the therapeutic milieu. These groups and a brief description of the functions they address are provided in Table 1. Other groups may be added and deleted from the program schedule based on the specific needs of the patients in the program at any given time. These groups tend to be impairment focused, and hence are more "discipline specific" and are offered when a critical mass of patients in the program at any one time could benefit from these interventions. These groups are briefly described in Table 2.

Discipline-Specific Therapies

Many patients require specific rehabilitation interventions, such as physical, occupational, and speech and language therapies to augment their overall treatment schedule. Patients may receive individual physical therapy to address impairments in motor or sensory functions

TABLE 1. "Core" Group Therapies

Group name	Description and intensity
Self-awareness	Awareness of impairments and spared functions, emotional reactions, relevance and meaning of short- and long-term rehabilitation goals; 4 hours/week
Self-regulation	Effects of cognitive, executive, and neurobehavioral impairments on social pragmatics and group interaction and process; 4 hours/week
Memory	Compensatory strategies for impairments of memory, utilization of organizational strategies and external mnemonic aids; 3hours/week
Problem-solving	Compensatory strategies for impairments of generating hypotheses and alternatives, anticipating, planning, and organizing for solving real-world problems; 3 hours/week
Independent living skills	Activities of daily living and community reentry skills; 2 hours/week
Language II	Effects of cognitive, executive, and neurobehavioral impairments on communication; 2 hours/week
Residential planning and outing	Planning and organizing for community-based group activities; 4 hours/week
Avocational	Identification of new or resumption of previous avocational/ recreational activities; 2 hours/week

and functional limitations in mobility, for example. Traumatic or vascular aphasic patients receive intensive individual language therapy. Patients often receive individual psychotherapy as well. Patients admitted more acutely to CNR may receive primarily discipline-specific therapies if they are not ready to participate in group therapies. These individual therapies may be supplemented by small discipline-specific groups, depending on the needs of the patient population at any one time.

Community-Based Interventions

A variety of group and individual therapies are provided outside of the clinical environment, consistent with the model presented in Fig. 2. These interventions are typically provided toward the latter phases of rehabilitation to promote generalization of compensatory strategies in the home and community. The rehabilitation goal identified by patients and families for participation in the program is generally successful reintegration into preinjury roles or environments. While clinic-based interventions can assist the patient with gaining awareness and identifying and learning appropriate strategies, the presence of neuropsychological impairments necessitates interventions in the community.

Rehabilitation therapists may address the communication abilities of aphasic patients in the community or the extent to which a patient with neglect can go grocery shopping. Community-based group activities may address neurobehavioral and executive impairments in planning and organizing outings to a local park or restaurant. CNR also has apartments located near the clinical facility and residential services at this site to allow for the rehabilitation of in-

TABLE 2. "Discipline-Specific" Group Therapies

Group name	Description and intensity
Orientation	Orientation to one's own injury history, current events, and utilization of personal orientation and memory aides, review of goals and progress; 4–5 hours/week
Visuospatial	Compensatory strategies for neglect, visual field defects, and impairments of visual perception; 2 hours/week
Dysarthria	Impairments of motor speech, utilization of motor speech strategies for functional communication; 3 hours/week
Language I	Impairments of receptive and expressive language, utilization of language strategies for functional communication; 3 hours/week
Exercise	Community-based group for strength, endurance, and exercise, facilitate patient participation in wellness and physical health; 2 hours/week

dependent living skills. Community-based interventions often continue after the patient has been discharged from clinically based rehabilitation therapies.

Individual Program Management

The patient's individual treatment program should reflect the dynamic changes characteristic of the recovery and rehabilitation process. Changes in medical status, psychological reactions, recovery of function, the family, or the environment all potentially contribute to or impede the rehabilitation process. To monitor and respond to these changes, CNR employs a variety of strategies to manage the individual's rehabilitation program. First, the primary therapist monitors progress and day-to-day fluctuations in the patient's functioning, and communicates with other relevant CNR staff as needed to adjust specific rehabilitation strategies or schedules. Second, monthly neuropsychology conferences, which are attended by the patient and family, the primary therapist, and the admitting neuropsychologist, serve to monitor overall progress and the extent to which short- and long-term rehabilitation goals are met. Third, the primary therapist and the admitting neuropsychologist conduct a staffing twice a month to obtain a comprehensive and detailed perspective of the patient's progress and need for changes in treatment schedule, location of services, need for family involvement, and readiness for discharge, among a host of other issues.

Family Involvement

Reintegration with the family and significant others is obviously an important dimension of holistic neuropsychological rehabilitation. CNR employs a variety of methods to involve the family in the rehabilitation process and outcome.

At admission, the primary therapist will establish a consistent and routine plan for communication with the family regarding the patient's goals, progress, and status in the program. This plan may include the frequency of contact and the type of information to be communicated. Some families desire weekly contact, while others only desire occasional contact. In general, it is best to "overcommunicate" and allow the families to indicate when to cut back. In some situations, weekly contact may be necessary to assure that goals and strategies are being appropriately generalized and the patient is consistently receiving the support and feedback that they require in their nontherapeutic environments. For example, if a patient has specific strategies identified regarding the use of his personal memory book–organizer, it may be necessary to routinely follow up with the family member for feedback regarding the success of these strategies in the home environment.

CNR also provides for a family education day once a month. Again, the specific contents of family education day varies as a function of the needs of the patients and their families who are receiving services at that time, but generally includes: (1) presentations by staff or visiting professionals on topics such as recovery of function and memory disorders, among others; (2) participation in individual and group sessions with the patient; (3) time with the primary therapist and family member to meet and discuss goals, progress, and specific issues as required; (4) family discussion and support group; and (5) lunch planned and prepared by the patients. Additionally, family education day usually includes a patient–family panel discussion. Three graduated patients and their family members, when able, are invited to return to CNR as a panel and share their experiences. The past patient is requested to prepare a short presentation of their injury, rehabilitation, and current activities and also share specific strategies–experiences they found helpful and useful. The clinical staff facilitates the panel, asking questions and encouraging discussion. Issues that may be specifically interesting to the patients currently in the program may be purposefully targeted. The presence of the family member also facilitates family participation and discussion. Not only is this panel highly valued by current patients, but those who return to share their story find participation on the panel to be a rewarding and therapeutic experience for them as well.

Professional Issues

CNR has maintained and developed its program integrity over its 15-year history and enjoyed an international reputation largely through adherence to well-established professional standards as well as through the support of Community Hospitals Indianapolis and the quality of all the staff. Discussion of all the professional issues that serve and affect the program go beyond the scope of the present chapter, but some of the more fundamental issues follow.

The Primary Therapist

Not all rehabilitation professionals want or are able to cope with the professional and emotional demands of the primary therapist model. Therefore, staff must be selected based on many personal and professional characteristics, including flexibility; ability to communicate and form meaningful therapeutic alliances; a certain curiosity to broaden one's professional repertoire as a function of each patient's needs; and the ability to ask for consultation, collaboration, and peer review, while still maintaining self-confidence in the multiple professional interactions that this model necessitates. This model, however, permits the therapist to directly address the patient's experience of their altered functioning, while remaining focused on the important neuropsychological and emotional issues in a professionally rewarding, holistic relationship. Because of the multiplicity of roles and functions inherent in the primary therapist model, at CNR all the therapists are referred to as a "rehabilitation therapist," rather than referring to staff based on their professional discipline. As such, CNR does not have a department of physical therapy or neuropsychology, for example. Moreover, this model necessitates a patient focus rather than on a discipline focus. In this way, the program and the functions of the staff are organized around the needs of the patient population served rather than around the discipline of the rehabilitation professional.

The Rehabilitation Team and the Therapeutic Milieu

The working relationships among the rehabilitation team are one of the most critical components of a holistic program. As previously discussed, the therapeutic milieu exists at CNR to serve the staff of CNR as well as the patients. The extent of team interaction and communication necessitates working relationships that are served by the values of the working culture, emphasizing a sense of value, acceptance, and support for the individual staff members. A culture with these values promotes professional growth and openness to feedback. In this context, one of the primary goals of the team is to care for and attend to the general health of the team, as a whole. Brain injury rehabilitation is a complex endeavor, professionally and intellectually, emotionally and existentially. The therapeutic milieu and the rehabilitation team at CNR function in a manner that supports these staff challenges. Toward these ends, CNR conducts a team meeting each week to focus on the team, the quality of our functioning, and the needs of the team and its constituent members. It is our belief that the best way to provide high-quality clinical care is to have professionally satisfied and highly skilled and trained staff who feel valued and well supported.

Education and Training

To maintain and advance the repertoire of clinical staff, CNR employs a variety of educational strategies. First, staff are encouraged and supported to develop specific areas of expertise that are of interest to them, whether this concerns memory disorders, hemispatial neglect, or executive disorders. Biweekly to monthly inservices address issues ranging from psychological reactions of staff to driving evaluations and are scheduled for all staff. As needed, staff frequently cotreat patients or colead groups to acquire new knowledge about treatment methodology, especially for new staff. Last, CNR provides training for physicians, neuropsychologists, and rehabilitation therapists from a variety of local universities, and frequently has visiting trainees from the United States or abroad, all serving to stimulate a culture of growth, stimulation, and professional development.

The Community Employment Services

The community employment services (CES) program at CNR is designed to enable the brain-injured patient to obtain and retain gainful employment. For patients who are able to be employed in either their previous job or in a new job with limited vocational intervention through the day treatment program, the CES program is not necessary. However, the CES program provides vocational services to patients who either by virtue of the severity of injury or lost opportunity will require extended vocational supports and the expertise of vocational specialists. CES services are often provided in concert with the involvement of the state vocational rehabilitation department. The CES program at CNR has various vocational services that are provided as a function of individual need.

Vocational assessment is provided through CES, and the general areas of assessment include but are not limited to: (1) review of patient and family goals and expectations; (2)

motivators and disincentives for employment; (3) vocational and educational history; (4) physical and neuropsychological status; (5) financial status, support, and benefits; (6) employment contacts; (7) substance use–abuse, or history thereof; (8) systems of support, including significant others, family, and friends; and (9) daily living abilities, including independence with daily routine, time management, community reentry, and transportation, among others. Given the results of this assessment, the parties involved (the patient, significant others, state vocational counselor, and CES assessment team) will determine needed CES services.

Based on the vocational assessment, career counseling is often required to assist the patient in the development of an individualized vocational plan. The patient will often require counseling to assist with the identification of short- and long-term career goals. These goals must reflect the meeting of the patient's abilities, desires, and limitations and the current labor market. Salary and benefit expectations also must be explored and formulated. The patient may be placed in a volunteer community-based situational assessment or may choose to participate in job shadowing. These opportunities provide an assessment of the patient's skills and strengths in a particular environment and allows the patient to gain knowledge of different job requirements and to explore vocational options.

Once a vocational plan has been developed, which identifies a specific competitive or noncompetitive job, vocational services prepare the patient for work reentry. Some patients require job search skills training, which serves to enhance verbal and written presentation skills, such as preparing a resume, practicing filling out job applications, or role-playing through a mock interview. Specific compensatory strategies can be introduced and practiced that will provide for higher success with ultimate job placement.

The CES program also offers job development and placement services. In this phase, the patient actively pursues employment by applying and interviewing for existing and unfilled positions in the community. Once hired, the patient and therapist integrate and apply necessary compensatory strategies to assist the patient in functioning in the vocational environment. The vocational specialist may recommend work site accommodations to allow the patient to meet employer performance standards, through the job development and placement phase. With the support of the CES staff, the patient learns the various components of the job to an extent that they become productive and independent.

For patients requiring more structure and vocational training, job-coaching services maybe recommended. Job-coaching services supplement the employers existing new employee orientation and training programs and assist the employee to implement compensatory strategies in the work environment and monitor progress and provide support as needed. The job coach should provide education to employers about the employee's strengths, skills, and special needs. Additionally, they should facilitate the work relationship by helping the supervisor feel comfortable in providing positive feedback and constructive criticism. Initially, the job coach will spend a considerable amount of time at the work site with the patient. As the patient's independence, accuracy, and feelings of confidence increase, the job coach begins to reduce the number of hours at the job site. Job-coaching intensity is individualized to each patient and the particular placement. Some patients may require intensive job coaching for an extended period of time, while other placements may have job coaching fading within several weeks of the placement. Once the patient requires only minimal job coaching and/or supportive services, only occasional monitoring occurs, and the patient transitions into a follow-along status. Follow-along services can be provided throughout the duration of employment. Generally, the job coach will have contact with the patient, family, and/or employer on a monthly basis for approximately 3 months. When the patient no longer requires monthly contacts, the patient will be discharged, with contacts made at another 3 months and 12 months postdischarge. Should the patient's status change, such as an increase in responsibilities or a change in supervisor, and require increasing amounts of monitoring or assistance, the patient can be readmitted into the program.

The ultimate goal of the CES program is to assist patients with acquired cerebral injuries to attain and retain competitive employment in a placement they find best meets their needs, skills, and interests.

References

Ben-Yishay, Y. (1996). Reflections on the evolution of the therapeutic milieu concept. *Neuropsychological Rehabilitation, 6,* 327–343.

Berquist, T. F., & Jacket, M. P. (1993). Awareness and goal setting with traumatically brain injured. *Brain Injury, 1993, 7,*275–282.

Goldstein, K. (1948). *Aftereffects of brain injury in war.* New York: Grune.

Hovarth, A. O. (1994). Research on the alliance. In A. O. Hovarth & L. S. Greenberg (Eds.), *The working alliance: Theory, research, and practice* (pp. 259–286). New York: Wiley.

Hovarth, A. O., & Symonds, B.D. (1991). Relation between working alliance and outcome in psychotherapy: A meta-analysis. *Journal of Counseling Psychology, 38,* 139–149.

Lubusko, A. A., Moore, A. D., Stambrook, M., & Gill, D. D. (1994). Cognitive beliefs following severe traumatic brain injury: Association with postinjury employment status. *Brain Injury, 8,* 65–70.

Mesulam, M.-M. (1985). *Principles of behavioral meurology.* Philadelphia: F. A. Davis.

Meltzer, M. L. (1983). Poor memory: A case report. *Journal of Clinical Psychology, 39,* 3–10.

Moore, A. D., & Stambrook, M. (1992). Coping strategies and locus of control following traumatic brain injury: Relationship to long-term outcome. *Brain Injury, 6,* 89–94.

Moore, A. D., & Stambrook, M. (1995). Cognitive moderators of outcome following traumatic brain injury: A conceptual model and implications for rehabilitation. *Brain Injury, 9,* 109–130.

Moore, A. D., Stambrook, M., & Wilson, K. G. (1991). Cognitive moderators in adjustment to chronic illness: Locus of control beliefs following traumatic brain injury. *Neuropsychological Rehabilitation, 1,* 185–198.

National Center for Medical Rehabilitation Research (NCMRR). (1993). *Research plan for the National Center for Medical Rehabilitation Research.* NIH Publication No. 93-3509. Washington. US Department of Health and Human Services, National Institutes of Health.

Prigatano, G.P., & Schacter, D.L. (1991). *Awareness of deficit after brain injury.* New York: Oxford University Press.

Raue, P. J., Goldfried, M. R., & Barkham, M. (1997). The therapeutic alliance in psychodynamic–interpersonal and cognitive–behavioral therapy. *Journal of Consulting and Clinical Psychology, 65,* 582–587.

Webb, P. M., & Glueckauf, R. L. (1994). The effects of direct involvement in goal setting on rehabilitation outcome for persons with traumatic brain injuries. *Rehabilitation Psychology, 39,* 179–189.

Wrightson, P. (1989). Management of disability and rehabilitation services after mild head injury. In H. S. Levin, H. M. Eisenberg, & A. L. Benton (Eds.), *Mild head injury* (pp. 245–256). New York: Oxford University Press.

15

The Oliver Zangwill Center for Neuropsychological Rehabilitation

A Partnership between Health Care and Rehabilitation Research

BARBARA A. WILSON, JONATHAN EVANS, SUE BRENTNALL, SHEILA BREMNER, CLARE KEOHANE, AND HUW WILLIAMS

Background and Introduction

The Oliver Zangwill Center (OZC) for Neuropsychological Rehabilitation officially opened in November 1996, following 3 years of negotiations between Lifespan Healthcare National Health Service (NHS) Trust, the Medical Research Council, and Anglia & Oxford Health Authority Research and Development Initiative. The center was named after Oliver Zangwill, Professor of Psychology at the University of Cambridge between 1954 and 1984, and a pioneer of brain injury rehabilitation in the 1940s, when he worked in Edinburgh helping soldiers wounded in World War II (Zangwill, 1947). The program is modeled on the work of the Adult Day Hospital for Neurological Rehabilitation in Phoenix, Arizona, which in turn grew out of an earlier program based in Oklahoma City (Prigatano *et al.*, 1986). Prigatano's program was heavily influenced by Ben-Yishay (1978) and adopted a holistic approach. Christensen opened a similar center in Copenhagen in 1985 (Christensen & Teasdale, 1995). The OZC follows many of the principles laid down by Ben-Yishay, Prigatano, and Christensen, although it probably has a stronger commitment to research than the centers established earlier.

BARBARA A. WILSON • MRC Cognition and Brain Sciences Unit, Addenbrooke's Hospital, Cambridge CB2 2QQ, and the Oliver Zangwill Center, The Princess of Wales Hospital, Ely, Cambs CB6 1DN, United Kingdom. **JONATHAN EVANS, SUE BRENTNALL, SHEILA BREMNER, CLARE KEOHANE, AND HUW WILLIAMS** • The Oliver Zangwill Center, The Princess of Wales Hospital, Ely, Cambs CB6 1DN, United Kingdom.

International Handbook of Neuropsychological Rehabilitation, edited by Christensen and Uzzell.
Kluwer Academic/ Plenum Publishers, New York, 2000.

Unfortunately, Oliver Zangwill died in 1987, but his widow, Shirley Zangwill, is alive and well. She was delighted to hear that the center was to be named after her late husband, came to the official opening, and hosted our first birthday party in November 1997.

A holistic approach brain injury rehabilitation "... consists of well integrated interventions that exceed in scope, as well as in kind, those highly specific and circumscribed interventions which are usually subsumed under the term 'cognitive remediation'" (Ben-Yishay & Prigatano, 1990, p. 400). Proponents of the holistic approach regard it as futile to separate the cognitive, psychiatric, and functional from the affective sequelae of brain injury (Ben-Yishay et al., 1985). Ben-Yishay's model follows a hierarchy of stages through which the patient must work in rehabilitation, namely, engagement, awareness, mastery, control, acceptance, and identity. Individual and group sessions are provided to enable patients to work through these stages and to help them achieve their optimal levels of functioning.

Prior to our opening we had goodwill messages from Anne-Lise Christensen and George Prigatano:

> The establishment of this nonresidential rehabilitation unit in the UK, providing postacute clinical service for people who have sustained a moderate to severe brain injury is an important step forward in the growing recognition of neuropsychological rehabilitation. Our experiences from the last 10 years have shown that the remediation of emotional problems gives the brain-injured person the understanding and insight into his or her problems that enables the person to take full advantage of cognitive training and promotes collaboration efforts and social adaptation. The development of neuropsychological rehabilitation has added to traditional medical and physical rehabilitation and made it possible for the brain-injured person to regain a life in which brain functions are used to the fullest. But the process of finding optimal rehabilitation methods is a continuing one. Therefore, it is particularly commendable that the new center will also have a strong research orientation. My warmest congratulations. (Anne-Lise Christensen, personal communication, Copenhagen, June 1996)
>
> First of all, let me congratulate you and your team for beginning what I am sure will be a successful rehabilitation program. I am delighted to hear that your program will be, in part, based on the model we have in Phoenix as well as the one in Copenhagen. It has been my experience that by focusing on both the cognitive as well as the emotional and motivational deficits of these clients, they make substantially better psychosocial adjustment.... It is clearly an extremely important venture for all countries, including the UK, to address clients in the manner that you seem to be approaching them. (George Prigatano, personal communication, Phoenix, June 1996)

The Mission Statement of the OZC

The mission of the Oliver Zangwill Center for Neuropsychological Rehabilitation is to provide high-quality rehabilitation for the individual cognitive, social, emotional, and physical needs of people with nonprogressive brain injury. We also aim to meet the needs of families of brain-injured people.

Our ultimate aim is to promote the maximum level of: (1)independent functioning in the home and community, and (2) productive work.

In partnership with clients, families, and other services and through our links with the Medical Research Council and the NHS Research and Development Initiative, we seek to apply the latest research findings, evaluate our service and investigate ways to improve neuropsychological rehabilitation.

Objectives of the Neuropsychological Rehabilitation Program at the OZC

1. Clients will be able to demonstrate understanding of their brain injury and its consequences for everyday life.

2. Clients will be able to demonstrate awareness of their individual strengths and weaknesses, relating to the consequences of their brain injury.
3. Clients will be able to demonstrate the ability to utilize strategies in order to compensate for the specific consequences of their brain injury.
4. Clients will be able to demonstrate the ability to monitor their own performance in using compensatory strategies.
5. Clients will be able to demonstrate carryover of objectives one to four from the group and individual settings of the program to their own community settings.
6. Relatives and significant others will be able to demonstrate an understanding of the relationship between brain injury and its consequences for the brain-injured individual and for themselves.
7. Relatives and significant others will be enabled to assist the individual in the use of strategies to compensate for the consequences of brain injury.

The OZC Structure

The Staff Team

The OZC has eight members of staff, three of whom are clinical psychologists who have specialized in neuropsychology, one occupational therapist, one physiotherapist, one speech and language therapist, one rehabilitation assistant (a psychology graduate), and one administrator/secretary. In addition, there is a consultant neurologist and a consultant neuropsychiatrist who attend as required.

The Clients

The OZC accepts up to 12 clients at a time; some of these clients will be on work trials for part of the week or attending college courses. All will have sustained a nonprogressive insult to the brain from one of the following:

1. A traumatic head injury.
2. A cerebral vascular accident.
3. A viral infection of the brain particularly encephalitis.
4. Hypoxic brain damage through, for example, heart attack, respiratory arrest, carbon monoxide poisoning, or anesthetic accident.

The OZC accepts people between the ages of 16 and 65 years of age, with the majority being under 50 years. They are typically at least 6 months postinsult, with some clients having sustained their brain injuries several years earlier.

The OZC Program

Each client has his or her own individual program coordinator (IPC). Any member of the staff team may be required to take on this role. Clients meet their own IPC at the beginning of the program to discuss their goals and ensure the program is coordinated to meet individual needs. The IPC acts as a link person between the client and other team members, relatives, significant others, and other agencies involved in the client's program.

Following referral (approximately half of all referrals are made by health authorities and half by personal injury lawyers), a 1-day preliminary assessment is arranged. The next stage is to offer a detailed 2-week assessment. Usually a member from each of the four main disciplines (psychology, occupational therapy, physiotherapy, and speech and language therapy) will be involved in the assessment. As well as assessing for the need for each discipline, clients are assessed on whether they are likely to benefit from and engage in the program and how they relate to other staff and clients in the center.

During the 2-week assessment, the OZC team begins the formal goal-planning process. The purpose of this system of setting goals and specifying how the goals are to be achieved is to provide a clear direction to each client's rehabilitation program and help individual clients and team members monitor the program. Appropriate goals are identified through discussion with the client and the relatives or significant others. Goals are extended or adjusted as necessary throughout the program. The full rehabilitation program typically lasts about 4 or 5 months. Goals are documented and reviewed weekly. Clients are given copies of the goals set and the progress made to keep in their personal files. Reports are written following (1) the initial 1-day assessment, (2) the 2-week assessment, (3) the intensive phase of the program, and (4) completion of the program. If necessary, additional reports may be required at various stages in the program. Examples of goal planning can be found in the case history of Barry presented later in the chapter.

The clients' day begins at 9:30 AM and finishes at 3:30 PM. Clients and staff are expected to be punctual and, as far as possible, clients are asked to arrange other appointments (for example, dental visits) after 3:30 PM. All clients are given an individual weekly timetable, which is reviewed and changed if necessary each week. An example of a typical timetable can be seen in Table 1.

The program is nonresidential and some patients travel in by train or bus or car each day. Transport is provided to and from the railway station. For others living farther afield, we help arrange accommodation in local bed-and-breakfasts or small hotels. A few patients reside elsewhere in the hospital. Almost all patients who require accommodation during the week return home at the weekends.

Content of the Program

Group Sessions

Cognitive Strategy Group. This group, run on a daily basis, helps clients to be aware of their cognitive problems such as processing speed, memory, attention, language, and visual scanning and how these affect their functioning on a variety of written and verbal tasks. Clients are taught about various compensatory strategies relevant to their needs and are given the opportunity to practice these strategies. They are encouraged to relate the tasks carried out within the cognitive strategy group to everyday activities. All members of the team help run this group.

Understanding Brain Injury Group. This group, run on a daily basis, encourages clients to develop and share their understanding of their own injuries. The group has an educational focus and clients are encouraged to take notes, learn from the handouts provided for them, and regularly review their progress.

Community Meeting. The purpose of this daily 15-minute meeting is to enable clients and staff to meet together to discuss matters of relevance to the smooth running of the program. It may include discussion of general program business or any specific issues that have

TABLE 1. A Typical Weekly Timetable[a]

Time	Monday	Tuesday	Wednesday	Thursday	Friday
9:30 AM to 10:00 AM	Cognitive strategy group	Cognitive strategy group	Cognitive strategy group	Cognitive strategy group	Cognitive strategy group
10:05 AM to 10:40 AM	Problem-solving group	Physiotherapy	Problem-solving group	Physiotherapy	Problem-solving group
10:40 AM to 10:55 AM	Coffee	Coffee	Coffee	Coffee	Coffee
10:55 AM to 11:20 AM	Communication group	Communication group	Communication group	Communiation group	Independent living skills
11:25 AM to 12:00 AM	Psychological support group	Individual psychological support	Psychological support group	Individual psychological support	Psychological support group
12:00 PM to 12: 15 PM	Community meeting group room	Community meeting group room	Community meeting group room	Community meeting group room	Community meet group room
12:15 PM to 1:15 PM	Lunch cm	Lunch cm	Lunch cm	Lunch cm	Lunch cm
1:15 PM to 1:50 PM	Speech and language therapy	Independent living skills	Discovery group	Speech and language therapy	Relatives and carers group
1:55 PM to 2:30 PM	Understanding brain injury group	Understanding brain injury group	Discovery group	Understanding brain injury group	Relatives and carers group
2:30 PM to 2:50 PM	Tea cm	Tea cm	—	Tea cm	Tea cm
2:50 PM to 3:30 PM	Memory group	Memory group	Discovery group	Memory group	Relatives and carers group
3:45 PM to 4:00 PM	Business of the day	Business of the day	Business of the day	Business of the day	Business of the day
4:00 PM to 5:00 PM	Goal planning meeting	Goal planning meeting	Goal planning meeting	Goal planning meeting	Goal planning meeting

[a]The last 2 meetings of the day are only attended by the staff members.
cm = common room

arisen. All clients and staff attend this meeting, which may be chaired by clients or staff members.

Memory Group. This group runs regularly to give clients the opportunity to develop ways of coping with memory problems. Clients learn about memory and how it works and the use of memory aids and techniques to make remembering easier. They learn compensatory strategies and how to use these in everyday life. This group is usually run by a psychologist or an occupational therapist.

Problem-Solving Group. This group helps clients develop their problem-solving abilities. They learn how to identify the process of problem solving and the use of strategies to compensate for difficulties in problem solving. They also learn how to transfer these compensatory strategies to everyday situations. This group is usually run by one of the psychologists.

Psychological Support Group. This group runs on a regular basis and provides clients with an opportunity to discuss emotional issues and draw emotional support from one another. Clients learn skills to overcome emotional difficulties. Examples of specific topics that may be covered are stress management, loss, mood and anger management, and interpersonal relationships. This group is always run by one of the psychologists.

Discovery Group. This group provides clients with the opportunity for social interaction, increased familiarity with community resources, and a chance to practice skills learned during other therapy sessions, particularly memory compensations. Clients are given an active role in planning, organizing, and implementing outings. These activities may include social, physical, cultural, sporting, and recreational activities that emphasize individual clients' strengths and also target areas of difficulty to try to overcome or bypass these. This group is usually run by the speech and language therapist and the occupational therapist.

Independent Living Skills Group. This group helps clients to become more independent in self-care activities (dressing, grooming, etc.) and also helps clients with other activities of daily living, such as money management and getting around the community safely. This group is usually run by the occupational therapist.

Communication Group. This group focuses on clients' communicative strengths and needs. The number of sessions varies according to individual needs. Clients are involved in deciding useful activities that enable them to develop their social communication skills and provide opportunities to practice in group sessions. This group is always run by the speech and language therapist.

Current Affairs and Newsletter Group. Through this group, which runs on a weekly basis, clients are encouraged to identify topical issues that form a basis for discussions. The group focuses on clients' language skills such as abstracting themes as well as summarizing and presenting information concisely to others.

A newsletter relating to events and issues about the unit is produced periodically. Clients may be involved in the production of the newsletter as part of their program. Reporting skills, editing skills, and information gathering skills form part of the focus along with keyboard, planning, and organization skills. This group is usually run by the occupational therapist and speech and language therapist. We say more about the newsletter later.

Relatives and Carers Group. This group runs on a weekly basis and provides education and emotional support to family members or significant others. It also provides an opportunity for feedback from (1) relatives to staff about progress or problems at home and (2) staff to relatives about progress or problems at the center. This group may be run by any member of the team.

Individual Sessions

Speech and Language Sessions. Clients receive individual sessions on any aspect of communication required. The sessions may be used to back up activities begun in the group setting, or as an opportunity to focus on specific communication problems. Individual sessions may continue throughout the program if necessary.

Occupational Therapy. Following a comprehensive assessment and thorough discussion with clients and their family members, the occupational therapist may formulate a treatment program that helps clients to become as independent as possible in as many areas of functional daily living skills as possible. The activities can range from self-care to work-related skills. Depending on clients' needs, therapy sessions can take place within the center, the community, and the home environment.

Physiotherapy. Physiotherapy is provided, where appropriate, as an integral part of clients rehabilitation programs. It can help clients address the following areas:

1. *Mobility.* This includes any difficulties or concerns clients may have about how to get around, both indoors and out in the community.
2. *Movement difficulties.* This refers to any specific movement difficulties that clients may have as a consequence of their brain injury. These may include such things as stiffness, pain, and difficulty with balance.
3. *General Fitness.* This refers to general stamina and exercise tolerance for everyday routines in addition to fitness for chosen leisure pursuits or sport. Here, physiotherapy can help clients address their level of fitness and plan their activities appropriately so that they make the best use of energy and avoid becoming fatigued.

Individual Psychological Support. Individual psychological support is provided, if required. Clients often have difficulties related to the experience of loss, radical change in lifestyle, and chronic frustration resulting from brain injury. They may need specific support to address particular emotional difficulties. If required, clients are offered psychological counseling to overcome depression and anxiety and to develop self-esteem and personal identity.

Other Individual Sessions

If required, additional individual sessions, such as individual memory therapy or social and studying skills, are offered.

Work Trials

During the intensive period of their program, clients are encouraged to think about how they see the future once the program has finished. If work reentry may be an option, a work trial will be arranged by their IPC. Prior to this, clients are encouraged to prepare for their work trial by devising or updating their curriculum vitae and completing a work trial application form (similar in format to a job application form). Once a specific work area has been established, the IPC will make contact with potential employers. If the employer is in agreement, specific goals are set and a contract signed by the client, the employer, and the IPC. Weekly feedback forms are completed separately by the employer and the client and then compared and discussed. The IPC monitors the work trial through regular contact with the employer.

Work trials can be used to assess a client's potential to work and to give clients experience of generalizing strategies developed with the OZC. If necessary, the client can be shadowed by a member of the OZC team in order to identify what skills are needed.

The length of time of work trials vary, depending on the needs of the client. Initially, clients will be engaged in work trials along with their attendance at the OZC; for example, 3 days work trial, 2 wo days at the OZC. At the OZC, clients have the opportunity to discuss any difficulties and to work on skills that need to be developed to make the work trial more successful.

On completion of the work trial a final assessment report is given by the employer to the client. From this, future plans are made regarding work opportunities and if necessary further work trials are arranged.

The Newsletter

Every 3 months the OZC clients produce a newsletter. There are reports of trips made by the discovery group, interviews with personalities, gardening tips, recipes, jokes, puzzles, and other topical items of interest. One personality profile was of Oliver Zangwill from his wife Shirley:

> Profile of Oliver Zangwill by his Wife Shirley Zangwill. On Wednesday, March 26, Alan and Barry interviewed Mrs. Shirley Zangwill:
>
> The name Zangwill comes from Latvia, as Oliver's grandparents lived in Riga. The family came to England in about 1860–1870 and lived in the East End of London.
>
> Oliver's father was a playwright and wrote comedies and tragedies about the Ghettoes. A murder mystery that Oliver's grandfather wrote was made into a silent film.
>
> A street in the East End is actually called Zangwill Road, named after Oliver's father Israel. Oliver's father married a lady called Eader Fartell, whose father was a Physicist and interested in electricity.
>
> Oliver's grandmother was one of the first women doctors who studied in France, purely because this country did not allow women to study in medicine at that time.
>
> Oliver had an older brother, who read chemistry and then went to work in South America. His sister Margaret studied French and then went to stay in Switzerland for some time before returning to the UK where she died 4 to 5 years ago.
>
> Oliver studied in a school in London and achieved his Starred First Degree in Cambridge in 1935. Oliver then went to work in Edinburgh at the Bangar Hospital with people who were brain injured due to war wounds received.
>
> Shirley was Oliver's second wife and they met on a train going to London and 6 years later were married. Oliver and Shirley came to live locally and Oliver worked at Cambridge University. He became the Chair at the age of 39 which was a young age to hold such a post.
>
> Oliver received two Honorary Degrees, one from St. Andrews and the other from Stirling University and he retired in 1984.
>
> Oliver was also very keen on animals and has had a range of animals from cats to monkeys.
>
> Shirley was very highly honored when Barbara telephoned to ask if the center could be named after Oliver. Shirley felt it was a mark of respect to have a unique center named after her husband.
>
> Shirley's main interests now include being involved with the East Anglian branch of Dentistry and she helps them to organize their two meetings a year. Shirley also is a very keen cook and enjoys cooking a wide range of dishes including Indian and Chinese food. Shirley has also been involved in the twinning of Isleham, a local village with a similar village in France. (Alan and Barry)

An account of a visit planned by the discovery group was written for the newsletter by one of our clients following a trip to Swaffham Prior Windmill:

Discovery Group Trip—4th June—Swaffham Prior Windmill

The group this week consisting of John, David, Gary, Sue and Jacqueline decided and organized to go to Swaffham Prior Windmill. John was selected as leader of the group. He also made the necessary phone call to confirm opening hours, costs and book a tour around the windmill. David was selected to be responsible for finances and time keeping. Jacqueline was selected to look into the directions and route needed to get to the windmill and John helped with this.

Friday arrived with very nice weather conditions. We left the center at approximately 1:15 PM and arrived at Swaffham Prior Windmill at 1:45 PM, driven by Sue. It was the same route as we went to Anglesey Abbey two weeks ago, just a bit closer.

Swaffham Prior Windmill is a nice, working windmill. It is scenic to look around and has four wings. We had a tour of the mill by the two owners which was very interesting and informative. As long as you are not afraid of heights and are flexible climbing up the windmill, you can get to see how the windmill works, grinding the corn to make flour. The only other problem would be if you are tall because the ceilings are low. It should be OK if you are under 6 foot!

At the base of the mill is a shop area to look around. It sells the flour the windmill produces. We bought a 1.5 kg packet for the center, costing us just £1.20. We also bought ourselves a postcard of the windmill for just 20 pence. The surprisingly good thing is that there are no admission charges for the windmill. However, as a group we put a donation into the donation pot. The only thing missing was a cafe or refreshment area but you could take your own refreshments or visit a cafe near by.

A very enjoyable trip was had by us all. It is in a suitable location to the center. Everybody fulfilled their tasks well. Sue brought the camera with her to take a picture of us all and John took a picture of the windmill. It was a good cheap trip which is worth considering in the future. (John)

As we have a number of visitors from overseas at the center, we sometimes ask our visitors to contribute to the newsletter. The following is an account from one of our German students:

A Stranger in Ely

When I came here to Ely, as a German psychology student, not used to English language and habits, I did not really know what awaited me. At the first glance the hospital at the very edge of the Fenland isle of Ely seemed to me a bit lost. At least it was not right in the middle of where the action is going on. But soon exactly this fact made my time here so enjoyable. The peacefulness of the place contributes a good deal to the day to day working atmosphere. I spend most of my time here with learning how to use neuropsychological tests mainly in order to assess higher cognitive abilities in patients with brain injuries. And of course I have to thank not only the psychologists who explained the tests to me but also the patients who agreed to let me take part in the test sessions. In addition to that I really enjoyed the work in the various groups, which gave me a good idea how neuropsychological rehab on a high cognitive level can be structured. This has very much to do with the thing I appreciated most in the Oliver Zangwill Center. And this is the interactive work between patients and a team of people of different professions, where the boundaries between the tasks of each person are very flexible. For me that allowed an insight not only into neuropsychologists' work but also into the work of related professions, like occupational therapy. Overall I had a very good time in Ely from the professional as well as from the social perspective for which I want to thank all the people here, professionals as well as patients. (Christian Muller)

Research at the OZC

The OZC represents a partnership between Lifespan Healthcare National Health Service (NHS) Trust, the Medical Research Council (MRC), and the Anglia and Oxford NHS Executive. This partnership fosters not only a high-quality clinical service, but an opportunity to evaluate the effectiveness of rehabilitation on a number of levels. At the most general level, we are evaluating the effectiveness of the service as a whole through collaborating with John

Stilwell, a health economist, who was in charge of the National Traumatic Brain Injury Study funded by the Department of Health.

At a more specific level, we are evaluating several treatment techniques and strategies, including: (1) attention-training strategies in collaboration with Ian Robertson and Tom Manly at the MRC—Applied Psychology Unit; (2) the effectiveness of errorless learning (Baddeley & Wilson, 1994; Wilson, Baddeley, Evans, & Shiel, 1994; Wilson & Evans, 1996) as a teaching method for brain-injured people (in collaboration with Linda Clare, John Hodges, and the late Kristin Breen in Cambridge; and (3) the evaluation of a new paging system (Wilson, Evans, Emslie, & Malinek, 1997a) for memory-impaired people.

In addition, we are developing new assessment procedures and outcome measures to assess response to rehabilitation as well as monitoring each client's progress.

Progress in the First Year

In the first year of operation we saw 60 people for assessment and treatment. We present a case study to illustrate one of the client's programs in greater detail.

Case Study: Barry

When Barry was 27 years old and working as a motorcycle courier, he was involved in a collision with a tractor and fell from his motorcycle. Although the reported length of coma was only 10 minutes, he remained in hospital for 7 days and appeared to have a posttraumatic amnesia of at least 1 month. Four years later he continues to have a retrograde amnesia of at least 8 weeks, as he does not remember the birth of his third child born 8 weeks before the accident.

Following discharge from hospital Barry attended outpatient physiotherapy at a local hospital for 6 weeks. He also attended an outpatient unit where he was seen by a clinical psychologist and an occupational therapist. This was followed by attendance at a sheltered workshop for 2 days a week for several weeks. He then went to horticultural college for a few weeks but, like the sheltered workshop, Barry appeared to be unable to "stick" to this activity.

In 1996, 3 years postinjury, Barry was referred to the OZC for a preliminary assessment of his suitability for our program. This assessment identified (1) problems with initiation, drive, memory, attention, and concentration; (2) difficulty completing any daily living task without prompting; (3) irritability and problems controlling anger; and (4) lack of confidence. Barry was considered suitable for our program of neuropsychological rehabilitation, and in January 1997, was admitted for a 2-week detailed assessment. The detailed assessment identified a number of impairments and disabilities or handicaps, which can be seen in Table 2.

Long-term goals were established following discussions between Barry and the rest of the OZC team. Long term in this context means goals Barry was expected to achieve by the time of his discharge. These goals were:

- Barry will plan and carry out his daily activities independently when at home on his own.
- Barry will attend a voluntary work placement.
- Barry will attend a part-time education course of his choice in the summer term.
- Barry will carry out gardening activities by himself when his wife does not wish to participate.
- Barry will carry out his personal exercise program independently and/or participate in a chosen leisure activity on a weekly basis.

TABLE 2. Summary of Barry's 2-Week Detailed Assessment

Impairments	Disabilities/Handicaps
Verbal and visual memory	Wandering aimlessly around the house; not being able to initiate or maintain any thing
Attention (broad impairment including selective and sustained attention)	Forgetting appointments
Planning	Forgetting child care procedures
Initiation and perseverance	Not answering the telephone
Insight	Not being able to read to the children
Anger control	Not being able to drive
Lack of confidence in communication	Not being able to play sport any more, particularly badminton
Coordination and use of intonation and stress patterns in speech	Not being able to do gardening or DIY because of physical limitations
Painful weak knee	Feeling angry all the time
Reduced exercise tolerance	

- Barry will feel more confident in his ability to communicate effectively, focusing on three main areas: reading to his children, speaking on the telephone, and managing his anger at home.
- Barry will demonstrate the ability to manage day-to-day finances (excluding bills).

An example of how the first goal was achieved can be seen in Table 3.

At the end of March, Barry's wife decided to leave him. We arranged for Barry to stay in Ely during the week and go home at weekends when his wife and children would be away. This arrangement would continue until his wife found alternative accommodation at which point Barry would live at home permanently.

Meanwhile, Barry had found a college place to study plumbing. He attended college 3 days a week and came to the OZC 1 day each week.

As a result of the changed domestic circumstances, Barry's goals were slightly adjusted to cope with the fact that he was now alone at home. Of eight long-term goals set for Barry to achieve at the end of rehabilitation, four were completely achieved and eight partially achieved.

Barry was discharged in June, following liaison between the OZC staff and Barry's local services, to ensure continued monitoring. He has a facilitator who visits him at home to help with his planning and he intends to complete the college course in plumbing.

Barry describes his time at the OZC in the following words:

> I had an accident on my motorbike 4 years ago, which is how I got my head injury. Before my injury, I was a confident, outgoing 27 year old. I was holding down a good job and supporting my family. When I arrived at the Oliver Zangwill Center in January of this year, my life was a bit of a mess. I used to sit at home all day doing nothing. I couldn't organize myself, far less anything in the house or the children and I couldn't remember things I had to do from one day to the next.
>
> During the 5 months I attended the Oliver Zangwill Center, the team developed a rehabilitation program which helped me to learn new ways of coping with my difficulties and to organize my life. My key worker helped to get me on a course at Norwich City College and the psychologist taught me strategies that I could use to compensate for my memory problems. The course has been really helpful and I am putting my new skills to good use in major "Do It Yourself" projects at home. I also damaged my knee in the accident and it was still very painful when I arrived at the center. I'd had to give up playing badminton which was one of my hobbies. The physiotherapist taught me how to strengthen my knee and now I'm playing badminton again and I only get an occasional twinge in my knee. The speech therapist helped me with some communication problems I had, which has helped me to feel much more confident about

TABLE 3. How One of the Long-Term Goals Was Achieved

Short-term goals	Plans of action
Barry will carry out his daily activities independently when he is at home on his own	
Step 1	
Barry will plan and carry out activities on 2 evenings each week consistently by 14.3.97	Barry will have timetabled a planning session early in the week to produce a lan of activity, then to check activity carried out the following day (Clare) Sheila to go to gym with Barry; Barry to make an appointment for gym assessment; use NeuroPage to act as reminder
Step 2	
Barry will plan and carry out domestic activities at the weekend (washing up, cleaning, etc.) With supervision for Easter weekend Using written plan/NeuroPage consistently	Discuss with Barry and his wife who plans the weekend activities (Clare) Discuss/produce a written plan (Sue); Barry will telephone NeuroPage messages required (Barry)
Step 3	
Barry will plan and carry out activities with the children over the weekend	Barry will attend individual and group planning sessions (Jacqueline/Sue) Barry will tie in both activities to produce a plan of activity for the whole weekend (Jacqueline/Sue)

myself and I've made new friends as a result. The occupational therapist taught me how to plan and to organize myself and now I live independently and can look after my three young children when they visit, which is really important to me. Attending the Oliver Zangwill Center has made a big difference to my life and I think the program at the center should be available to more people who have suffered a brain injury.

Is Rehabilitation Effective?

There is no doubt that units like the OZC are sorely needed in the United Kingdom. A report commissioned by the Department of Health (Greenwood & McMillan, 1993) stated that "... the absence of a specialist rehabilitation service for victims of brain injury has been the norm" (p. 250). While the authors of the report regard this situation as "woefully inadequate," there remains the question as to whether rehabilitation, such as that to be offered by the OZC is indeed effective? In fact there is mounting evidence that the answer to this question is "yes": yes economically, yes clinically, and yes in terms of quality of life for brain-injured people.

Is Rehabilitation Economically Effective?

In one American study of 145 brain-injured patients (Cope, Cole, Hall, & Barkan, 1991) the estimated savings in care costs following rehabilitation for severely brain-injured people was over £27,000 per year. A Danish study (Mehlbye & Larsen, 1994) reported that spendings in health and social care for patients attending a nonresidential program were recouped in 5 years. The costs of not rehabilitating brain-injured people are also considerable, given the fact that many are young with a relatively normal life expectancy (Greenwood & McMillan, 1993).

In a review of rehabilitation effectiveness, Cope (1994) believed that postacute rehabilitation programs can produce sufficient savings to justify their support on a cost-benefit basis. He also suggested they could be run even more efficiently in the future.

Is Rehabilitation Clinically Effective?

Numerous studies have shown clinical improvement or reduction in disability and handicap following rehabilitation. One study (Aronow, 1987) showed no difference between a group of brain-injured patients receiving rehabilitation and a control group not receiving rehabilitation. However, the group receiving rehabilitation was more impaired to start with and thus caught up with the others through rehabilitation. Two studies (Fryer & Haffey, 1987; Mills, Nesbeda, Katz, & Alexander, 1992) found that training in real-life activities yielded more positive results than trying to address underlying impairment. Two other studies (Blackerby, 1990; Spivack, Spettell, Ellis, & Ross, 1992) found high levels of treatment delivered in a relatively short time were associated with better outcome. A recent follow-up study of head-injured patients (Shiel, 1999) found those who received rehabilitation were far less likely to show physical aggression than those who did not.

An interesting study from the United States (Rattok *et al.*, 1992) compared different intensity of treatments for three groups of brain-injured patients. All three groups achieved the same success rate in terms of employment at 6-month follow-up. The groups differed, however, in that those who spent most time in cognitive rehabilitation did better on cognitive tasks, those who spent more time on interpersonal skill training did better on tasks involving interpersonal skills and those trained in both improved on both.

Does Rehabilitation Improve Quality of Life?

A British study (Johnson, 1987) found the employment rate of brain-injured people could be tripled following individualized and intensive work reentry programs. Prigatano *et al.* (1986) found that patients undergoing treatment were less emotionally distressed than control group patients. More recently, Prigatano *et al.* (1994) reported greater productivity in those patients undergoing a holistic rehabilitation program.

General Comments

A recent review of recovery of cognitive functioning following nonprogressive brain injury (Wilson, 1998) looks both at natural recovery and at changes in cognitive functioning following intervention or rehabilitation.

There is increasing evidence that rehabilitation can improve cognitive functioning (Katz & Wetz, 1997; Merzenich *et al.*, 1996; Ponsford, 1995; Robertson, in press; Tallal *et al.*, 1996). Rehabilitation programs may work through people to compensate for their difficulties (Wilson & Watson, 1996), or through achieving restoration (or partial restoration) of functioning through plasticity and exercising. Robertson (in press) suggests that repetition may be possible after relatively small lesions, while compensatory processes are more likely to underlie recovery from larger lesions. Kolb (1995) believes language skills show a greater propensity for recovery than other cognitive functions. Attention deficits also may respond to specific training in certain circumstances (Sturm, Willmes, Orgass, & Hartje, 1997), particularly with regard to unilateral neglect (Robertson, Tegnér, Tham, Lo, & Nimmo-Smith, 1995).

There is considerable evidence that teaching the use of compensatory strategies results in improved cognitive functioning (Bergman & Kemmerer, 1991; Evans, Emslie, & Wilson, 1998; Kirsch, Levine, Fallon-Krueger, & Jaros,1987; Wilson, J. C., & Hughes, 1997b). There is also evidence that learning can be enhanced through the use of certain strategies (Alderman, 1996; Baddeley & Wilson, 1994; Clare, Wilson, Breen, & Hodges, 1999;; Downes *et al.*, 1997; Wilson & Evans, 1996; Wilson, 1997; Wilson *et al.*, 1994).

Conclusions

We have selected just a few of the many studies attempting to answer the question, "Is rehabilitation effective?" Despite some methodological problems, "strong evidence of the overall effectiveness of rehabilitation on general measures of handicap has emerged in the past 5 years" (Cope, 1994, p. 216). We have mounting evidence that rehabilitation reduces the effect of cognitive, social, and emotional problems, leading to greater independence on the part of the patient, reduction in family stress, and eventual employability for many brain-injured people. This situation can only improve with the establishment of centers such as the Oliver Zangwill Center, where outcomes and research into effectiveness will be monitored in order to achieve maximum results.

References

Alderman, N. (1996). Central executive deficit and response to operant conditioning methods. *Neuropsychological Rehabilitation, 6,* 161–186.

Aronow, H. U. (1987). Rehabilitation effectiveness with severe brain injury: Translating research into policy. *Journal of Head Trauma Rehabilitation, 2,* 24–36.

Baddeley, A. D., & Wilson, B. A. (1994). When implicit learning fails: Amnesia and the problem of error elimination. *Neuropsychologia, 32,* 53–68.

Ben-Yishay, Y. (1978). *Working approaches to remediation of cognitive deficits in brain damaged persons. Rehabilitation Monograph No. 59.* New York: New York University Medical Center.

Ben-Yishay, Y., & Prigatano, G. P. (1990). Cognitive remediation. In M. Rosenthal, E. R. Griffith, M. R. Bond, & J. D. Miller (Eds.), *Rehabilitation of the adult and child with traumatic brain injury* (2nd ed, pp. 393–409). Philadelphia: F.A. Davis.

Ben-Yishay, Y., Rattok, J., Lakin, P., Piasetsky, E. G., Ross, B., Silver, S., Zide, E., & Ezrachi, P. (1985). Neuropsychologic rehabilitation: Quest for a holistic approach. *Seminars in Neurology, 5,* 252–259.

Bergman, M. M., & Kemmerer, A. G. (1991). Computer-enhanced self sufficiency: Part 2. Uses and subjective benefits of a text writer for an individual with traumatic brain injury. *Neuropsychology, 5,* 25–28.

Blackerby, W. F. (1990). Intensity of rehabilitation and length of stay. *Brain Injury, 4,* 167–173.

Christensen, A-L., & Teasdale, T. W. (1995). A clinical and neuropsychological led postacute rehabilitation programme. In M. A. Chamberlain, V. C. Newman, & A. Tennant (Eds.), *Traumatic brain injury rehabilitation: Initiatives in service delivery, treatment and measuring outcome* (pp. 88–98). New York: Chapman & Hall.

Clare, L., Wilson, B. A., Breen, E. K., & Hodges, J. R. (1999). Learning face–name associations in early Alzheimer's disease. *Neurocase, 5,* 37–46.

Cope, D. N., Cole, J. R., Hall, K. M., & Barkan, H. (1991). Brain injury: Analysis of outcome in a post-acute rehabilitation system. Part 1: General analysis. *Brain Injury, 5,* 111–125.

Cope, N. (1994). Traumatic brain injury rehabilitation outcome studies in the United States. In A.-L. Christensen & B.P. Uzzell (Eds.), *Brain injury and neuropsychological rehabilitation: International perspectives* (pp. 201–220). Hillsdale, NJ: Lawrence Erlbaum.

Downes, J. J., Kalla, T., Davies, A. D. M., Flynn, A., Ali, H., & Mayes, A. R. (1997). The preexposure technique: A novel method for enhancing the effects of imagery in face–name association learning. *Neuropsychological Rehabilitation, 7,* 195–214.

Evans, J. J., Emslie, H., & Wilson, B. A. (1998). External cueing systems in the rehabilitation of executive impairments of action. *Journal of the International Neuropsychological Society, 1,* 399–408.

Fryer, J., & Haffey, W. (1987). Cognitive rehabilitation and community readaptation: Outcomes from two program models. *Journal of Head Trauma Rehabilitation, 2,* 51–63.

Greenwood, R. J., & McMillan, T. M. (1993). Models of rehabilitation programmes for the brain-injured adult—I: Current provision, efficacy and good practice. *Clinical Rehabilitation, 7,* 248–255.

Johnson, R. (1987). Return to work after severe head injury. *International Disability Studies, 9,* 49–54.

Katz, R. C., & Wetz, R. T. (1997). The efficacy of computer-provided reading treatment for chronic aphasic adults. *Journal of Speech, Language and Hearing Research, 40,* 493–507.

Kirsch, N. L., Levine, S. P., Fallon-Krueger, M., & Jaros, L. A. (1987). The microcomputer as an "orthotic" device for patients with cognitive deficits. *Journal of Head Trauma Rehabilitation, 2,* 77–86.

Kolb, B. (1995). *Brain plasticity and behaviour.* Hillsdale, NJ: Lawrence Erlbaum.

Mehlbye, J., & Larsen, A. (1994). Social and economic consequences of brain damage in Denmark. In A.-L. Christensen & B. P. Uzzell (Eds.), *Brain injury and neuropsychological rehabilitation: International perspectives* (pp. 257–267). Hillsdale, NJ: Lawrence Erlbaum.

Merzenich, M. M., Jenkins, W. M., Johnston, P., Schreiner, C., Miller, S. L., & Tallal, P. (1996). Temporal processing deficits of language-learning impaired children ameliorated by training. *Science, 271,* 77–80.

Mills, V. M., Nesbeda, T., Katz, D. I., & Alexander, M. P. (1992). Outcomes for traumatically brain injured patients following post acute rehabilitation programmes. *Brain Injury, 6,* 219–228.

Ponsford, J. (1995). Mechanisms, recovery and sequelae of traumatic brain injury: A foundation for the REAL approach. In J. Ponsford, S. Sloan, & P. Snow (Eds.), *Traumatic brain injury: Rehabilitation for everyday adaptive living* (pp. 1–31). Hove, Lawrence Erlbaum Associates.

Prigatano, G. P., Fordyce, D. J., Zeiner, H. K., Roueche, J. R., Pepping, M., & Wood, B. C. (Eds.). (1986). *Neuropsychological rehabilitation after brain injury.* Baltimore: The Johns Hopkins University Press.

Prigatano, G. P., Klonoff, P. S., O'Brien, K. P., Altman, I. M., Amin, K., Chiapello, D., Shepherd, J., Cunningham, M., & Mora, M. (1994). Productivity after neuropsychologically oriented milieu rehabilitation. *Journal of Head Trauma Rehabilitation, 9,* 91–102.

Rattok, J., Ben-Yishay, Y., Ezrachi, O., Lakin, P., Piasetsky, E., Ross, B., Silver, S., Vakil, E., Zide, E., & Diller, L. (1992). Outcome of different treatment mixes in a multidimensional neuropsychological rehabilitation programme. *Neuropsychology, 6,* 395–416.

Robertson, I. H. (in press). Theory-driven neuropsychological rehabilitation: The role of attention and competition in recovery of function after brain damage. In D. Gopher & A. Koriat (Eds.), *Attention and performance XVII.* Cambridge, MA: MIT Press.

Robertson, I. H., Tegnér, R., Tham, K., Lo, A., & Nimmo-Smith, I. (1995). Sustained attention training for unilateral neglect: Theoretical and rehabilitation implications. *Journal of Clinical and Experimental Neuropsychology, 17,* 416–430.

Shiel, A. (1999) The effect of rehabilitation on violent behaviour after severe head injury. Unpublished Ph.D. thesis, University of Southampton, England.

Spivack, G., Spettell, C. M., Ellis, D. W., & Ross, S. E. (1992). Effects of intensity of treatment and lengths of stay on rehabilitation outcomes. *Brain Injury, 6,* 419–439.

Sturm, W., Willmes, K., Orgass, B., & Hartje, W. (1997). Do specific attention deficits need specific training? *Neuropsychological Rehabilitation, 7,* 81–103.

Tallal, P., Miller, S. L., Bedi, G., Byma, G., Wang, X., Nagarajan, S. S., Schreiner, C., Jenkins, W. M., & Merzenich, M. M. (1996). Language comprehension in language-learning impaired children improved with acoustically modified speech. *Science, 271,* 81–84.

Wilson, B. A. (1997). Cognitive rehabilitation: How it is and how it might be. *Journal of the International Neuropsychological Society, 3,* 487–496.

Wilson, B. A. (1998). Recovery of cognitive functions following non-progressive brain injury. *Current Opinion in Neurobiology, 8,* 281–287.

Wilson, B. A. & Evans, J. J. (1996). Error free learning in the rehabilitation of individuals with memory impairments. *Journal of Head Trauma Rehabilitation, 11,* 54–64.

Wilson, B. A., & Watson, P. C. (1996). A practical framework for understanding compensatory behaviour in people with organic memory impairment. *Memory, 4,* 465–486.

Wilson, B. A., Baddeley, A. D., Evans, J. J., & Shiel, A. (1994). Errorless learning in the rehabilitation of memory impaired people. *Neuropsychological Rehabilitation, 4,* 307–326.
Wilson, B. A., Evans, J. J., Emslie, H., & Malinek, V. (1997a). Evaluation of NeuroPage: A new memory aid. *Journal of Neurology, Neurosurgery, and Psychiatry, 63,* 113–115.
Wilson, B. A., J. C., & Hughes, E. (1997b). Coping with amnesia: The natural history of a compensatory memory system. *Neuropsychological Rehabilitation, 7,* 43–56.
Zangwill, O. L. (1947). Psychological aspects of rehabilitation in cases of brain injury. *British Journal of Psychology, 37,* 60–69.

16

The INSURE Program and Modifications in Finland

MARJA-LIISA KAIPIO, JAANA SARAJUURI, AND SANNA KOSKINEN

"The trouble with using experience as a guide is that the final exam often comes first and then the lesson."

—Unknown

Background

INSURE (Individualized Neuropsychological Subgroup Rehabilitation Program) is a 6-week rehabilitation program tailored to the special needs of selected subgroups of traumatically brain injured (TBI) patients (Kaipio, Sarajuuri, & Koskinen, 1997) and based on neuroscientific research findings. The basic program costs $350 (US) per day. INSURE has been developed taking into account the overall care and management system needs. At the moment, while INSURE is being run only in the Käpylä Rehabilitation Centre, demand exceeds supply.

For the patient, the procedure is an intensive course in dealing with TBI and related human, social, and economic aspects, to allow TBI patients and all concerned (relatives, friends, employers, etc.) to continue with their lives and cope with the injury-related changes. For the finance providers and the health care system, INSURE is a flexible component that can be used as a specific part of the continuum of rehabilitation and management. It is also used as a diagnostic procedure in TBI patients, for formulating long-term rehabilitation plans, for engaging a short work trial, and for educating professionals and next of kin.

The INSURE program is recommended for patients for whom there are realistic possibilities of achieving productivity and psychological balance by this means. Selection for the program is undertaken with care. The medical and psychological assessment and the therapeutic procedures in INSURE take account of both the mild injuries (Kaipio, Sarajuuri, &

MARJA-LIISA KAIPIO, JAANA SARAJUURI, AND SANNA KOSKINEN • Käpylä Rehabilitation Center, Department of Clinical Neuropsychology, 00610 Helsinki, Finland.

International Handbook of Neuropsychological Rehabilitation, edited by Christensen and Uzzell. Kluwer Academic/ Plenum Publishers, New York, 2000.

Koskinen, 1995) and the differences between real-life and laboratory tasks and demands that Damasio (1994) has illustrated so delicately. Sophisticated neuropsychological rehabilitation and neuropsychological psychotherapeutic techniques, undertaken contemporaneously with multiple forms of vocational and medical rehabilitation, lie at the core of the program. Expertise, responsibility, caring, and persistence are emphasized in the work of the professional team.

INSURE has been under development since 1991, and has been used in its present form since 1993 (Kaipio, Sarajuuri, & Koskinen, 1993; Kaipio *et al.*, 1995, 1997). The INSURE population forms a subgroup of the 170 TBI patients treated annually in the Käpylä Rehabilitation Centre in Helsinki. For other subgroups of TBI patients (Eames & Wood, 1989), various other kinds of rehabilitation services are available in the Käpylä Rehabilitation Centre.

Referrals for the inclusion in the program come from hospitals, insurance companies, the public health care system, and private clinics throughout Finland. Neurologically, injuries range from fairly mild to severe from which there has been good recovery. Selected patients begin treatment anytime from 2 months to many years following injury. Chronicity is not perceived as any hinderance to potential benefit from INSURE intervention. Participants have stated that such an intensive course of powerful true-to-life psychotherapy would have been beneficial even had they not suffered TBI.

The ideological and theoretical bases of the INSURE program spring from the enthusiastic and pioneering work of Professors George P. Prigatano, Yehuda Ben-Yishay, and Anne-Lise Christensen (Ben-Yishay *et al.*, 1985; Christensen, Pinner, Moller, Teasdale, & Trexler, 1992; Prigatano & Wood, 1985, 1994; Prigatano, & Schacter, 1991). The profoundly human and professional approaches to psychotherapy and neurorehabilitation of Professor George P. Prigatano are evident in the content of the program.

INSURE Subgroups

Different subgroups, each with special needs, can be clearly defined among applicants. Some patients are in a late subacute/early postacute phase, and no previous rehabilitation has been undertaken. Other patients are in a later postacute phase and they have histories of consistent, sound treatment, and rehabilitation, but simply need more. Another special subgroup often seen consists of patients in whom the neuropsychological or mental sequelae of injury and their functional and psychosocial implications have been under- or misdiagnosed, resulting in confusion and delay in treatment and recovery. Another subgroup is formed by patients whose TBI-related mental direct or reactive symptoms have solely or for the most part been interpreted and treated as if they were of psychiatric origin. Medication has in many such cases been variable and requires extremely careful reassessment. Of utmost importance is to assess the TBI in detail, and devise a specific and practical plan of rehabilitation, particularly since some of the patients have not previously been properly assessed.

The diagnostic confusion mentioned above can lead to and is traditionally closely connected with litigation and extra psychological suffering and reactive symptoms. Such patients are therefore carefully assessed, treated, and supported in the INSURE program. Patients whose injuries are "mild," a term that can nevertheless span a wide range, are referred for inclusion in the INSURE program often for obtaining a second opinion concerning their injuries and sequelae, or for rehabilitation. Particular attention is paid to associated injuries or symptoms, such as cervical injuries, pain, sleep disturbance, and true or suspected posttraumatic stress disorders.

Selection of Participants

Applicants whose behavior is socially normal and constructive and who have evident needs and desires to obtain information, understand, and cope in relation to their lives and injuries are selected for participation in the INSURE program. They are independent as regards daily life, and physical disabilities are slight or absent. Patients who have had psychiatric, alcohol-, or drug-abuse problems before injury are excluded. Applicants are from 20 to 50 years of age.

The critical nature of personal commitment is emphasized during the neuropsychological recruitment interview. It is crucial for patients to be flexible, able to absorb information, and receptive to coaching with regard to the injury and life situation. Subjects' awareness (Prigatano & Schacter, 1991) about their disabilities and the program rationale jointly form a basis for motivation and attitude to program work, during and after participation in the program.

The selection period is used to establish motivation and commitment. If appropriate, applicants may be asked to take part in therapy groups or an INSURE seminar to assess their responsiveness and suitability for inclusion in the program. They are given the opportunity to study INSURE educational material on videotape or meet a previous member of the INSURE program to allow them to gain a clear idea of how the groups work, the general atmosphere, and the rationale of the program. After they have received detailed information about the procedure and the ideology behind it, applicants are asked to assess how the program might meet their needs and help them achieve their goals in the context of their current life situations.

In assessing applicants, we bear in mind that this procedure is beneficial only for members of particular subgroups, and not for all individuals who have suffered TBI. The basic principle of learning to cope with TBI, however, can be applied generally in the rehabilitation of injuries with a wide range of complications and severity. We also see individuals who do not need or like to work in groups and programs. Such individuals, in fact, benefit most from intensive individual therapy and coaching. Applicants unsuited to the program receive information and recommendations regarding appropriate rehabilitation.

The INSURE Professional Team

Members of the INSURE team are selected for their professionalism, to ensure consistency of standards. In selecting and training the team, the same aspects are emphasized and criteria applied are the same as in selection of patients. Devotion is one of the most important qualities. The program is directed by a clinical neuropsychologist. Three expert clinical neuropsychologists work closely and intensively with the group and individual participants in the program. Participants have individual neuropsychological psychotherapy sessions daily, with the primary therapist. The primary therapist organizes the rehabilitation at the individual level. The INSURE team meets as a group once a week to discuss the patients formally.

Members of the INSURE team are trained in the use of modern therapeutic and medical facilities in neurorehabilitation. The multiprofessional team includes professionals of clinical neuropsychology, neurology, rehabilitation nursing, social work, speech and language therapy, and occupational and physical therapy. Medical consultations are arranged, most often with specialists in neuropsychiatry, neuroradiology, and physiatry.

Structure of the Basic Program

INSURE is an outpatient program. However, patients living a far distance from the center can stay in the clinic. The daily schedule runs from 8:30 AM to 4:00 PM. The program simulates the stress of working days. Accordingly, it can be regarded as a brief simulated work trial. Typical postinjury phenomena and disabilities, such as fatigue and sleep disturbances and impairments in organizing effectively and withstanding stress, become evident, which would not be achievable if only conventional neuropsychological assessment in polyclinic were used. Participants partly plan their weekly schedule independently, as they would in their real jobs.

The INSURE groups are small, consisting of five–eight members, which ensures intense working conditions. The program is open to relatives and those concerned, applicants, lecturers, and to a limited extent other professionals and students, in particular, psychotherapy groups. Participants coach and inform such visitors as necessary.

The day begin with a group in which members and neuropsychologists determine individual goals for the day and the program. As the program continues, long-term goals are set. Achievement of goals is discussed and progress is followed. Records are kept by the group chairman and secretary.

Neuropsychological Psychotherapy Group

The neuropsychological psychotherapy group is the heart of the program; it meets from Mondays to Thursdays. Group sessions involve lessons and workshops in which injury-related pathophysiological, neurobehavioral, and neuropsychological aspects of TBI are discussed in detail. Neurological, neuropsychological, psychological and neuropsychiatric findings and considerations, psychosocial predictors, and possible risk factors are thoroughly examined and debated. Diagnostic indicators and methods used in evaluating TBI and their limitations are studied. The most intensive and popular lessons and workshops in which members of neuropsychological psychotherapy group take part deal with injury-related and reactive changes in personality, behavior, emotion, and life as a whole. Special care is taken to secure a high standard of presentations in the therapy groups. The presentations have to be scientific and inspiring.

Former INSURE participants also give lectures and lead discussions in psychotherapy groups. These give patients perspective in relation to coping with all the changes that can follow injury. Primary therapists review lectures during subsequent individual therapy sessions, taking account of individual injuries to enhance understanding and capability of coping. The lessons and workshops take place during the first 3 weeks of the program.

During the fourth week of the INSURE program the patients in the neuropsychological psychotherapy group give personal presentations, as summaries or posters. Each puts together the medical facts and details about his or her injury. They interpret and discuss their observations and experiences and those of their relatives, friends, and employers concerning injury-related changes and functional limitations imposed by them. These presentations, like many other aspects of the program, are videotaped for review.

Realistic, relevant, and consistent information given to the group helps patients create personal tools for assessing recovery and symptoms. Control is enhanced and stress related to TBI relieved. Patients also need to become cognizant, because understanding is poor in general. Psychological balance and well-being depend greatly on availability of information and therapeutic support.

Only if the patient is sufficiently knowledgeable about injury phenomenology, personal reactions, and probabilistic prognostics can he or she understand what is happening and why and distinguish between self-related, injury-related, and reactive phenomena. An ability to see oneself apart from the injury relieves uncertainty, confusion, shame, fears, and feelings of lack of control arising from altered and partly unpredictable functioning of the brain and mind.

Overlapping Multidimensional Feedback in Groups

Group activities of various kinds are used to reinforce and enrich the program. Group activities mimic meetings and negotiation during a working day. Many typical symptoms reveal themselves only in group settings, during interaction with others. Enjoyment of life, motivation, and the pleasures of friendship and society are emphasized in planning activities and in forming relationships.

Practical significance of classic, well-known, injury-related changes in relation, for example, to information processing, persistence, energy, attention, and reasoning are calibrated from the point of recovery, compensation, and personal functional obstacles in cognitive groups. Recommendations are made regarding possible limitations in working ability and impending trials of work. The ideology behind the cognitive group is not the remedying of cognitive symptomatology, but demonstration and learning its rationale. The goal is to facilitate subjects' compensation for their cognitive symptoms. Treatment software and lectures are used to operationalize cognitive changes and make their logic clearly understandable. The significance of subtle changes, such as fatigue or slowness, that are not evident from any kind of test are studied.

Thus, sports group involves riding, swimming, playing tennis or golf, or wall climbing for fun, simply for joy of mastery of the body and the pleasure of physical exercise. Patients are encouraged to start or restart sporting activities. The activities in the sports group also reveal subtle physical disabilities experienced by many participants. Relaxation and jogging groups are also popular.

Even mild traumatic brain injury can subtly influence psychosocial behavior. A pragmatic approach is the key to achievement of satisfactory social relationships. Adaptation of such an approach is therefore central to successful rehabilitation. Changes in figurative language, focusing and understanding of humor and sarcasm and so on can restrict possibilities of TBI victims for socializing, negotiating, and expressing themselves. The optimal goal of the pragmatic group is to coach the patient in awareness of mastery on a pragmatic basis of altered circumstances (Söderholm & Kaipio, 1997).

The pictures of self group is a workshop where the patients study and express their emotions, experiences, visions of themselves, and their lives through photography. These will include images of childhood, achievements, family, the accident, the losses resulting from the injury, pain and sorrow related to the injury, and increases in understanding and control over life. During the final week of the INSURE program, the group sets up an exhibition.

The sociodrama group aims to express lessons, experiences, and questions in the language of drama. This group meets once a week.

The quality-of-life group meets at the end of each week. It tackles social and material issues relating to everyday life, for example, problems finding work or financing a trial of work, hobbies, and good health practices. Participants in the program are also advised on how to deal with insurance and the health care systems. The infrastructures and customs of health care, compensation, and insurance systems are complicated even for those unaffected by injury.

The INSURE Seminar

After 4 weeks of intensive study a 2-day INSURE seminar is held. Employers, relatives, friends, and professionals from insurance companies and the public health care system are encouraged to take part, to share information, and to learn about experience following traumatic brain injury. During the seminar, INSURE program professionals and participants give presentations dealing with a wide range of topics, from neuropathology and neuroradiology to personal experience. All are intended to shed light on TBI and its human and social aspects. On the second day of the seminar, former participants in INSURE programs and their relatives and employers take part. Their presentations are mostly straightforward descriptions of experience from which lessons can be learned. Presentations are often moving and sometimes lighthearted. They encourage new thinking. During the seminar, each participant attends a meeting where a plan for continuation of his or her rehabilitation is reviewed and adjusted. The meetings are with members of the rehabilitation team, but also involve relatives and those concerned with reimbursement and employers.

Conclusion of the INSURE Program

During the sixth week of the INSURE program, participants assess what they have learned and new outlooks they have established. They share experiences and discuss and refine future plans, making practical arrangements for their realization. Therapy, management of the situation, and work trials and education will have been worked out during the program. Most clients continue with intensive neuropsychological psychotherapy and coaching for different periods following completion of the basic program. Neuropsychological coaching and support generally seems to be a prerequisite for success in trials of work and education and for achievement of good psychosocial and psychological balance. Individual neuropsychological therapy following the INSURE program is arranged through public or private health care services.

Recommendations are prepared for those concerned with reimbursement as far as future rehabilitation is needed. After completion of the INSURE program, follow-up and coaching can be arranged in the TBI polyclinic in the Käpylä Rehabilitation Centre. On completion of the basic program, when necessary, the subjects can participate in the INSURE work and school program described below. This supports work trial and education.

On completion of an INSURE program, patients should have substantial knowledge about TBI, giving them a sound basis for understanding and coping with TBI-related changes and for participating in coached work trials.

The INSURE Work and School Modifications

The INSURE work and school programs complement the basic program. One modification is for patients who want to continue with coached trials of work and education of different lengths and natures after completing the basic INSURE program. In most cases, lengthy, individually tailored trials of work and education are needed to find an optimal level of functioning. The other INSURE work and school modification is for young adults. The latter cannot benefit from a short 6-week procedure as adults can. Younger patients need more intensive coaching to find the functional stamina and psychological balance.

The INSURE work and school programs are directed by the neuropsychologist. Adjustment of working circumstances and management of neuropsychological limitations at work necessitate professional neuropsychological coaching. TBI symptomatology and the patients' education and personal histories and qualities must be taken into account. Trials of work are encouraged and carried out within the general market, usually with a neuropsychologist collaborating with the patient. A coached trial of work with a period of therapy is often the only way to get and keep a permanent job.

Work should not restrict the time for recreation to the extent that no energy remains for activities outside working hours. Jobs that are too simple, too mechanical, or too artificial are not recommended. Having a job is not an end in itself, but can help patients regain functionality and solve psychosocial problems, giving them meaningful and satisfying lives once more (Handy, 1997). Patients are taught to assess goals concerning work and studies realistically, with regard to changes relating to TBI rather than advising abandonment of career goals and dreams. Much effort is made to find ways of achieving goals and making dreams come true in realistic ways.

The 16-month INSURE work and school program is for patients who have been injured during chidlhood or early adulthood. The program focuses on neuropsychological psychotherapy and trials of work and education. TBI-related behavioral, emotional, and functional mental limitations may become evident only as a person gets older and needs to meet the psychosocial demands of grown-up life and work. Participants are mostly from 20 to 25 years of age.

In this program for young adults, participants attend a 3-week booster INSURE procedure twice a year. Otherwise, they attend the INSURE psychotherapy group and individual neuropsychological therapy once a week while participating in trials of work or education. The overall procedure and the neuropsychological psychotherapy provided meet needs of members of this age group well. Patients can enter the program during the first 3-week booster in October or the second 3-week booster in February. The INSURE work and school program has been under continual development since 1995.

Follow-up Study

The INSURE program is based on expertise and a culture of assessment, study, and development. A controlled 2-year follow-up study is being conducted (Sarajuuri, Kaipio, & Koskinen, 1997). Psychosocial outcomes are being assessed. Matched controls are drawn from patients of the neurosurgical department of the Helsinki University Central Hospital undergoing traditional forms of rehabilitation. Preliminary findings are encouraging (Sarajuuri *et al.*, 1997). A further publication will appear in a year.

Beyond Routine Assessment and Treatment

> *"Good judgment comes from experience and experience comes from bad judgment"*
>
> —Barry LePatner

Judgment of TBI-related neurobehavioral changes in brain functioning and rehabilitation of the sufferers from them necessitate fresh approaches rather than just routine assessment and treatment. As is now well-known, an examiner can fall into a number of traps in determining TBI sequelae and the rehabilitational needs of the patient. The emergency unit may not have recorded in detail initial findings such as mechanism of injury, loss of consciousness, Glasgow Coma Scale score or posttraumatic amnesia. Loss of consciousness may have been misleadingly brief or nonexistent. There may be an absence of structural neuroimaging findings even though mechanism of injury is indisputable with TBI sequelae. Scanning may have been performed too late to reveal all of the acute changes in the brain. It is also not rare for a patient to have been discharged in a confused state a few hours after the injury or before they have become confused. The latter circumstances may subsequently be misinterpreted or cited as evidence that there has been no confusion following injury. The significance of neurobehavioral findings and results of functional imaging may then be underestimated or regarded as not objective or not hard evidence.

Although it is known that a blow to the head will result in diffuse axonal injury, the entire extent of which cannot be revealed by structural imaging, results of scanning tend to be regarded as objective measures of the injury. In cases in which symptoms have been interpreted as relatively severe in relation to an apparently minor mechanism of injury, care is needed if a true picture of the injury is to be obtained and the patient helped. There are no operational definitions of what forces and mechanisms are sufficient to cause TBI. In addition, not enough is known about physiological and neurochemical variables for a critical injury level to be identifiable. In every program we see patients who have been in extremely severe accidents, and despite this their symptoms have been interpreted as psychiatric because there has been not marked loss of consciousness and no findings in structural neuroimaging, which leads in many cases to medicolegal dilemmas.

Patients referred to the program who are assessed as suffering from minor or mild injuries in fact, are often found to have suffered moderate or severe injuries but to exhibit no marked neurological status symptoms. It must be borne in mind that there is no exclusive definition of mild injury. The neuropsychological sequelae of the traumatic brain injury is easily underestimated. In some patients results of routine neuropsychological assessment will be normal. Some patients will find no difficulty in completing neuropsychological tests that primarily measure the operational level of mental functions. Despite this, the neuropsychology still seems to rely heavily on tests that do not necessarily identify the problems such as fatigue, slowness, problems of attention, problems of mental programming and initiative, and problems relating to personality and any kind of emotion. If the problems are severe enough, they will be seen in a polyclinical examination. If not, they typically become evident only long term or during a trial of work. Ability to conduct good neuropsychodiagnostics is invaluable, and much expertise and experience of incorrect judgment is needed. It can also be beneficial if an examiner undertakes long-term psychotherapy and coaching with TBI patients.

Many of the neurobehavioral symptoms related to TBI mimic classic, psychiatric states such as depression, aggression, posttraumatic stress disorder, personality disorders, or aggravation. Patients whose symptoms have been interpreted and treated as psychiatric, despite their organic nature, form a specific subgroup. TBI patients tend in any case to be fragile and confused because of inablity to control and understand altered mental functioning. Incorrect neuropsychiatric diagnosis and treatment easily leads to worsening of patient´s condition, possibly to reactive psychological problems, exacerbating the problem of obtaining a clear picture of symptoms. Emotional qualities, personality, and behavior before injury should be carefully differentiated from predictable reactive changes and neurobehavioral symptoms. Problems relating to any cervical injuries, pain, or suspected psychodynamic factors underlying symptoms require careful examination. Again, a trial of treatment is often a good way to determining the origins of symptoms.

Marked neurobehavioral findings also may be neglected or underestimated by medical specialists hoping for spontaneous recovery (and lesser costs) if a patient otherwise appears "normal." A patient will not usually be aware of problems in the early phases of recovery. He or she will readily agree with an optimistic or nonknowledgeable examiner, and will often be eager to return to work prematurely. Trying to return to work too early can in any case prejudice possibilities of finding and keeping a job. A patient should not be released into the labor market to test his or her working ability before thorough evaluation of the injury and associated risks. Failure in trials of work and in social settings can often provoke secondary psychological problems. In the INSURE program many of the patients have previously tried a rapid return to work. Medical practitioners may believe a rapid return to work will be therapeutic and promise recovery. They may support rapid return, even when risk of failure is evident. Such errors could be prevented if treatment is extended beyond routine, careful prediction conforming to severity of injury and the person concerned were made, and support and coaching systems were set up for patients.

Sophisticated interpretation of the many indicators of TBI is the means of good judgment and relevant rehabilitation. What is needed is an ability to go beyond routine assessment so that psychodiagnostic findings make sense in relation to patients' symptoms, and not just differences in medical opinion. Common sense should not be forgotten in neuropsychodiagnostics. TBI is not a state appropriate to judgment within the framework of rigid, operational definitions. Application of fuzzy logic is always needed to some extent. In many cases diagnostic dilemmas can be resolved through trials of treatments. Such trials need to be undertaken rather than leaving patients unrehabilitated. It is often easier and more humane and economic to undertake a trial of treatment than perpetuate diagnostic procedures and discussions.

If a patient needs physiotherapy or speech therapy, there is usually no problem. The need for professional neuropsychological rehabilitation and, to an even greater extent, neuropsychologically based psychotherapy is more difficult to meet. Long-term needs for them may not be acknowledged, even though it is now known at the most fundamental level that neurobehavioral and psychological changes and related rehabilitation are the keys to recovery, achievement of good psychological balance, and restoration of normal life. Neuropsychological rehabilitation is often not organized until major problems have arisen or there have been failures in trials of work. Failure to organize neuropsychological rehabilitation may occur because there has been hope of spontaneous recovery, because ideas regarding the possibilities of neuropsychological treatment procedures have been restricted, or because neurobehavioral sequelae have been underestimated. Neglect of neuropsychological treatment is undesirable. In many cases it leads to exacerbation of a patient's condition.

Rehabilitation needs to be preventive in nature. Patients need information, coaching, and rehabilitation early or during recovery. Need for rehabilitation increases and accordingly so does expense, if organization of rehabilitation is initially inadequate. Delay in rehabilitation can seriously prejudice long-term recovery und outcome.

In general, the need to undertake more than just routine assessment and treatment means that special attention is paid in the INSURE program to the subgroup of minor or apparently minor injuries and to modern methods of neuropsychodiagnosis and therapy. Emphasis is laid on tailoring trials of work to meet patient's needs and in coaching the patient during such trials. Great attention is paid to patient's descriptions of problems following the TBI, to the history of treatment of the latter, and to symptomatology. This is particularly important in the case of patients who have undergone lengthy and onerous medicolegal investigation procedures. Assessment procedures often replace rehabilitation. The recommendation is that medical disputation should be set aside and treatment initiated instead.

Ethical and Economic Aspects of INSURE

"Tradition is what you resort to when you don't have the time or the money to do it right"

—Kurt Herbert Adler (1905–1988)

In Finland, at least, there is not much in the way of tradition regarding neurorehabilitation following TBI. Patients are therefore liable to receive less than optimal treatment and rehabilitation. Economic practices also may be deficient (Haas & Prince, 1997), thanks to faulty thinking. Victims have to face up to alteration in their mental functions and consequently their modes of life. Each needs to appreciate the probability of recovery in his or her particular case. Those responsible for reimbursement have to deal with financial matters. Providers of rehabilitation services have to resolve problems of access to the services on the basis of the medical needs of patients. They also have to make judgments on the basis of scientific debates and assess likely outcomes realistically.

Rehabilitation and management of TBI victims is perceived as time consuming and expensive. Costs of rehabilitation following TBI are disputed. TBI victims tend to be young, however, with many years of working life ahead of them. Rehabilitation services need to be available for patients to be treated aggressively and successfully in the acute phase. Much money is spent on acute care, but subsequent expenses are queried. However, lack of acute care but not of rehabilitation and long-term services might be regarded as unethical. Hesitation about paying for rehabilitation easily ends in greater needs for rehabilitation, poorer outcomes, and greater ultimate expense.

It may sometimes be thought that if the needs for acute care have been minor, the injury is mild and effective neurorehabilitation is unnecessary. This is, however, a misconception. The reverse may be true. Neuropsychological tools are most effective in the rehabilitation of less obviously severe TBIs. Mild injury may also be equated with no injury, with no need for rehabilitation. Patients with injuries at the less severe end of the spectrum are nevertheless exactly those people with realistic possibilities of returning to productive life and regaining working ability at some level via focused neuropsychological and psychotherapeutic rehabilitation and supported work trial. In polyclinics this subgroup is often undertreated or not treated at all. From the ethical and medicolegal points of view, problems therefore arise.

There are no ethical grounds for pressing for uniformity of outcome following TBI. If two patients have similar kinds of injury, the fact that one experiences more severe neurobehavioral problems than the other does not necessarily mean that this patient is feigning illness or that the symptoms are unrelated to the injury. Differences in extent of recovery or in outcome may simply reflect individual differences in injury mechanism, in brain tissue, genetic and hormonal makeup, and coping abilities. The risks of TBI are also greater in individuals in whom psychological and psychosocial risk factors exist. They are also greater in those who lack the support and exposure to caring others that are predictive of good outcomes, when combined with medical realism and use of appropriate medical procedures.

The INSURE program is designed to be reasonable in cost, length, and effectiveness, to make it appealing in relation to subjects with different kinds of sources of reimbursement, patients going to work, or patients in litigation. The structure and content of the INSURE program are under continual developement, with emphasis on both the biological and human aspects of rehabilitation medicine. Modern methods of neuropsychodiagnosis are used and particular attention is paid to the economic and legal aspects of the practice of rehabilitation medicine. Members of the team executing the INSURE program are continually trained in modern neurosciences to meet the needs of TBI subgroups.

The atmosphere within the program is open and human. No conflict is seen between exhibition of humanity and professionalism, nor between humanity and accuracy of medical diagnosis and effective treatment. The INSURE program is subject to continual adjustment as neuroscience develops. It is also adjusted to take account of ideas and criticism from participants and follow-up information regarding psychosocial outcomes. The less serious a TBI, the more talented a victim, and the greater the demands of actual or potential employment, the greater are the expectations of rehabilitation procedures.

Demands for "objective" findings (e.g., structural changes in brain tissue demonstrable by scanning for symptoms relevant to those a patient is suffering) are balanced against the necessity for good outcome of treatment in the INSURE program. The victims in the middle of medicolegal controversy are treated not as opponents but as patients with real problems. Subjects affected by differential diagnostic problems are particularly welcome in the INSURE program. Scientific evidence suggests that outcome following TBI is worse, if there has been no specialized rehabilitation (Hall & Cope, 1995). Different subgroups of TBI patients need different kinds of treatment and rehabilitation. The problems that stem from TBI are real and need to be taken seriously.

Concluding Words

"Victory goes to the player who makes the next-to-last mistake"
—Savielly Grigorievitch Tartakover (1887–1956)

The experience of TBI as a victim, a relative, those concerned, or as a professional represents a major challenge of human life (Kapur, 1997). The effects of TBI are more far-reaching than is usually imagined. Even experienced professionals can underestimate TBI and overestimate their expertise.

"The soul breathes through the body, and suffering, whether it starts in the skin or in a mental image, happens in the flesh" (Damasio, 1994). Human and socioeconomic effects of TBI are substantial. Humanity owes much to the victims and professionals who have raised awareness about TBI and advanced neuropsychological rehabilitation.

References

Ben-Yishay, Y., Rattok, J., Lakin, P., Piasetsky, E. D., Ross, B., Silver, S., Zide, E., & Errachi, O. (1985). Neuropsychological rehabilitation: Quest for a holistic approach. *Seminars in Neurology, 5(3),* 252–259.

Christensen, A. L., Pinner, E. M., Moller, P. P., Teasdale, T. W., & Trexler, L. E. (1992). Psychosocial outcome following individualized neuropsychological rehabilitation of brain damage. *Acta Neurol Scandinavia, 85,* 32–38.

Damasio, A. R. (1994). *Descartes'error. Emotion, reason and the human brain.* New York: Avon Books.

Eames, P., & Wood, R. L. (1989). The structure and content of a head injury rehabilitation service. In R. L. Wood & P. Eames (Eds.), *Models of brain injury rehabilitation,* (pp. 34–37). London: Chapman and Hall.

Haas, J. F. & Prince, J. M. (1997). Ethics and management care in rehabilitation medicine. *Journal of* Head Trauma Rehabil*itation,* 12 (1)., vii–xiii.

Hall, K. M., & Cope, D. N. (1995). The benefit of rehabilitation in traumatic brain injury: A literature review. *Journal of Head Trauma Rehabilitation, 10*(1), 1–13.

Handy, C. (1997). *The hungry spirit. Beyond capitalism—A Quest for purpose in the modern world.* London: Hutchinson.

Kaipio, M-L., Sarajuuri, J., & Koskinen, S. (1993). Rehabilitation Program for Subgroups of Young Traumatically Brain Injured Patients. International Symposium on Neurorehabilitation. A perspective for the future. May 13th–15th. Klinik Bavaria. Germany.

Kaipio, M-L., Sarajuuri, J., & Koskinen, S. (1995). A need to go beyond reliance on routine assessment and treatment. 5th Nordic Meeting on Neuropsychology, August 17–19, Uppsala, Sweden.

Kaipio, M-L., Sarajuuri, J., & Koskinen, S. (1997). Insure—Program and modifications. Second World Congress on Brain Injury, May 9–14, Seville, Spain.

Kapur, N. (1997). *Injured brains of medical minds.* Oxford: Oxford University Press.

Prigatano, G. P., & Schacter, D. L. (1991). *Awareness of deficit after brain injury. Clinical and theoretical issues.* Oxford: Oxford University Press.

Prigatano, G. P., Fordyce, D. J., Zeiner, H. K., Roueche, J. R., Pepping, M., & Wood, P. C. (1985). *Neuropsychological rehabilitation after brain injury.* Baltimore: The Johns Hopkins University Press.

Prigatano, G. P., Klonoff, P. S., O'Brien, K. P., Altman, I. M., Amin, K., Chiapello, D., Shepherd, J., Cunningham, M., & Mora, M. (1994). Productivity after neuropsychologically oriented milieu rehabilitation. *Journal of Head Trauma Rehabilitation, 9,* 91–102.

Sarajuuri, J., Kaipio, M-L., & Koskinen, S. (1997). Psychosocial outcome following INSURE program. Second World Congress on Brain Injury, May 9–14, Seville, Spain.

Söderholm, S., & Kaipio, M-L. (1997). Pragmatic groups in the INSURE program. Second World Congress on Brain Injury, May 9–14, Seville, Spain.

17

The CRBI at the University of Copenhagen

A Participant–Therapist Perspective

CARLA CAETANO AND ANNE-LISE CHRISTENSEN

Introduction

The Center for Rehabilitation of Brain Injury (CRBI) is a postacute, holistic rehabilitation day program, of approximately 4 months duration, where 15 patients (referred to as students) participate in a combination of individual and group activities. The program is holistic and neuropsychological in orientation, allows for individualized goal setting, uses interdisciplinary planning and treatment, and provides a therapeutic milieu that addresses cognitive, emotional, and social concerns. See Christensen and Caetano (1999), Christensen and Teasdale (1998), and Trexler and Helmke (1996), for an extensive description of these types of programs.

As detailed descriptions of the theoretical background and practical elements of the program have previously been described, for example, Christensen and Teasdale (1993), and outcome data presented as in Christensen, Pinner, Møller Pedersen, Teasdale, and Trexler (1992), Teasdale, Christensen, and Pinner (1993), Teasdale and Christensen (1994), and Larsen, Mehlbye and Gørtz (1991), the rehabilitation process will be presented in this chapter as a case study, that is, from the point of view of a young woman (LL) whose career and personal life was drastically altered by brain injury. The purpose of the presentation will be to describe the process of rehabilitation from referral to follow-up in a qualitative manner, so as to highlight the dynamic nature of development and change that take place during such a process.

CARLA CAETANO AND ANNE-LISE CHRISTENSEN • Center for Rehabilitation of Brain Injury, University of Copenhagen, 2300 Copenhagen S, Denmark.

International Handbook of Neuropsychological Rehabilitation, edited by Christensen and Uzzell.
Kluwer Academic/ Plenum Publishers, New York, 2000.

The Referral Phase

LL was referred to the CRBI by her social worker; in Denmark, each individual is automatically allocated a social worker, based on the municipality he or she lives in. Thus, should a referral not come directly from the health services (as, for example, after discharge from inpatient treatment, or by the student's own general practitioner), referrals can be made via social services. As treatment is paid by state, county, municipal, health and social services, a representative from one these sectors is always involved in the referral phase. (See Chapter 23, this volume, for a further description of the Danish rehabilitation system.) Irrespective of the referral source, the student's own physician is always informed.

Ideally, the following information is obtained from the institutions previously involved in the student's care, namely: (1) a discharge summary from the hospital (2) neuroradiological results, (3) neuropsychological reports, (4) other relevant medical records and summaries, (5) physiotherapy status reports, (6) speech and language therapy reports, (7) social information pertaining to rehabilitation possibilities, and (8) psychosocial information, with particular reference being made to family and other forms of social support.

A referral is first reviewed by the CRBI's internal committee, consisting of the referral secretary, the director, and a neuropsychologist, to evaluate appropriateness for the program. Once approved at this preliminary level, the student along with other referrals is reviewed by the CRBI's external referral committee, at one of its five annual meetings. This committee consists of four physicians (from departments of neurosurgery, neuromedicine, physiatry, and psychiatry), a representative from the Social Services Department, and members of the CRBI's internal review committee.

A primary consideration is that the referred person meets the criteria for treatment (refer to Appendix A for detailed description of these criteria). In terms of LL, she was in her early 20s, with no history of chronic physical or psychiatric illness, substance abuse, or congenital brain dysfunction. Her medical records indicated that she was in excellent health prior to the rupture of two aneurysms: the first of the left internal carotid artery, which included a small left anterior choroidal artery being patched, 1 $^1/_2$ years prior to referral, and an aneurysm of the right anterior choroidal artery, approximately 7 months prior to referral. Each aneurysm was clipped, and at the time of her second surgery, computerized tomography (CT) scanning showed bilateral basal ganglia damage, left greater than right. At discharge, neurological examination indicated that she was alert, oriented, with equal and reactive pupils. Reflexes and sensory functioning were intact with only minimal motor asymmetry noted for the right hand. The physical therapy discharge evaluation was that she was independent in self-care, although there was indications of decreased right extremity strength especially for the upper extremity, with minimal impairment of balance and decreased fitness. Neuropsychological difficulties were described as impairments in verbal memory, word finding, and aspects of executive function. It was recommended that she receive outpatient neuropsychological rehabilitation and physical therapy that included exercise to increase strength and aerobic training.

Before final acceptance into the program, a date was set for her to undergo a preliminary evaluation by a neuropsychologist at the CRBI to determine her current level of functioning, resources, and motivation for program participation. This evaluation consists of an interview with the student and typically their significant other(s) and a neuropsychological evaluation, using the Luria Neuropsychological Investigation (LNI) (Christensen, 1975, 1989), supplemented by Ravens Progressive Matrices, Set 1 (see also Christenen and Caetano, 1997;

Christensen, Jensen, & Risberg, 1990, for a description of this approach to evaluation). In addition, if there are specific motor or speech problems, the physical therapist and speech therapist are involved in the preliminary evaluation.

A written report of the findings, combined with the previous history, results, and so forth, is made and rehabilitation recommendations given. The recommendation may either be acceptance into the day program (or variations thereof, such as a reduced program or individual therapy) or referral to an alternate setting. Typically, the written report is given and discussed with the student before a copy is sent to the referral source and to the general practitioner.

LL came to the interview and preliminary investigation with her spouse. LL had been in the process of completing a university degree prior to the onset of the aneurysms, and had had no treatment subsequent to the first surgery and only a brief period of outpatient rehabilitation (10 sessions) after the second surgery. A neuropsychological evaluation conducted 1 month after the second surgery described her status as follows: Visual perception, visual construction, and visual memory were intact. However, mild attentional disturbances with moderately severe impairments of verbal memory, executive function, and word finding were present. She was, therefore, interested in receiving further rehabilitation so that she possibly could continue her studies (a degree in art history, although she was unclear about a specific career choice). She appeared rather passive regarding future planning and the means by which she could achieve her goals.

Her spouse was highly motivated for her to receive the treatment needed to continue with her education, and indicated that he would support her. While both LL and her spouse appeared friendly, cooperative, and supportive, the couple stated that they had always had a close but turbulent relationship and contributed some information pertaining to the cause of their difficulties, for example, problems in communicating and frequent separations due to her husband's business travels. Recently, however, they had undergone additional stress due to relocation. As a result, they had a somewhat limited social network, and tended to be more dependent on each other. However, both felt they received support from the family and friends they had previously known.

As part of the preliminary conversation of the LNI is to evaluate motivation, insight, and learning capacity, both student and significant other are asked to comment on functioning. Both LL and her spouse were in agreement concerning the complaints regarding function subsequent to her brain injury, namely, (1) "slowness," that is, slowed reaction time and information processing, (2) "mixing up words," that is, as evidenced by paraphasia, (3) difficulties in sustaining attention when reading, (4) difficulties with spelling, (5) "slow in writing," that is, right-sided motoric slowness and weakness most noticeable for reduced handwriting speed, and (6) "being more introverted," that is, while previously regarded as outgoing and socially active, both LL and her spouse agreed that she had become more secluded, choosing to be alone more. The latter appeared due more to her own lack of initiative for which she she did not appear to be concerned.

Once the interview phase was completed, higher cortical functions were evaluated using the LNI, directed by the hypotheses formed during the interview phase and from previous data. LL appeared cooperative and friendly but somewhat restricted in affect and slow both verbally and in task completion, the latter being consistent with the student's own report of functioning in the interview. Difficulties were noted on attentional and simple problem-solving tasks, with LL becoming easily overwhelmed. Memory performance was aided by the use of a previously learned visualization strategy, which she spontaneously employed. Overt language comprehension and expression appeared intact and writing/spelling of familiar material was remarkable only for very slow printing of the material. Of note, however, was that when given additional time, tasks could be completed adequately. Visual–spatial constructional tasks were intact but significant for perfectionistic tendencies, for example, dissatisfaction with adequately completed tasks and negative evaluation of performance. Performance on the Ravens was slow, that is, indicative of accurate problem solving but confirming that information-processing speed was reduced. Thus, although generally having difficulty in processing speed, task completion was adversely affected by poor awareness of time management such that LL felt overwhelmed and anxious, resulting in diminished functioning. However, when time pressure was removed or LL asked to increase time estimations for task completion, performance improved.

Thus, the current findings in combination with previous history and her acceptance of treatment suggested that LL was in need of assistance in dealing with a brain injury not only for understanding the nature of her difficulties and their effects on her and others both emotionally and socially, but also for learning to compensate for these difficulties while recognizing strengths and the resources available. Thus, it was recommended that she be admitted into the day program for treatment.

Preprogram Evaluation and Planning

Once accepted into the program, each student is given a primary therapist, that is, a psychologist who is responsible for the student throughout the program, for developing a close, collaborative relationship with the student, providing feedback, and for ensuring that the rehabilitation process occurs in a dynamic, interactive manner so that the student may participate as actively as possible. The primary therapist conducts the preprogram evaluation, which consists of (1) a semistructured interview, concerning information regarding educational, occupational, and social history; (2) a questionnaire to be completed by the student and a significant other, namely, the 63-item European Brain Injury Questionnaire (EBIQ), which evaluates difficulties related to brain injury experienced in the past month (see Teasdale *et al.*, 1997, for a comprehensive description of this measure; see also Deloche *et al.*, 1996); and (3) neuropsychological tests, predominantly quantitative in nature (see Caetano & Christensen, 1997, for a detailed description of the evaluation measures used at the CRBI). These results, taken together with the LNI and previously acquired data from various sources, provide the context from which to summarize functioning and to create an individualized rehabilitation plan.

LL's preprogram evaluation confirmed previous findings of slowed reaction time and decreased information-processing speed, which resulted in difficulties of visual–motor and complex sustained attentional tasks and right-sided weakness. Her passivity, and lack of attention were partially responsible for verbal learning disturbances (as, for example, of a simple list of words) and recall was therefore below average. Recall of contextual verbal information, however, was less adversely affected, consistent with LL's self-report that in conversation or watching a film, she would often experience brief comprehension difficulties, but was able to "catch up" by understanding the context (due to her generally high level of intellectual functioning). On formal speech and language evaluation, no difficulties in verbal comprehension were noted, reading was adequate but slow, word-finding difficulties were minor, but word generation was delayed. Finally, mild disturbances in executive functioning were noted.

Thus, LL evidenced difficulties primarily due to lack of initiative and consequently disturbances in attention, which resulted in impaired verbal information processing and recall. Further difficulties in executive functioning were, for example, in the selection and execution of cognitive plans, where not only the generation and selection of appropriate goals but also the initiation, sequencing, and completion of multitask activities posed difficulty.

In terms of psychosocial functioning, questionnaire and interview results indicated that both LL and her spouse perceived that she needed interests outside of the home, and that decisions were made with difficulty and task completion was slow. Her spouse noted difficulties in taking initiative and in being organized She, in turn, described herself as isolated, having lowered self-esteem and getting her feelings easily hurt. Physical functioning was described as unremarkable for balance and mobility. Running, however, was hampered by pain in the knee joint. Hand coordination and grip strength were intact but concerning the latter, the right hand was weaker than expected. Endurance was in the low-average range, due to decreased aerobic functioning.

The above-mentioned data are then presented by the primary therapist at the interdisciplinary team conference so as to finalize rehabilitation planning. The team at the CRBI consists of clinical and neuropsychologists, a speech and language therapist, special education teachers, and physiotherapists, with each team member contributing to the rehabilitation planning of each student.

In LL's case, the following rehabilitation goals were agreed upon :

1. *Cognitive:* To train attention, verbal memory, executive functioning. LL would be matched to a cognitive group, with others of similar educational/occupational background and cognitive difficulties.
2. *Psychosocial:* To address lack of initiative, social isolation, lowered self-esteem, and self criticism. This would be achieved in individual psychotherapy, group psychotherapy, and a project group consisting of tasks that met some of LL prior (and possibly future) interests in artistic activities.
3. *Physical Training:* As for all program participants, a fitness and endurance training program would be individually tailored for LL by the physical therapists. In LL's case, emphasis was also placed on increasing right arm and hand strength and right leg strength to ensure that running could be accomplished without knee pain. LL's goal of improving right-sided weakness was also addressed by participation in a dance group, playing squash, and cycling. These latter activities were selected to also address social isolation.

Treatment Phase

At the start of the introductory week, which consists of project activities, a welcoming party is given to the students and their significant others. At this event, the student's family members and staff meet in an informal manner. Once the students and their families have been welcomed by the director, the staff, students, and their significant others formally introduce themselves to one another. Thereafter, a brief description of the structure of the program is given by the staff. The evening concludes with the staff, students, and their families conversing and sharing a light meal together.

During the introductory project week, the 15 group members are divided into three smaller groups of five, all of whom are to plan and execute a joint project, for example, "defining life quality," and they participate in physical training. Emphasis is on allowing the students to take the initiative, with the therapists acting as consultants. The goal is to create a finished product by a specific deadline (usually within 3 days) and to present the project as a group to the entire staff and other students. This activity provides the opportunity for the students to become acquainted with one another and for therapists to further evaluate functioning in more naturalistic settings. It also provides an opportunity for ascertaining how the students can most appropriately be divided into various group activities (i.e., cognitive, specialized project, psychotherapy, and physical training groups). As a result of the introductory project week, the content of these groups also will be modified to meet the specific needs of program participants.

The formal day program starts after the project week, where the various program elements and close collaboration of the staff creates a milieu essential for effective treatment. (See Appendix B for an example of a typical day in the program.) Once the day program has started, there is daily contact between staff concerning program participants and a weekly student meeting is held with all staff present to evaluate progress being made and revise treatment goals. During the initial treatment period, LL was engaged, although she showed little initiative. She could identify difficulties and was motivated to compensate for them, but lacked the initiative to do so. She was less likely, however, to acknowledge her strengths and tended to be highly self-critical, which explained, in part, her passivity and is indicative of what Goldstein (1952) terms the development of protective mechanisms in the face of overwhelming anxiety.

At the midpoint of treatment (i.e., after approximately 2 months), a summary of functioning is presented and treatment goals are evaluated. LL's status in terms of cognitive, physical, and emotional–social functioning were as follows.

Cognitive Functioning

Generally, feedback from the staff suggested that LL was well able to manage the tasks required in the various program activities, namely, the morning meetings, project groups, cognitive training groups and physical training, although encouragement and support was still needed. For example, in the morning meeting she had been the chairperson, gymnastics leader, and had been responsible for providing information on current news items and the daily lexicon. She did, however, have difficulty in self-presentation, that is, appearing shy, avoiding eye contact, and speaking very softly. Regarding the latter, individual voice training was given and subsequently she received direct feedback from staff in individual and group activities to make her aware of these tendencies. Furthermore, in individual therapy, emphasis was placed on time management and preparation of tasks.

Attention–Concentration

LL sustained attention adequately when completing task requirements. She became aware, however, that she became more easily fatigued in the late afternoon and evenings. As LL was intelligent and creative, repetitive easy tasks bored her and resulted in less than optimal performance. The treatment plan was therefore adjusted to evaluate performance on tasks she regarded as more stimulating. Her affect and performance were found to improve under these conditions. This tendency was discussed with her and she was asked to identify which tasks she considered being boring–creative so as to self-monitor performance and to encourage initiative. With divided attention tasks, pace slowed but was relatively error free. Although these tasks were completed without becoming distracted, she became anxious under time pressure, which adversely affected performance. The latter difficulty she attributed, in part, to a premorbid tendency for anxiety to impede abilities.

This pattern of response was discussed in individual therapy and subsequent rehabilitation goals for her were: (1) to continue working under time pressure, to help cope with anxieties by adopting a more realistic time management approach; (2) to identify easy tasks and alternate between difficult and easy tasks during a given day in order to minimize fatigue; and (3) due to complaints of sleep disturbances (i.e., sleeping approximately 5 hours per night), it was recommended that 15-minute breaks be taken after each activity at home and during the program, in order to prevent overstimulation and excessive fatigue in the late evening.

Memory Function

LL had difficulty in planning for or recalling events without external aids and/or prompts. While in the program, she was encouraged to use a day planner, and subsequently developed this skill extremely well. With this aid, she completed all task requirements requested independently. It was suggested that the day planner be expanded to include important points in a discussion, since some difficulty in recall of conversations and difficulty remembering peoples' faces (the latter appeared due, in part, to her shyness and lack of interest, resulting in poor eye contact and interest in others) were reported. However, while at the CRBI, these difficulties were not evident.

Subsequent rehabilitation goals were to continue expanding the use of the day planner, as needed. Additional strategies such as (1) visualization techniques (due to creativity and interest in art), and (2) study techniques (such as the preview, question, read state, test, i.e., PQRST method) were to be introduced, practiced, and evaluated for effectiveness.

Executive Function

LL had difficulties in certain aspects of executive functioning. While she was well able to evaluate task requirements and to generate plans for completing them, difficulty appeared when keeping track of multiple task elements, which resulted in becoming overwhelmed and anxious. Rehabilitation focused on increasing awareness of this difficulty and decreasing anxiety by allowing for more preparation time for tasks. When material was of a more simple verbal nature, a checking off technique for completed items was practiced, which proved to be effective. For more complex material, "mind maps" were presented and discussed as a possible aid, and examples were given of its uses. LL found the latter useful, as a more visual orientation allowed for a creative expression of material. Thus, this approach was tried out for note taking and summarizing written material.

Subsequent rehabilitation goals were to develop strategies in planning for more complex tasks, stressing adequate preparation for optimal functioning. This created awareness of defensive mechanisms, for example, an extremely self-critical attitude regarding slow performances, which led to anxiety and depression.

Verbal Function

In daily functioning, LL expressed herself with only minor and infrequent word-finding difficulties, of which she was nonetheless greatly aware and found troubling. She experienced a slower reading pace than premorbidly. On observation, the difficulty appeared to be due to reduced tempo rather than difficulties in letter–word recognition. Similarly, when slowly executed, she wrote well (especially when printing), although with minor spelling difficulties (due more to overcautiousness than linguistic problems), which were embarrassing to her. Noted spelling difficulties were explained by slower writing and some lost automaticity in spelling words, as well as errors due to "slips of attention."

Subsequent rehabilitation goals were to (1) use a word-processing program as an aid in writing, as this increased speed, as well as (2) to practice cursive writing skills (which had not previously been attempted, due to avoidance rather than confronting the difficulty). Practicing reading and spelling were to be conducted in a more naturalistic manner, that is, by providing "assignments" simulating university course requirements.

Physical Functioning

LL participated with increasing enthusiasm in the physical training. She complied with the aerobic and weight training program with ease and was motivated to train outside program hours. Similarly, she participated in the dance group and weekly squash activities with great interest. As she was interested in pursuing bicycling as a hobby, cycling lessons were started, guided by the physical therapists. The concluding physical therapy evaluation indicated that right-sided fine motor control and strength, running speed, and general strength and endurance were improved. The subsequent goals of rehabilitation were to support interest in these activities and encourage continued participation after treatment.

Emotional and Social Functioning

While finding the day program interesting and challenging, LL reported difficulties outside of the program, that is, adjustment difficulties in a new environment. As the program progressed, marital difficulties were apparent. She was able to cope, however, by expressing feelings of sadness, frustration, and anger and seeking and receiving emotional support in treatment and from a former social network. Joint therapy was provided by the primary therapist to offer the couple an opportunity to deal with their marital conflict (as both had expressed a desire to clarify concerns with the therapist). It appeared, however, that while amicable in dealing with their frustrations, the couple saw separation as likely.

LL also viewed herself as a person who liked to work independently and found it difficult to adapt to some of the goals of the project group, for example, in making a video in collaboration with others in the group. Her difficulties were due, in part, to her high expectations of the project, which she initially thought should match previous training in film making and frustration in having to compromise expectations because of the relative lack of training of the other group members. She was able to openly discuss these difficulties, however, with the primary therapist, that is, as premorbid tendencies and an expression of a critical attitude toward herself, which allowed for a constructive problem-solving approach with the other group members. In addition, because of the interdisciplinary nature of the treatment team, these difficulties were discussed with other staff members who were able to supplement the primary therapists interventions. In time, LL was also able to recognize various group activities as beneficial in overcoming passivity.

In the group psychotherapy sessions, emphasis is on self-expression and support of each other's life experiences prior and subsequent to brain injury, rather than on group cooperation for task completion, as in the project group. LL showed concern for others and was able to benefit from the group in terms of receiving emotional support. She was particularly concerned about future career choice, feeling uncertain as to whether to continue with her original plans. She maintained an interest in the arts, but even prior to injury had been contemplating a career in photojournalism. Rehabilitation therefore consisted of encouraging LL to explore creative interests, which she had completely abandoned postinjury.

Subsequent rehabilitation goals were: (1) to work on two art projects per week and present them in individual therapy (one musical, one visual); (2) to give a 30-minute weekly musical lesson to the therapist; (3) to access art studios; and (4) to continue marital therapy.

LL also showed increasing self-confidence over time. She was an active participant in the various activities and increased social interaction both within the group and outside of the program, trying to establish new friendships.

Final Phases of Treatment and Follow-up

In the latter part of the rehabilitation, greater emphasis was placed on developing studying skills, as LL was considering returning to university and/or furthering education within the arts, as she became more confident regarding her strengths. Thus, the following was focused upon: (1) planning for use of extra time to compensate for slower speed of processing, and (2) self-evaluation of study methods and "test" results. Specifically, when taking these "tests," she was encouraged to plan ahead for the amount of time to be spent on the various questions to compensate for poor time management. She allowed more time to review answers afterwards, as this improved accuracy.

Trial tests (reading of literature and answering questions about the text and practical application) were held on topics pertinent to future studies. As she had difficulties in managing complex activities (e.g., cooking, planning daily activities, etc.), allowing an extra "half-an-hour" to plan more specifically for them significantly increased efficacy. Continued use was made of the day planner as a memory aid, for example, noting what personally significant events had transpired during the day (especially in conversation). Practice of cursive writing had not been effective in improving speed in this task, and thus use of a computer (typing) proved to be more helpful. This was decided as the approach to be used in the future. When studying, practiced use of the PQRST technique improved encoding and retrieval.

In terms of psychosocial functioning, continued emphasis was placed on encouraging activities outside the home, for example, physical activities and participation in artistic events of interest. Creative projects were continued on a weekly basis. In the latter part of the program, LL was more active socially and showed more interest in others, which was manifested by, for example, maintaining eye contact and strengthening voice projection, and resulted in improved communication skills.

Thus, considerable improvement was noted and self-reported in these areas. Unfortunately, however, just prior to completion of the program her husband requested a divorce, for which LL was distressed but somewhat prepared. Therefore, in the final weeks marital therapy was replaced by individual psychotherapy, which focused on helping LL manage this stressful event. After much discussion of various educational, occupational, and social possibilities, LL decided to travel for a period and to continue studying full time when she returned.

At the time of program completion, although there had been improvements in most areas of cognitive functioning, information-processing speed was still slower than would be expected premorbidly, particularly when exacerbated by task complexity and psychomotor constraints. When fatigued, performance declined. Consequently, the following options were reviewed: (1) continued adequate advance planning for such tasks (as was emphasized in cognitive training), and (2) continued brief rest breaks during the day, as was modeled in the program particularly when working on demanding tasks.

Verbal memory deficits persisted, but if a day planner were consistently used as in the program, functioning was most effective. Study techniques and examination-taking behavior were reviewed for future execution. It was strongly recommended that should she return to university, (1) a laptop computer be used to increase writing speed, and (2) extra time be allowed to complete examinations.

Of particular significance was LL's creative ability. She enjoyed playing the flute and showed excellent abilities in the visual arts. With increasing awareness of these abilities, she decided to pursue these activities in the future. The art projects completed during the program were of a high quality, and artistic skills likely could provide a means of employment. She considered art courses as a means to achieving this end and wanted to continue taking courses and working in the field.

As for psychosocial functioning, in the light of the divorce, she chose to travel with a friend for a period until the university semester started. Her mood was at times dysthymic and she was understandably anxious about the future. She nonetheless evidenced improved self-esteem and a positive attitude toward the challenges ahead. Subsequent to program completion, follow-up treatment was available in the form of monthly group sessions for 6 months and individual sessions (as needed) up until 8 months or more with the primary therapist. For LL, individual follow-up would be made available on return from her travels. Continued physical training was also encouraged because it generated feelings of alertness and relaxation, and allowed for the development of social contacts.

At the 2-year follow-up, LL had completed her university studies (received a BA) and had passed examinations with excellent results. Because of success in this regard, she is currently furthering her education and is planning to work in graphic design. She reports that effective management of cognitive problems also has resulted in improving social contacts and self-confidence.

Thus, 2 years subsequent to treatment, LL described her experience of the program as follows:

> I really liked the way the program was structured . . . each day started out with a general all-person meeting with one talking about a hot topic of news and ending with a stretching exercises. [The program] . . . made us work our brain and body as well as on our communication skills . . . the daily changes in the schedule made it seem varied and less likely for me to get bored or to set myself up in a tight schedule with little or no variation. I started running in the program and it is something that I still do today as it makes me feel well rounded. I especially liked the talks I had with my primary therapist. She made me think hard about what I wanted and ways to go about getting it . . . the treatment I received at the Center was so beneficial and meaningful to the way I live today. When I joined the program I was a person who had serious problems with memory, attention, and executive functions. The Center had me realize [that I had] these problems and found a way for me to reach out and organize my life in thought and practice. I finished my degree with the highest marks possible. Without the Center, I don't think this would have happened. The Center made me feel good about myself as well as giving me the best treatment possible.

In conclusion, LL came to rehabilitation with deficits related to brain injury and with unclear goals for the future, lacking self-confidence and vacillating between anxiety and passivity. The rehabilitation received at the CRBI, rather than being the conclusion of a process, was instead a stepping stone for LL to regain confidence, by identifying strengths and weaknesses, and compensating for them and planning for the future. As such, social isolation decreased and she has been able to take the initiative needed for the future.

Conclusion

LL's case has served as an example of how rehabilitation can be individualized within a structured day program. First, it is important to note that the theoretical foundation of the program provides a structure that is flexible enough for treatment to be individualized. While individual treatment is stressed to ensure that (1) unique needs are addressed, (2) personal support is provided, and (3) development of self-confidence is encouraged, group activities provide a naturalistic setting for broader interaction, enabling students to develop awareness and receive feedback. Furthermore, group participation provides a context of social support and camaraderie for some, while for others it provides a safe social setting in which to explore emerging skills and accuracy of self-evaluation. The rehabilitation process therefore is one in which interventions are modified suitably for the evolution of functioning of each individual, alone and with groups.

Second, and of particular relevance, is to address the cognitive and psychosocial interactions of the individual as comprehensively as possible. This is achieved by not only addressing the student's state prior to injury, but also by exploring resources, limitations, and opportunities within the current context, and by identifying individual hopes of achievement in the present and future.

Third, treatment takes place in a dynamic manner, that is, based on the close collaboration between (1) the student and primary therapist, (2) the primary therapist and the interdisciplinary team, and (3) the primary therapist and the student's broader network, in order to make ongoing feedback consistently available concerning the status of the student. Often in the initial phases of treatment, emphasis is on creating awareness and clarifying experiences, while later in treatment the focus shifts to future planning and the means to achieve these ends. Irrespective of the phase of treatment, however, the relationship with the primary therapist remains one of critical importance, as it provides continuity across the various phases of treatment and between the varied, interactive treatment.

Ultimately, the goal for students of the day program is to develop a satisfying quality of life through continued education, occupation, and improved psychosocial adjustment and physical well-being. As such, it appears that this type of program is an effective means for achieving this end.

References

Caetano, C. & Christensen, A-L. (1997). The design of neuropsychological rehabilitation: The role of neuropsychological assessment. In J. León-Carrión (Ed.), *Neuropsychological rehabilitation—Fundamentals, innovations and directions* (pp. 63–72). Delray Beach, FL: St. Lucie Press.

Christensen, A. L. (1975). *Luria's neuropsychological investigation. Manual and test materials* (1st ed.). New York: Spectrum.

Christensen, A. L. (1989). The neuropsychological investigation as a therapeutic and rehabilitative technique. In D.W. Ellis and A.L. Christensen (Eds.), *Neuropsychological treatment after brain injury* (pp. 127–153). Boston: Kluwer.

Christensen, A-L. & Caetano, C. (1997). Alexander Romanovitsch Luria (1902–1977): Contributions to neuropsychological rehabilitation. *Neuropsychological Rehabilitation, Special Issue 6*, 279–303.

Christensen, A-L. & Caetano, C. (1999). Cognitive neurorehabilitation: A comprehensive approach. In D. T. Stuss, G. Winour, & I. H. Robertson (Eds.) *Neuropsychological rehabilitation in the interdisciplinary team: The postacute stage* (pp. 188–199).

Christensen, A. L. & Teasdale, T. W. (1993). A comprehensive and intensive program for cognitive and psychosocial rehabilitation. In F. J. Stachowiak (Ed.), *Developments in the assessment and rehabilitation of brain-damaged patients* (pp. 465–467) Tubingen, Germany: Gunter Narr Verlag.

Christensen, A. L. & Teasdale, T. W. (1998). Rehabilitation assessment and planning for head trauma rehabilitation. In G. Goldstein and S. R. Beers (Eds.), *Rehabilitation* (pp.171–180). New York: Plenum Press.

Christensen, A. L., Jensen, L. R., & Risberg, J. (1990). Luria's neuropsychological and neurolinguistic theory. *Journal of Neurolinguistics, 4*, 137–154.

Christensen, A. L., Pinner, E. M., Moller Pedersen, P., Teasdale, T. W., & Trexler, L. E. (1992). Psychosocial outcome following individualized neuropsychological rehabilitation of brain damage. *Acta Neurologica Scandinavica, 85*, 32–38.

Deloche, G., North, P., Dellatolas, G., Christensen, A.L., Cremel, N., Passador, A., Dordain, M., & Hannequin, D. (1996). Le handicap des adultes cérébrolésés: le point de vue des patients et de leur entourage. (Point of view of patients and their close relatives on the handicap of brain damaged adults). *Annales de Réadaptation et de Médicine Physique., 39*, 21–29.

Goldstein, K. (1952). Effects of brain damage on personality. *Psychiatry, 15*, 245–260.

Larsen, A., Mehlbye J., & Gortz, M. (1991). *Kan genoptræning betale sig? En analyse af de sociale og okonomiske aspekter ved genoptræning af hjerneskadede. (Does rehabilitation pay? An anaysis of the social and economic aspects of brain injury rehabilitation)* Copenhagen: AKF Forlaget.

Teasdale, T. W., & Christensen, A. L. (1994). Psychosocial outcome in Denmark. In A. L. Christensen and B. P. Uzzell (Eds.), *Brain injury and neuropsychological rehabilitation: International perspectives* (pp. 235–244). Hillsdale, NJ: Lawrence Erlbaum.

Teasdale, T. W., Christensen, A. L. & Pinner, M. (1993). Psychosocial rehabilitation of cranial trauma and stroke patients. *Brain Injury, 7*, 535–542.

Teasdale, T. W., Christensen, A-L., Willmes, K , Deloche, G, Braga, L, Stachowiak, F., Vendrell, J. M., Castro-Caldas, A., Laaksonen, R. K., & Leclercq, M. (1997). Subjective experience in brain injured patients and their close relatives: A European Brain Injury Questionnaire study. *Brain Injury, 11*, 543–563.

Trexler, L. E. & and Helmke, C. (1996). Efficacy of holistic neuropsychological rehabilitation: Progran characertistics and outcome research. In W. Fries (Ed.), *Ambulante und teilstationär Rerehabilitation von hirnverletzten* (pp. 25–39). *(Outpatient rehabilitation for brain injury)* München: W. Zuckschwerdt Verlag.

Appendix A

CRBI Admission and Exclusion Criteria

Admission requirements

- At least 16 years of age
- Brain injury of known etiology
- Completion of the necessary medical treatment for brain injury
- Physical independence (as regards transport and personal hygiene)
- Some possibility of communicating
- Potential for work/education/improvement in life quality

Exclusion criteria

- Current substance abuse
- Chronic, severe, psychiatric condition
- Chronic, severe physical illness

Appendix B

Example of CRBI Day Program Structure

	Tuesday				
9:00–10:00	Morning meeting 1 psychologist, 1 physical therapist, all 15 participants				
10:00–10:15	Break				
10:15–11:00	Physical training group 1 3 physical therapists 5 participants	Cognitive training group 1 1 psychologist 4 participants	Communication group 1 speech and language therapist 4 participants	Individual hour with primary therapist 1 psychologist 1 participant	Individual special education 1 special education therapist 1 participant
11:00–11:15	Break				
11:15–12:00		Group psychotherapy 1 2 psychologists 7 participants	Voice training 1 voice therapist 1 participant	Individual hour with primary therapist 1 psychologist 1 participant	
12:00–1:00	Lunch				
1:00–1:45	Physical training group 2 3 physical therapists 4 participants	Project group 1 2 psychologists 7 participants	Special education: math group 1 special education teacher 3 participants	Individual speech and language therapy 1 speech and language therapist 1 participant	
1:45–2:00	Break				
2:00–2:45		Project group 1 (cont.) 2 psychologists 7 participants	Individual hour with primary therapist 1 psychologist 1 participant		

18

The Delta Group Experience

TBI in France

PIERRE NORTH, ANNE PASSADORI,
AND PAUL MILLEMANN

The Delta Groups

In France a good system exists for the early care of head injuries, thanks to an efficient emergency ambulance service created 20 years ago and a network of neurosurgical departments to receive patients. The rehabilitation and long-term care of such patients has lagged behind developments in some other countries. Few specialized units for head injury patients exist, particularly to assure their follow-up and to facilitate home return (social outcome) and work return.

In the last 10 years or so, with the rapid growth of cognitive neuroscience and behavioral neurology, there has been a movement in neurology in France away from academic studies and toward cognitive, emotional, and behavioral concerns, a development already well established in America and Northern Europe. A group of French neurosurgeons and neurologists—Cohadon, Held, Laplane, Mazaux, and Truelle—who founded "France Traumatisme Cranien," has been of influence, bringing together professionals and families of the patient in this initiative toward assuring a better outcome for head injury patients. Thanks to the aid of the European Brain Injury Society (EBIS), at present presided by Neil Brooks, Great Britain, and of all our European partners, France has been able finally to make progress in this area. We have been able to benefit from an ensemble of programs (BIOMED), initiated by the European Union, that permits meetings, exchanges, and development of measurement tools, workshops, and specialized education for the care of head injury patients.

In essence, a transitional program was born in a structure created 50 years ago to care for victims of World War II. This structure, unique in France and intended to aid the integration of war victims, was designed from its conception to receive head injury patients with the aid

PIERRE NORTH, ANNE PASSADORI, AND PAUL MILLEMANN • The Mulhouse Center for Readaptation, 68093 Mulhouse, Cedex, France.

International Handbook of Neuropsychological Rehabilitation, edited by Christensen and Uzzell. Kluwer Academic/ Plenum Publishers, New York, 2000.

of three services: functional rehabilitation, professional counseling, and further education, working together in a coordinated manner in conjunction with special knowledge of rehabilitation neurology.

The Mulhouse Rehabilitation Center

The experience acquired at the Mulhouse Rehabilitation Center has served with others as a basis for the creation and design of 17 experimental evaluation units for social rehabilitation and professional orientation [Unité d'Evaluation, de Réinsertion et d'Orientation Sociale et Professionnelle (UEROS)], distributed across France and benefiting from government support, since 1996. One of the experimental evaluation units is the transitional program, named Delta by the patients, the elaboration of which has as its objective the medical independence and social autonomy of the patients with the aid of their families and a team of professionals. In order to achieve this, priority has been given, not to the elementary activities of daily life (eating, dressing, washing) or to medical care, but to cognitive troubles, psychoaffective difficulties, and behavioral problems.

The Delta programs were intended to be transitional in the sense of assisting the transition from medical dependence to social, familial independence. In other words, the patient was no longer considered as a clinical entity, but as a person to whom one must listen, in order to help him or her find a place once more in the family, the neighborhood, and the workplace, both as a person and as a citizen belonging to a community. For this, it was necessary to evaluate the repercussions of trauma on his or her cerebral condition, to analyze the cognitive disorders due to lesions, to evaluate psychoaffective problems (any behavioral modifications observed in different contexts), to note handicaps, to study at the same time premorbid personality, present personality, potential motivation, and strengths and weaknesses, in order to create a sense of life and to assist in acceptance of the current condition; that is, to counsel him or her in accepting long-term disability and to build a new life, compatible with his or her hopes and to make available the potential for carrying out a realistic project (Christensen, 1994).

Thus, the objective of the Delta program was to withdraw the patient from a purely medical context in order to reinsert the individual in the family, giving once again the personal dimension to relations with others (Mazaux & Destaillats, 1994).

The Delta program functions as a support group, the structure of which is as close as possible to the patient's family, with its rules of solidarity, values, responsibility, and rituals. The patient works in small groups on problems of behavior, practicing community living skills, cognitive remediation, and training in activities of daily living. He or she learns to interract, to forge a new relationship with others, and to discover potential to rebuild existence, in order to face the unexpected problems of life.

Selection Criteria

The patients entered the pilot study on average 28 months after injury (range, 12–36 months), and the patients and their families were selected and evaluated according to the following criteria :

1. Patient selection characteristics :
   a. General guidelines: individuals who are confused in their cognitive functioning, but are fairly cooperative and require only daytime supervision.

b. Specific admission criteria :
   - Glasgow Coma Scale, ≤ 8; Glasgow Outcome Coma Scale, 1–3.
   - Adolescent and predominantly young adult patients (16 to 50 years of age) who require assistance in learning to become functionally independent in the home.

c. Patients have previous evidence of continued and progressive improvement in functional areas (i.e., speech, cognition). Patients have sufficient cognitive and personality skills to be able to participate in small group interaction within four weeks of entry into the program. Educational levels are between 9 to 16 years of schooling with a mean of 11½ years.

2. Family involvement :
   a. At least one family member who is in close contact with the patient postdischarge must agree to actively participate in the program. Active participation means monthly attendance at group meetings and regular attendance at family consultation meetings.
   b. Families and patients sign a contract and:
      - Are contacted weekly by a call from the case manager.
      - Are given monthly program reports.
      - Are provided with an education program.

Patients are evaluated over a period of 3 days, 3 months before their enrollment in the Delta program, and over a 3-day period, 3 months after the end of the program. The program lasts 3 months, with patients being treated 5 days a week.

Patient Population

We have followed 38 head injury patients who have been included in the Delta programs between 1993 and 1997, of whom 32 had traumatic brain injury (TBI). In the interest of having a more homogeneous group, five patients with stroke and one with a tumor were excluded from the present study.

The 32 TBI patients included in this report consisted of 31 males and 1 female, aged 20 to 45, years with a mean age of 28 years and the following age ranges: 60% were between 20 to 25 years of age; 30% were between 26 to 45 years of age; and less than 10% were between 46 to 50 years of age.

Patient Evaluation

The evaluation covers a number of fields.

Medical

Evaluation was per the EBIS document (Truelle, Brooks, Potagas, & Joseph, 1994) and consisted of analysis of the parameters of the gravity of the trauma (Glasgow scale, duration of the post traumatic amnesia, of coma, and of cerebral lesions), the topography of the lesions, the evaluation of the neurological sequelae (sensation, motor, cerebellar, linguistic, epileptic), the orthopedic and pulmonary sequelae, evaluation of the current pharmacological treatments, and the examination of factors involved in functional restoration (prelesional, lesional and postlesional) (Stein, Brailowsky, & Will, 1995).

Functional Capacities

Basic activity of daily living was evaluated by application of a purpose-designed questionnaire devised by the occupational therapists. Practical daily life skills were assessed with the competency rating scale (Prigatano, 1986); a tool designed for judging very practical skills given to the patient and the relatives (this scale is scored on a six-point scale on 30 items) before and after the Delta program.

The McAuley outcome scale developed by Girard *et al.,* (1996) defined the level of productivity based on the amount of independence demonstrated in the given activity setting versus the amount of assistance required. Outcome was operationally defined for two activity settings (home or work) with six levels of productivity for each (see Table 1).

Cognitive

The focus has been the objective specification of cognitive functioning. Neuropsychological tests have been employed to explore areas such as attention and concentration, memory, language, problem solving, and executive functions (Lezak, 1987).

The evaluation of the different cognitive functions (Brooks, 1989) is carried out by means of a relatively detailed neuropsychological assessment (Table 2), in order not only to understand the degree of the problems but to help choose the compensatory strategies for restoration of the individual in the retraining workshops. It also is used to select prognostic factors for social reintegration and return to work and to evaluate cognitive troubles in the genesis of the psychoaffective problems and the adaptive capacity of the patient.

In the present study, neuropsychological evaluation took place about 28 months after the brain injury, when spontaneous recovery had more or less finished. Whatever the domain under exploration, all patients were evaluated just before their entry into the care of the Delta group and reevaluated 6 months later (see Table 2). This procedure, apart from its clinical feasability, avoided more or less the effect of test–retest and spontaneous recovery that may interfere with therapeutic treatment. These objective specifications have been completed by subjective reports and behavior ratings as a means of investigating cognitive dysfunction.

TABLE 1. Evaluation Scales for Neurological Status and Outcome after TBI with McAuley Rehabilitation Institute Outcome Scale

Level	Home	Work
1	Does not perform any household duties	Does not perform volunteer work activities
2	Performs at least 5–25 % of household duties	Volunteer or sheltered workshop
3	Performs at least 26–69 % of household duties; supervised living, i.e., foster care	Supported employment, i.e., paid employment with on site vocational assistance or job coach
4	Performs at least 70–89% of household duties; structured independent living, i. e., apartment	Independent paid employment at lower than premorbid level
5	Performs household duties independent at premorbid level (90–100 %)	Employed at premorbid vocational level
6	Performs household duties independent at greater than premorbid level	Employed at higher than premorbid level

TABLE 2. Results of the Neuropsychological Evaluation of the Patients Before Entry into Study and at Study Completion

Neuropsychological measure	Number of patients	Mean before Delta program	Mean after Delta program	Significance P value of differences
Cognition (WAIS-R)				
Verbal IQ	16	83.5	86.5	< 0.01
Performance	16	69.6	76.38	< 0.001
General IQ	16	76.61	81.31	< 0.01
Information	16	6.0	7.6	< 0.01
Comprehension	16	7.4	8.3	< 0.05
Pictures Arrangement	16	5.50	7.84	< 0.001
Memory Verbal (WMS-R)				
Verbal	19	73.4	89.5	< 0.01
Visual	19	9.7	100.1	< 0.001
General	19	78.8	86.6	< 0.01
Rivermead	22	17.1	18.6	NS
Grober and Bushke free recall words	19	48.88	54.11	NS
Rey's 15 words (total of the 5 trials)	26	39.4	45.3	< 0.001
Rey's 15 signs (total of the 5 trials)	23	28.7	33.4	< 0.05
Benton Recognition	22	11.3	12.5	< 0.001
Attention				
Trail making test A	17	76.8 sec	71.3 sec	NS
Trail making test B	17	158.1 sec	139.3 sec	NS
Executive functions				
Tower of London, Series 5 (normal)	13	9.75	8.00	< 0.05
Tower of London, Series 5 (negative cue)	13	11.9	9.2	< 0.05
Stroop test	22	46.8	55.7	< 0.001
Wisconsin (series)	14	5.35	5.50	NS

Clearly, neuropsychological tests do not fully reflect the significance of the disorders as felt by the patient in everyday environment or their effect on daily life. For this reason, in addition to these tests, we have used questionnaires that were submitted to the patient and to a close family member who witnesses day-to-day life. Using these questionnaires, one can often uncover situations in which a cognitive or memory deficit may exist that would not be revealed by other means of evaluation. The questionnaires are:

1. The Van der Linden memory questionnaire (Van der Linden, Wyns, Coyette, von Frenckell, & Seron, 1988) is a French language adaptation, consisting of 64 questions subdivided into 10 sections, with values from 0 to 6.
2. The Newcastle Questionnaire (Bradley, Welch, & Skilbeck, 1993) is divided into four sections investigating cognitive ability, affective response, involvement in social activities, and role in the family. Both the patient and a close relative are asked to complete the questionnaire before and after discharge.

Psychoaffective

Anxiety, emotional troubles, mood changes, behavior, and subjective experience of well-being have been investigated with the Hamilton scales (Hamilton, 1960) (anxiety and depression), the Neurobehavioral Rating Scale (NRS) (Levin *et al.,* 1987), whose purpose is to assess behavioral sequelae (this scale is scored on a seven point scale on 27 items), and the European Brain Injury Questionnaire (EBIQ) for patients and relatives (Teasdale *et al.,* 1997). The EBIQ is a self-report questionnaire concerning subjective experience of cognitive, emotional, and social difficulties scales relating to eight specific areas of functioning, together with a global scale of 63 items that proved to be reliable and valid for brain-injured groups.

Patient Program

After carrying out this evaluation with different team members, a "Life Project" was elaborated. This is an expression of the patients' goals, which are regarded as important and possible to achieve reintegration. A program of cognitive training for the development of compensation strategies is then devised.

The basic part of the individual patient training consists of an intensive, personalized cognitive stimulation with memory, attention, and ability-to-reason workshops. The time devoted to each per week is as follows :

1. Memory training, two $1^1/_2$-hour sessions.
2. Attention training, two 30-minute sessions.
3. Problem solving, one 2-hour session.

Group training is essentially devoted to daily life activities (social independence, communication, and reintegration into real life), sport activities (group and individual), and creative activities such as theatre, music, and puppets. The time devoted to each sector per week is:

1. Daily life activities, one $2^1/_2$-hour session.
2. Social independence, one 2-hour session.
3. Communication, one 2-hour session.
4. Sport, two $1^1/_2$-hour sessions.
5. Creative activities, three 2-hour sessions.

Psychotherapy constitutes the heart of the treatment (Prigatano, 1986) and is conceived as the work of a community. The group functions as a unique psychic entity. The therapist manages the interaction and the communication between group members in a therapeutic process. Inadequate behavior is considered as a disorder of social interaction. These sessions have the following components: scenarios, role-plays, simulations, allowing patients to express their emotions, and observation of their coping strategy, which is analyzed, explained, and reinforced. Different familial roles such as self-image, autocriticism, and self-esteem are also treated. Most of the sessions are filmed and conducted by two therapists. As these sessions progress, we attempt to determine the psychopathological factors that play a role in the social and professional reintegration.

In addition to this basic program, individual support activities are offered as a function of the patients' needs: physiotherapy, occupational therapy, speech therapy, individual psychotherapy, computer-assisted reinforcement of attention, logical reasoning, and problem resolution are available.

During the program, the patient is confronted with the following situations, either in the center, in an independent apartment, or with his or her family on weekends:

1. Managment of daily life (budgeting, shopping, preparing meals, hygiene, housework).
2. Managment of social life (administrative tasks, mail, telephone, diaries, information devices).
3. Adaptation to the urban environment (use of public transport, train, bus, shopping in town, driving a car).

The desired goal of these different model situations is to confront the patient with the realities of the environment with the support of the group and the professionals. One team member is designated as "case manager," with the responsibility of following the project of a patient and its adjustment as a function of difficulties encountered in different situations. A contract is signed between the different parties engaging the participants to work toward the realization of the project, for the duration of the project, which is 3 months. The program takes place over 5-day periods, with an average of 5 to 7 hours of intensive work per day, over the 3 months.

This transdisciplinary team working with each patient is composed of the following personnel:

1. Full time: a physician and a physical therapist.
2. Part time: a neuropsychiatrist, three physical therapists, two speech therapists, a vocational psychotherapist, a neuropsychologist, a clinical psychologist, four recreational therapists, and three nurses.
3. Case management is for a variable period of time, with a possibility of follow-up at 1 to 2 years for patients who have returned home, 2 to 4 years for patients who have returned to work, and more if behavioral problems persist.

Results

The results provide information about neuropsychological functioning and adjustment in the home and work environment.

(See Table 2 regarding the neuropsychological outcome.) Not all the patients were subjected to the totality of the evaluation tests. Rather, these were applied as a function of the individual needs of each patient to construct his or her personal project. The analysis of the data was carried out using the Student test for paired samples when the variances were homogeneous. When the variances were heterogeneous, the Wilcoxon *T*-test was applied. For the analysis of qualitative data (Wisconsin Card Sorting Test [WCST-]Tower of London), the Sign test was used.

The analysis of the results indicate significant progress in the following categories: speed of information processing, verbal and visual learning, planning strategies, and the control of impulsive behavior. These observed results are above and beyond spontaneous recovery (evaluations were carried out on average 18 months after the trauma). Certain results, such as WCST and Grober and Bushke free word recall, are not significant because the values were near to normal at the time of evaluation for study entry. The memory performance results need perhaps to be treated with caution due to implicit memory effects (probable test–retest in the Wechsler Memory Scale-Revised [WMS-R] and Rey's 15 signs). Progress in learning tasks, however, is seen thanks to the use of an alternate version of the test: Rey's 15 words and the Benton test.

Return Home Outcome

The data for the McAuley outcome scale were obtained for 32 TBI subjects. These data demonstrate a clear positive result. Before the initiation of care, most of the patients were dependent and capable of carrying out only a few domestic tasks: 5–25% (level 2) for 12 patients, 26–69 % (level 3) for 11 patients. After 3 months of stimulation and care, 11 patients progressed to categories 2 to 3, and 9 patients progressed to category 5, an illustration of a flexibility and an adaptation to the environment and of a certain learning transfer from one group to another.

Marital status changed during the study. At the beginning, there were 23 unmarried patients, 5 married patients, 2 divorced patients, and 2 patients with common-law partner. At the end of the program, the following changes were noted: one unmarried patient married, one patient entered a relationship with a common-law partner, one of the married patients divorced, and two patients separated from common law partners. The two divorced patients were still divorced.

Return to Work Outcome

The results of the return to work of this group (see Table 3) are particularly favorable, since 25% started working again full time and 20% started part-time work, for a total of 45% of patients working. Only 30% or so did not work at all. Twenty-five percent are being evaluated for their professional orientation, following new job training courses or work in protected workshops.

Discussion

One must interpret these results with caution, for they depend on many variables,. Overall, however, the data show improvement with the Delta group experience.

The neuropsychological findings show improvement in areas of intellectual, memory, and executive function, but not in attention–concentration. This could be due to the emphasis on functional and social factors in the program structure. Both home and work situations become more satisfactory. After treatment, patients perform more household and work activities. The findings also show a tendency of patients to move to a higher functional level in the home, sug-

TABLE 3. Professional Reintegration, Return to Work (RTW) of Patients at Study Completion

RTW Catergory	Number
Full time	8
Part time	7
Work training	3
Sheltered workshop	2
Prevocational assessment program	3
No work	9
Total	32

gesting a likelihood of returning to employment at or near a premorbid level. Changes in marital status were minimal.

Almost three quarters of the patients returned to work, and remarkably, 25% of those were employed full time. This is especially remarkable since the employment laws in France at present favor part-time work in order to reduce unemployment. However, the last Delta group has been evaluated only for 4 months. Normally, a year is required to judge the success of a continued work return. Early work (Oppenheim-Gluckmann *et al.,* 1997) has provided evidence that a number of issues (physical limitations, family support, psychosocial factors) influence evaluations for social reintegration and return to work. Despite these factors, the Delta group experience demonstrates evidence of what can be accomplished with integration of cognitive, emotional, and behavioral concerns when patients, families, and professionals work together toward the same goals.

This work is the product of numerous contacts mentioned in the introduction, but also the result of visits to H. Levin and G. Prigatano in the United States, of discussions with D. Stein, and of a continuous participation within the European Standardized Computerized Assessment Procedure for the Evaluation and Rehabilitation of Brain-Damaged Patients (ESCAPE) program. None of it would ever have happened, however, without the understanding and ever-friendly help of Professor A.-L. Christensen and her team in Copenhagen.

References

Bradley, V.-A., Welch, J.-L., & Skilbeck, C.-E. (1993). The Newcastle Study: Background, Subject, and Method. In *Cognitive retraining using microcomputers* (pp. 210–227) Hillsdale, NJ: Lawrence Erlbaum.

Brooks, N. (1989). Closed head trauma: Assessing the common cognitive problems. In M. D. Lezak (Ed.), *Assessment of the behavioral consequences of head trauma* (pp. 61–85). New York: Alan R. Liss.

Christensen, A. L. (1994). Visions for rehabilitation. In A. L. Christensen & B. P. Uzzell (Eds.), *Brain injury and neuropsychological rehabilitation* (pp. 293–299) Hillsdale, NJ: Lawrence Erlbaum.

Girard, D., Brown, J., Burnett-Stolnack, M., Hashimoto, N., Hier-Wellmer, S., Perlman, O. Z., & Siegerman, C. (1996). The relationship of neuropsychological status and outcome following traumatic brain injury. *Brain Injury, 10,* 663–676.

Hamilton, M. (1960). A rating scale for depression. *Journal of Neurology NeuroSurgery and Psychiatry, 23,* 56–62.

Levin, H.-S., High, W.-M., Goethe, K.-E., Sisson, R.-A., Overall, J.-E., Rhoades, H.-M., Eisenberg, H.-M., Kalisky, Z., & Gary, H.-E., (1987). The neurobehavioral rating scale: Assessment of the behavioral sequelae of head injury by the clinician. *Journal of Neurology NeuroSurgery and Psychiatry, 50,* 183–193

Lezak, M. (1987). Assessment for rehabilitation planning. In M. J. Meier, A. L. Benton, & L. Diller (Eds.), *Neuropsychological rehabilitation* (pp. 41–58). New-York: Churchill Livingstone.

Mazaux, J. M., & Destaillats, J. M. (1994). Des troubles cognitifs aux troubles comportementaux, problèmes d'évaluation. In C. Bergego & Ph. Azouvi (Eds.), *Neuropsychologie des traumatismes crâniens graves de l'adulte* (pp. 207–221) Paris: Les Ateliers de Garches.

Oppenheim-Gluckman, H., North, P., Dumond, J. J., Fayol, P., Bouvat, M. F., & Missonnier, P. (1997). Psychopathology, professional and social reinsertion in brain injury. *Poster Session Second World Congress on TBI.* Seville.

Prigatano, G. (1986). *Neuropsychological rehabilitation after brain injury.* Baltimore: The Johns Hopkins University Press.

Stein, D. G., Brailowsky, S., & Will, B. (1995). *Brain repair.* New York: Oxford University Press.

Teasdale, T. W., Christensen, A.-L., Willmes, K., Deloche, G., Braga, L., Stachowiak, F., Vendrell, J.-M., Castro-Caldas, A., Laaksonen, R.-K., & Leclercq, M. (1997) Subjective experience in brain–injured patients and their close relatives: A European Brain Injury Questionnaire study. *Brain Injury, 11,* 543–563.

Truelle, J. L., Brooks, N., Potagas, C., & Joseph P. A. (1994). A European chart for evaluation of patients with traumatic brain injury. In A. L. Christensen & B. P. Uzzell (Eds.), *Brain injury and neuropsychological rehabilitation* (pp. 281–291). Hillsdale, NJ: Lawrence Erlbaum.

Van der Linden, M., Wyns, C., Coyette, F., von Frenckell, R., & Seron, X. (1989). Editest Bruxelles. Le Q.A. M. Questionnaire d'Auto-Evaluation de la Mémoire (pp 1–28). Personal communication.

19

Neuropsychological Pediatric Rehabilitation

LÚCIA WILLADINO BRAGA
AND ALOYSIO CAMPOS DA PAZ, JR.

Background

The child is not a miniature adult. Decades after Piaget proved this elementary yet revolutionary discovery, many areas of medicine still struggle to view the child as a singular, unique patient with needs and problems that are specific to the stages of development long ago surpassed by the adult. Highly significant differences, not only from neuroanatomical and neurophysiological perspectives, but familial, social, and cultural as well, contribute to the fundamental need for treating the child within a global perspective that encompasses the elements essential to this specialized focus.

Studies conducted with adults generate parameters and help delineate and establish methods that fail to adequately serve the brain, which is in the initial phases of development. The central nervous system's (CNS) patterns of recovery and compensation differ greatly between adult and child; thus, the consequences of a malformation or trauma to the CNS in the maturation process impacts on that young brain in vastly different ways.

Anatomical Aspects

The Brain

The brain of a newborn accounts for 15% of the infant's total body weight; in adulthood, it is only 3%. At birth, the brain generally weighs between 350 and 400 grams (24% of the size of an adult brain), and it grows rapidly until attaining maturity, reaching 1000 grams during the first year of life; 75% of the total weight of an adult brain by the end of the second year of life;

LÚCIA WILLADINO BRAGA AND ALOYSIO CAMPOS DA PAZ, JR. • The SARAH Network of Hospitals for the Locomotor System, 70.330-150 Brasilia, Brazil.

International Handbook of Neuropsychological Rehabilitation, edited by Christensen and Uzzell.
Kluwer Academic/ Plenum Publishers, New York, 2000.

and by the sixth year of life, the brain arrives at 90% of its adult weight (Parker, 1990). During its first year, the brain's anatomical development includes increase in size, branching out of neuroprocesses, production of glial cells, and the growth of myelin (Peacock, 1986).

Myelinization

At birth, myelin exists in posterior, frontal, and parietal lobes; in the immediate neonatal period, it spreads to the occipital lobes (geniculocalcarine system). The frontal and parietal lobes myelinate throughout the course of the first year of postnatal life. The largest part of the brain's myelinization is completed at the end of the second year of life (Parker, 1990). The prefrontal cortex matures relatively late. A small part of the myelinization continues and is completed at the end of the second decade of life (Katzman & Pippius, 1973). The brain continues to mature anatomically and physiologically throughout the development process; it becomes increasingly complex and undergoes biochemical changes linked to its maturity (Norton, 1972), as well as synaptic and dendritic changes.

Neuroimaging and the Developing Brain

Over the last few years, the advancements in neuroimaging have permitted a greater understanding of some of the neuropsychological and/or motor disturbances in children. If we view the higher mental functions as a complex functional system, the relation between brain imaging and clinical findings are very different from those found in an adult brain, with respect to both malformation and trauma, even outside of a direct anatomoclinical correlation.

The cases we have chosen to describe may provide justification. The computed tomographic (CT) scan of a 14-year-old girl reveals a significant poroencephaly in the right hemisphere, with an absence of a large area of the brain (Fig. 1). Although this adolescent has mild hemiplegia on the right, she managed to achieve all of the milestones of gross motor development within the standard time period, had normal speech development, and has been well adapted in a regular school. A detailed neuropsychological exam revealed mild problems in concentration and difficulties in dealing with complexities. However, these disturbances are at a level that, at the time have not affected the child's scholastic and social performance.

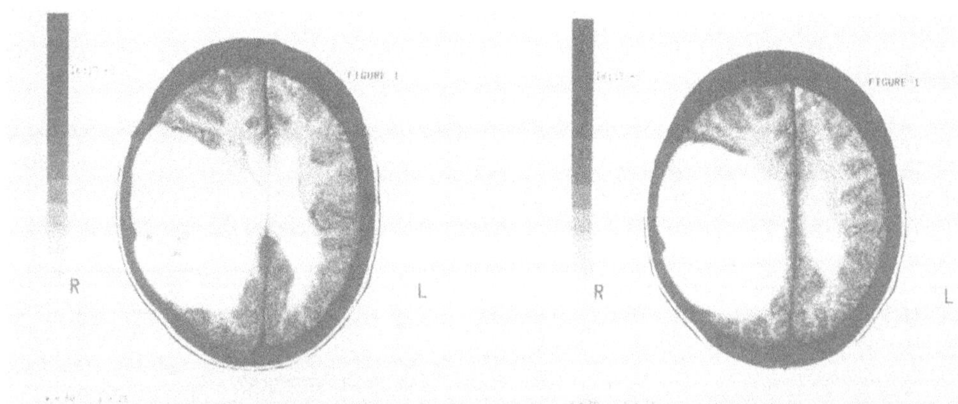

FIGURE 1. Axial CT image: Extensive right frontal parietal cavitation, in ample contact with the lateral ventricle. Presentation of gray and white matter in borders (porencephaly).

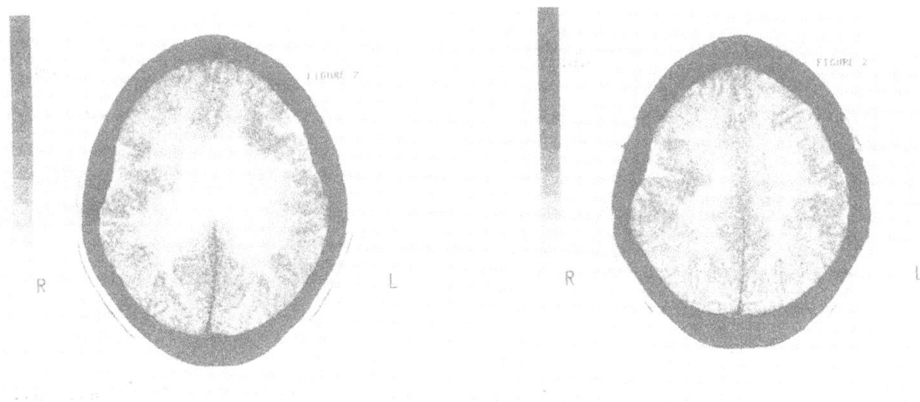

FIGURE 2. Axial CT image: Plane that extends from the cortex to the ventricular wall, covered with gray matter (schizencephaly) in right frontal parietal and left frontal regions.

On the other hand, we can observe in this case of neuronal migration error in a 15-year-old boy with schizencephaly in the right frontal parietal and left frontal regions (Fig. 2), who despite an injury that in neuroimaging exams appears smaller than the aforementioned case, presents notable delays in language acquisition, spastic tetraplegia, and significant mental retardation.

A vast majority of children who are born with poroencephaly or schizencephaly present hemiplegia and some degree of neuropsychological disturbance. Nevertheless, motor and neuropsychological involvement occurs in varying degrees of severity and are not directly related to the extent of the injury.

In children with cerebral palsy due to perinatal anoxia, CT scans were found that did not have any radiological findings and a clinical state of severe spastic tetraplegia, with an absence of voluntary movements, speech, and verbal comprehension.

Nine cases of schizencephaly and 12 of poroencephaly were analyzed. It was observed that the cognitive and motor sequelae were greater in schizencephaly, although in poroencephaly there is absence of a larger area of the brain.

These are but some of the examples that show that although neuroimaging findings in traumatic brain injury (TBI) cases could be correlated with repercussions in the child's daily life, they do not apply in a majority of the cases.

Neuronal Plasticity

Part 1 of this volume addresses neuronal plasticity and its mechanisms at length. Thus, in this chapter, we will make but a few comments on the effects of plasticity on the initial phases of the development process.

The main transformations that occur during the brain's embryonic and fetal development have been recognized for almost a century. However, studies on the subadjacent cellular occurrences in specific segments of the brain, their interconnections, and neuronal plasticity are far more recent.

The nervous system begins with a flat, thin plane of cells on the dorsal surface of the developing embryo (the neural plate); this tissue then forms an elongated and hollow structure (the neural tube). Three protuberances emerge from the edge of the tube, which are the genesis of the three main parts of the brain: the forebrain, midbrain, and endbrain (Jacobson, 1978).

The development of the brain takes place in eight main stages: (1) the induction of the neural plate, (2) the localized proliferation of the cells, (3) the migration of the cells from the location at which they were generated to the region where they will stay, (4) the aggregation of the cells that will come to form the identifiable parts of the brain, (5) the differentiation of immature neurons, (6) the establishment of connections between neurons, (7) the selective death of specific cells, and (8) the elimination of some of the connections established initially in exchange for the creation of new connections (Finger, 1978).

Once the boundaries of the developing nervous system's principal regions have been demarcated, its plasticity becomes progressively limited with each new stage of development. For example, every neural plate's upper cephalic extremity initially starts out as a primitive field-ocular area from which the forebrain and the eye's neural region will eventually develop. If a small portion of the ectodermal tissue is removed during this stage, the defect is quickly corrected by the proliferation of neighboring cells, and the development of both the forebrain and the eye continues normally. However, if the same were to occur during a more advanced stage, a permanent defect would result in either the forebrain or the eye's neural region, depending on the exact location where the tissue was extracted (Porter, 1988). Plasticity and functional recovery are much more effective during the early stages (Kujala *et al.*, 1997). The notion that time was the key element in the correlation between damage and development of the CNS evolved. In other words, the length of time lapsed from the onset of the problem came to be seen as the essential link between the injury and its consequences.

Rapin (1989) affirms that pre- and perinatal injury to the left hemisphere rarely results in aphasia in the child, yet adults suffering a lesion in the same area frequently sustain permanent aphasia as a consequence. She also stresses that plasticity is generally limited, even during early childhood, and is proportionally related to the importance of the location and the extent of the injury. Various authors (Parker, 1990; Maegaki *et al.*, 1997) state that the postinjury changes occur more freely in infancy and probably lessen with age; nevertheless, he emphasizes the importance of recognizing the limits of plasticity.

Life Experiences and Familial, Social, and Cultural Relationships of the Child

Head injury could affect the most varied human functions, such as the bases of action, adaptation, knowledge acquisition, communication, memory, concentration, judgment, and emotion. When a child sustains a trauma to the brain, he or she has had less life experience, learning bases, and social interaction, although still in the stages of acquiring knowledge and broadening his or her social relationships.

The child's place within the family structure is also different from that of an adult's. From the moment the child is born, his or her parents begin to discover ways of relating to that son or daughter, and thus in one form or another stimulate his or her development. During their child's infancy, the parents are involved in the teaching–learning process and each new acquisition is on some level mutually gratifying. Head injury abruptly interrupts the development process and leads to the loss of skills that were already acquired. For the family, the acute phase postinjury is usually a stressful period. However, time, commitment, meaningful interaction, and a degree of disposition for the stimulation of neurodevelopment should continue among the family members, especially when the family is given some type of emotional support.

These variables are relevant in the rehabilitation of the child with head injury because in addition to the organic compensation that might occur in the brain (neuroplasticity), the child can develop strategies of action for the attainment of functional objectives (Rapin, 1989; Posner, Digirolano & Fernandez-Duquel, 1997). Vygotsky (1993) argued that development that has been complicated by a deficiency may result in a creative process (physical and psychological). A restructuring of the adaptive functions, such as transposition, substitution, and equalization, prompted by the disadvantage, could lead to the creation of roundabout paths to development. This does not mean, however, that the child is capable of overcoming all of his or her difficulties. The degree of compensatory mechanisms depends on the organic injury and the success of his or her subsequent social adaptation, and the results range from excellent to very poor (Vygotsky, 1993).

Traumatic Brain Injury in the Child

Throughout the period of growth and development, the child may sustain varying degrees of TBI. Most head injuries are often not noticed during infancy; incidents of mild trauma frequently result in an overemphasis on physiological functioning, so much so that with a considerable improvement in the sensory and motor areas doctors may ignore cognitive problems that will become more accentuated in the future.

Head injury might also affect the acquisition of new skills. An evaluation conducted at a given age often fails to take into account those functions that are not ordinarily developed at that specific age. Abilities that are still being evolved, such as reading, could suffer greater damage than those that have already been well consolidated. If the injury occurs at an age when the child is not yet expected to be able to read, then systematic evaluations must be conducted continuously to ascertain whether or not the child will have developmental problems with this skill at a later date. Many of the neuropsychological deficits resulting from mild injuries are only perceived later in the development, when poor performance in school signals that something is wrong.

Trauma to the brain could, in varying degrees, affect diverse functions that have repercussions on the child's daily life. Depending on the location of the injury, changes in the muscular tonus could result with the emergence of spasticity or hypotonia of hemiplegic, diplegic, or tetraplegic distribution. In some instances, the child may suffer gait limitations, complete loss of walking, or the need for support apparatuses (such as walkers or crutches). Primitive reflexes could become impaired.

With injuries affecting the cerebellum, balance difficulties, tremors, and dysarthric speech generally occur. Even in children who present no apparent severe motor problems (such as loss of walking, difficulties in tasks of construction) an inability to pick up a ball, clumsiness, poor fine motor coordination, slowness in using a pencil, and mild balance disturbances can be observed.

When they are not evaluated with precision, motor deficits could oftentimes lead to the impression that the child has impaired mental abilities or sensory deficiencies, even if he or she does not. Movement deficits could affect social relationships and self-esteem, in addition to possibly having a negative bearing on school adaptation or scholastic performance. Hearing and sight disturbances, or even total loss of either function, could result from TBI; thus, the learning process, on a global scope, may be seriously affected.

The child with brain injury is generally slower in reacting to visuomotor, visuospatial, spatial dexterity, and tasks involving the processing of visual and verbal information. They also experience difficulties in dealing with information of greater complexity; consequently, as the child advances from one school grade to the next and the quantity of information and breadth of learning stimuli increases, a decline in performance in relation to his or her peers is often observed.

The concept of cognition is very broad and is given varying definitions by the numerous schools of thought within neuropsychology. Nevertheless, it is observed that even children with mild TBI have greater difficulties in problem-solving activities and do not acquire knowledge with the same ease as do other children. The administration of a broad and all-encompassing neuropsychological exam immediately following the injury is crucial in order to obtain a baseline for the follow-up on and accompaniment of future performance.

According to Ylvisaker (1989), memory deficit is the most common cognitive alteration resulting from mild head injury. Concentration problems are also significant. Learning difficulties could be partially attributed to distractibility, lack of persistence, and impulsiveness (Ewing-Cobbs, Fletcher, Landry, & Levin, 1985).

If the injury occurs before the child is 2 years of age, regardless of the hemisphere, the child will nevertheless be able to speak, albeit with possible delays. The diffuse injuries that occur during an early stage are more impairing than the focal ones. In the preschool child, head injury could lead to delay or impairment of language acquisition and development. However, adolescents who suffer injury after having acquired more substantial knowledge and skills have deficit patterns that could be considered similar to those of adults (Jordan, Ozanne, & Murdoch, 1988), although recovery appears to be swifter than that of the adult (Parker, 1990). Deficits in communication and comprehension should be meticulously analyzed.

A vast majority of children who sustain a head injury after having completed 3 years of age present emotional problems. Psychiatric disturbances are more common after a severe or moderate injury than after a mild one (Rutter, Chadwick, & Shaffer, 1983). Personality changes in general are more pronounced in the child than in the adult. The inability to carry out certain activities, coupled with problems in social acceptance, could contribute to the onset of depression.

Head injury could lead to lack of inhibitions and socially unacceptable behavior, irritability, impulsiveness, aggressiveness, low frustration threshold, poor motivation, lack of initiative, and poor goal orientation. Members of the family and school community should be given tools for dealing with this type of problem; support and assistance are also necessary.

Neuropsychological Pediatric Rehabilitation at the SARAH Network in Brazil

The SARAH Network

The SARAH Network of Hospitals for the Locomotor System is a fully federally funded institution that cares for patients with diseases of the locomotor system and has four large hospital complexes in full operation. They are located throughout metropolitan regions in Brazil: Brasília, Salvador, Belo Horizonte, and São Luís. Four additional facilities are presently under construction or in the final stages of planning. An architectonic proposal dominates the physical structure of all the network hospitals. At SARAH, the person is treated first as an individual, *then* as a patient. This humanistic approach is applied within an environment that is designed to serve as a parallel support for the work conducted by the staff.

The SARAH network also has a university for graduate work in rehabilitation sciences and a technology center for the construction of hospital facilities and the development of hospital and rehabilitation equipment. The network houses 800 beds and conducts over 9 million procedures annually. It treats all of the diseases of the locomotor system and consequently a large number of children and adults with brain injury.

Over the course of the last 5 years, the SARAH-Brasília hospital admitted 2386 children with brain injury. Some of these began their treatment at SARAH while still in the acute stage; however, since the SARAH Network is primarily focused is on rehabilitation, the majority of these cases are referred to the network after the initial phase at intensive care units of general hospitals. All of the children treated have some type of motor deficit and generally are severe or moderate cases of TBI.

Rehabilitation of the Child with Brain Injury

Principles

The SARAH Network has guiding principles that govern its rehabilitation work:

- **Understand** that child as a human being who is still in the stages of discovery; a small "researcher" learning about the world, who, at a given moment, was forced to confront an injury.
- **Create** a pediatric rehabilitation program based on a perception of the child as both the subject and object of his or her own recovery process and not as the object on which techniques and methods are applied.
- **Improve** the quality of life of the child undergoing rehabilitation, with a program that merges different areas of knowledge, aimed at the primary goal of offering the child a greater chance to actively partake of community and society.
- **Simplify** techniques and procedures; simplification is the synthesis of complexity: "one cannot simplify that which one does not understand."
- **Act** upon the attainable objective that correspond to each child's possibilities in order that he or she can benefit from a better quality of life.

The search for a humanistic and holistic approach demands an intense interaction among all of the professionals who will participate in the evaluation and rehabilitation of the child, requiring the family's understanding and an in-depth comprehension of the sociocultural context within which the child lives (including school and the community).

Evaluation and Rehabilitation as an Integrated Process

A neuropsychological evaluation must be elaborated in conjunction with a global evaluation of the child, which should be conducted by all of the professionals participating in the case. The methodology used at the SARAH network in the initial stages consists of an evaluation is also conducted of each of the following areas: neuropediatrics, functional therapy (physical therapy and occupational therapy), neuropsychology, speech therapy, social work, and nursing. When necessary, an analysis by the neurosurgeon, orthopedist, nutritionist, and/or other specialists who come into contact with the child and family.

Each one of these different professionals analyzes quantitative data for the control of the child's development postinjury; nevertheless, qualitative data are also registered on each child, since every individual is unique. Requisite neurophysiological and neuroimaging exams, as well as movement and balance analysis tests (conducted by the movement laboratory in accordance with each case's necessities), are also added to the data accumulated on the patient. At the end of the technical evaluation in each area, the team meets to elaborate a preliminary conclusion and a global baseline for the child and to define realistic goals to be attained; two case managers who will coordinate the rehabilitation process are also selected at this time.

The conclusion of the evaluation involves the case managers conducting a home visit, establishing closer ties with the family, and consequently returning to the hospital with complementary data that will be incorporated into the evaluation and rehabilitation process.

Within the SARAH Network approach, evaluation and rehabilitation are one and the same process. The first evaluation will reveal the child's initial deficits and strong points, in addition to discovering the learning strategies that he or she employs, thus supplying the necessary information to begin rehabilitation. Subsequently, each stage of rehabilitation will help to define the evaluation instruments and methodology to be used next, provoking changes and adjustments in the rehabilitation process. Of course, all of the professionals have a group of tools or fixed variables (which are utilized in all the evaluations) for a comparative analysis that is based on standard parameters, in this way ensuring that a trend analysis be conducted for every case.

The neuropsychological evaluation is based on Luria's (1970) view of the cognitive and visuopraxic functions as being a complex functional system composed of various subcomponents. In the clinical assessment, these subcomponents are studied separately, with the aim of determining the principle deficits that underlie disturbances of complex functions (Luria, 1970; Christensen, 1978).

Based on the evaluation proposed by Christensen (1978), as well as the theories developed by Piaget (1954, 1966, 1975, 1978, 1979) and Vygotsky (1981, 1987a, b, 1989, 1993), qualitative data are gathered in the domain of language, memory, learning, visual–spatial processing, sensory–motor functions, attention, and executive functions. In this evaluation, Vygotsky's (1989) theory on proximal development zone is applied; in other words, what the child does on his or her own is assessed (as a first reference), but also what he or she is able to do with some sort of assistance (as a second reference). This allows for the verification of not only what is mature, but also what is still in the process of maturation. All of this is essential to the rehabilitation program.

It is important that the team be thoroughly acquainted with the theories of development and neuropsychology in order to obtain reliable qualitative data on the child's functioning, with information on his or her strengths and weaknesses. This is fundamental to the elaboration of a rehabilitation program that has viable, attainable goals that will have a realistic impact on the child's daily life.

The Rehabilitation Program

Initially, the child is treated in an intensive daily program; in accordance with the progress made, the treatment activities are sequentially spread to twice a week, once a week, once every 2 weeks, and eventually monthly, for control purposes.

The program is coordinated by two case managers, one from each area of specialization; selection is made by the team itself and in accordance with the strengths and weaknesses of the child. The reason for selecting two individuals for each case resides in the goal of establishing a constant critical discussion about the progress of the rehabilitation, integrating the objectives of each learning–teaching activity, facilitating the interconsultations with the other professionals, in addition to ensuring that there is always at least one reference professional available to the child and family, should the other need to be absent (due to illness, seminars, vacation, etc.). Each one of the cases is very specific and has its goals well defined; each child's rehabilitation program is individualized.

To ensure that the perspective of the child as a *whole* is not lost, the rehabilitation activities are always structured in a playful way, integrating goals from different specialties. For example, if the functional therapist aims to improve the balance of the knees' positioning and the neuropsychologist intends to work with the mental operation of classification (Piaget, 1978), the case managers will create a "game" in which the child will separate objects while in the kneeling position. The family participates in all of the rehabilitation sessions. The presence of a family member helps the child adapt to a new environment. In addition, the parents are given an opportunity to learn the necessary rehabilitation activities and include them in the daily routine of the home.

The family members are given information on the disease, as well as the evaluation and rehabilitation that will be conducted. The principle is one of "***demedicalization***"; the team ceases to be the proprietor of the knowledge once it shares that information with the parents, and the rehabilitation activities will gradually shift from the hospital to the home, eventually becoming part of the games played among siblings or between parent and child. The intention is to attain functional objectives of neuropsychological and motor rehabilitation through enjoyable activities that are part of the home's day-to-day routine.

In order to facilitate the family's learning process, the team created 300 loose drawings (such as those in Figs. 3 and 4), which are selected and grouped according to the specifics of each case; this will become an individualized manual that is given to the parents. This manual is in turn modified and updated in accordance with the child's progress (Campos da Paz, Burnett, & Nomura, 1996).

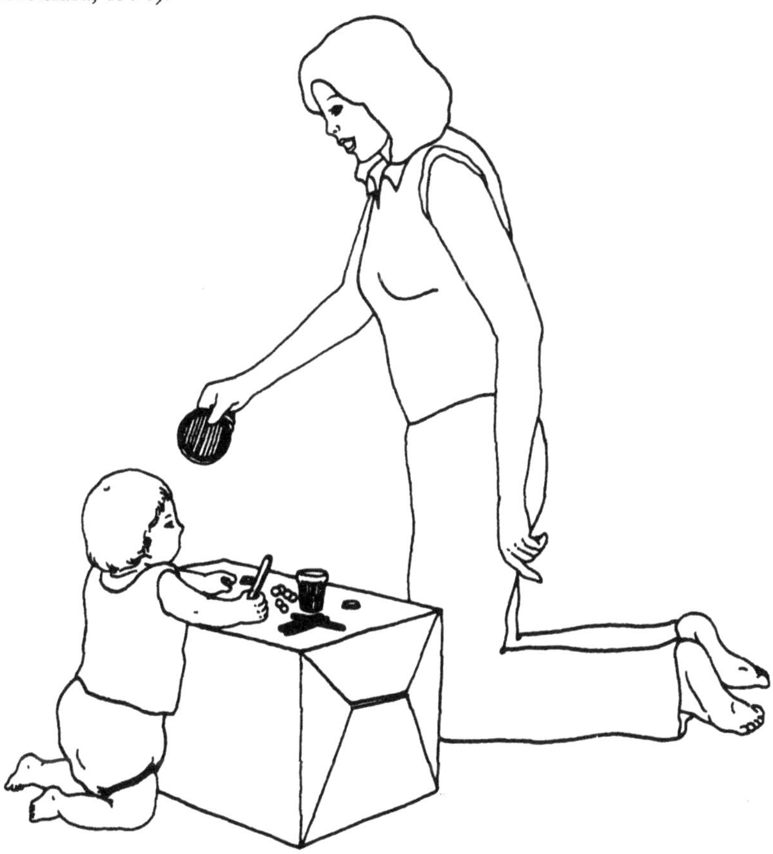

FIGURE 3. Motor and neuropsychological development could be simultaneously stimulated by playful activities which come naturally to the child. *SARAH's Parent Guide to Child Development, Brazil, 1984.* Edited by The SARAH Network of Hospitals for the Locomotor System. Designed by Paulo Roberto de Freitas Guimaraes.

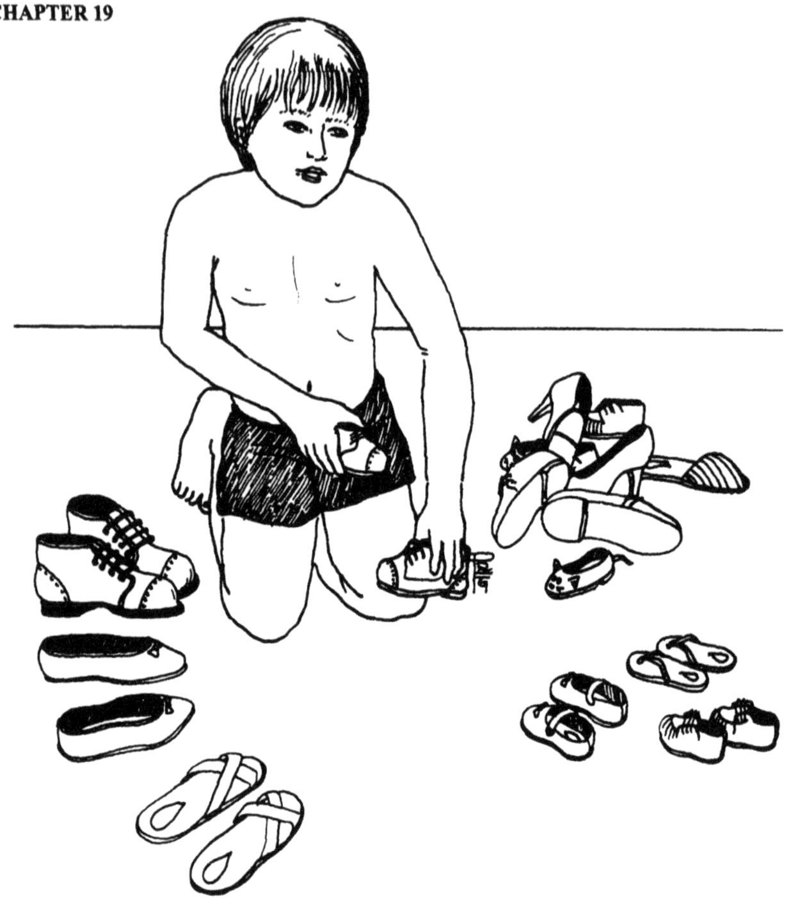

FIGURE 4. Cognitive development can be worked through the use of simple materials found at home. *SARAH's Parent Guide to Child Development, Brazil, 1984.* Edited by The SARAH Network of Hospitals for the Locomotor System. Designed by Paulo Roberto de Freitas Guimarães.

An ecological approach governs the selection of the materials that are used in the rehabilitation activities. The objects chosen could be found in the home of each child (in accordance with information gathered during a previous home visit) and to which a playful meaning is attached; after all, in infancy, playing is the most effective way to learn. The materials and their uses could be very simple, such using shoes (Fig. 4) to work the cognitive capacity of pairing like objects (Piaget, 1979). The simplification of the material ensures that the activities could be performed at home; in addition, they will be accessible to all socioeconomic classes. Whenever possible, hospital activities are conducted outside; this stimulates the child's natural spontaneity and facilitates interaction.

Rehabilitation is based on the interaction between the child and the family and medical–paramedical team. The higher mental functions initially develop on the social plane (interpsychological) and subsequently as an intrapsychological category (Vygotsky, 1993). Rehabilitation *is* development. According to Bruner (1989), the manner in which adults or older children structure their interactions is fundamental to their development. If these allow the child participate in more complex activities in which he or she normally would not do so alone, the child will then begin to increase his or her independence in that activity, resulting in increased learning and autonomy. Furthermore, as stated by Posner *et al.* (1997), the size or number of brain areas involved may be affected by practice, consequently altering the pathways utilized by a given skill.

The Parents

The participation and involvement of the parents in their child's rehabilitation is not a simple process (Campos da Paz *et al.*, 1996). The team must fully understand that TBI causes an abrupt, serious disruption in family life and activates a wide spectrum of emotions such as loss, uncertainty about the child's future, guilt, and fear. Cases in which the TBI occurred in a traffic accident or in such situations involving other family members who may have been wounded or killed are even more complex.

Thus, immediately following the injury, the family generally is not yet capable of participating in rehabilitation, and so information about the disease is passed on in an extremely gradual manner, as a response to the questions posed by the parents or other family members. The team's role in relation to the family during these initial moments is primarily one of lending support and assistance in handling this new situation. A majority of parents require individualized psychological assistance during this phase.

The rehabilitation model developed at the SARAH network includes parent groups, coordinated by a team psychologist, which start off as daily meetings, but are gradually scheduled at greater intervals in accordance with the needs of each group. While the parents participate in these group meetings, the children are involved in socializing activities. In cases where the parents cannot participate in rehabilitation, the team tries to work with other family members, siblings, or a primary caregivers at home.

The rehabilitation model based on the participation of the family has had very positive results. Research conducted at the SARAH network (Braga, 1983) show that children with brain injury who are stimulated by the trained family had statistically more significant neuropsychological and motor development in 1 year than the group stimulated only by specialists ($P < 0.001$). It is important to bear in mind that this rehabilitation model is compatible with the Brazilian reality and culture, and that perhaps such an extensive family commitment might not be a realistic proposal within the context of other cultural realities. Nevertheless, a degree of family attention and involvement is essential when the child is injured, especially in moderate and severe cases of brain injury. At the very least, parents must be given orientation on how to deal, in their day-to-day routine, with problems such as lack of concentration, irritability, depression, impulsiveness, lack of initiative, or other problems that could be present in the daily life of a child with TBI.

School

School is the child's main route back to social reintegration. Consequently, the child's placement in or return to school should be done with the utmost care and attention, to avoid a reversal of the expectations of the child, the family, and the school's own team of professionals.

The child who suffers a TBI during preschool age generally has an easier time adapting to the school environment, since he or she could be placed in a regular class with children who have the same cognitive level and also because there isn't yet an excess of curricular content. An important task for the rehabilitation team is to instruct the teachers on how to deal with the child's problems, propose necessary adaptations, and accompany month by month the child's development and scholastic performance. The return to regular school for those children with moderate or severe TBI who already know how to read and write, especially in the advanced grades, can be much more complex.

The rehabilitation team should make detailed evaluations not only of the neuropsychological functions, but also the child's responses to the diverse academic situations that he or she must face. The neuropsychologist could help the child discover strategies for bypassing these difficulties, co-constructing with the child roundabout paths, in addition to helping the child interact with other children, the family, and his or her community.

It is important not to rush the return to scholastic activities; it is fundamental that frustration, one of the variables that greatly impairs scholastic performance, be avoided. Since the child already has neuropsychological deficits that must be overcome, low self-esteem cannot be allowed to aggravate the situation.

The tendency at SARAH is to integrate the child or adolescent in a regular school whenever possible. In some cases, the child is not yet in a condition to return to the same grade he or she was in before the injury and therefore must begin again in a lower grade. Many times this is extremely difficult on the parents, because it could be taken to signify a regression. Therefore, it is essential that the family be given support, because their positive involvement in the child's return to academic life is fundamental to his or her integration.

During any stage of development the rehabilitation team should stay very close to the family and the school, not only at the moment of reintegration, but in an involved follow-up throughout the child's entire academic development as well.

When the return to school is conducted in the midst of all of this attention and concern, school ends up becoming "the best therapy," and generally the child is able to make significant developmental leaps in a short period of time.

The aim of neuropsychological rehabilitation is not solely the recovery of higher mental functions, but is primarily the rendering of assistance in the search for an improvement in the child's quality of life postinjury. This involves the family, school, friends, community, and leisure activities. Above all, neuropsychology should be actively engaged in assisting the child develop ways of coping and forms of participating in his or her community so that he or she can experience the best quality of life possible.

Outcomes

In May 1998, the SARAH network began a survey of 83 randomly selected children and adolescents who had sustained TBI and had undergone rehabilitation with the humanistic approach based on Luria's theories. Three preliminary questionnaires were created on quality of life and social reinsertion: one was answered by the children, another by the mothers, and the third by the school teachers. The study is presently being further elaborated, and will be submitted for publication upon its completion. The initial results were very promising, with positive response from the three groups questioned regarding the integration of the child with TBI in the schools and the community, as well as the child's quality of life postinjury. These results support the relevance of a humanistic rehabilitation, one that views the child as a being undergoing a process of development, a "researcher" capable of actively participating in his or her growth process, helping to establish viable functional goals, coping strategies, and roundabout paths in the quest for social reintegration.

In conclusion, the aim of neuropsychological rehabilitation is not solely the recovery of the higher mental functions, but is primarily the rendering of assistance in the search for an improvement in the child's quality of life postinjury. This involves the family, school, friends, community, and leisure activitie. Above all, neuropsychology should be actively engaged in helping the child to develop ways of coping and forms of participating in his or her community so that he or she can experience the best quality of life possible.

ACKNOWLEDGMENTS The authors would like to extend their gratitude to Anne-Lise Christensen, PhD, for her very valuable support and assistance; to Barbara Uzzell, PhD, for her orientation; and to Gylse-Anne de Souza Lima, MD, and Paula Azevedo.

References

Braga, L. W. (1983). *O desenvolvimento cognitivo na paralisia cerebral: Um estudo exploratório*. Unpublished master's thesis, Universidade de Brasília, Brazil.

Bruner, J. (1989). Vygotsky: A historical and conceptual perspective. In J. Wertsch (Ed.), *Culture communication and cognition: Vygotskian perspectives*. New York: Cambridge University Press.

Campos da Paz, A., Jr., Burnett, S. M., & Nomura, A. M. (1996). Cerebral Palsy. In R. Duthie & G. Bentley (Eds.), *Mercer's orthopaedic surgery*, (9th ed., pp. 444–473). New York: Oxford University Press.

Christensen, A. L. (1978). *El diagnostico neuropsicologico de Luria*. Madrid: Pablo del Rio.

Ewing-Cobs, L., Fletcher, J. M., Landry, S. H., & Levin, H. S. (1985). Language disorders after pediatric head injury. In J. Darby (Ed.), *Speech and language evaluation in neurology: Childhood disorders* (pp. 97–111). New York: Grune & Stratton.

Finger, S. (1978). *Recovery from brain damage: Research and theory*. New York: Plenum Press.

Jacobson, M. (1978). *Developmental neurobiology*. New York: Plenum Press.

Jordan, F. M., Ozanne, A E., & Murdoch, B. E. (1988). Long-term speech and language disorders subsequent to closed head injury in children. *Brain Injury*, 2, 179–185.

Katzman, R., & Pappius, H. M. (1973). *Brain electrolytes and fluid metabolism*. Baltimore: Williams & Wilkins.

Kujala, T., Alho, K., Huotilainen, M., Ilmoniemi, R. J., Lehtokoski, A., Leinonen, A., Rinne, T., Salonen, O., Sinkkonen, J., Standertskjold Nordenstam, C. G., & Naatanen, R. (1997). Electrophysiological evidence for cross-modal plasticity in humans with early and late onset blindness. *Psychophysiology, 34*, 213–216.

Luria, A.R. (1970). *Higher cortical functions in man* (3rd printing). New York: Basic Books.

Maegaki, Y., Maeoka, Y., Ishi, S., Shiota, M., Takeuchi, A., Yoshino, K., & Takeshita, K. (1997). Mechanisms of central motor reorganization in pediatric hemiplegic patients. *Neuropediatrics, 28*, 168–174.

Norton, W. T., (1972). Formation, structure and biochemistry of myelin. In G. J. Siegel, *et al.* (Eds.), *Basic neurochemistry* (pp. 74–99). Boston: Little, Brown.

Parker, R. S. (1990). *Traumatic brain injury and neuropsychological impairment*. New York: Springer-Verlag.

Peacock, W. J. (1986). The posnatal development of the brain and its coverings. In A. J. Raimondi, M. Choux, & C. Di Rocco (Eds.), *Head injuries in the newborn and infant* (pp. 53–66). New York: Springer-Verlag.

Piaget, J. (1954). *The construction of reality in the child*. New York: Basic Books.

Piaget, J. (1966). *L'image mentale chez l'enfant*. Neuchâtel: Delachaux & Niestlé.

Piaget, J. (1975). *O nascimento da inteligência na criança*. (A. Cabral, Trans.). Rio de Janeiro: Zahar.

Piaget, J. (1978). *Seis estudos em psicologia*. (M. A. .D. Amorim, Trans.). Rio de Janeiro: Forense-Universitária.

Piaget, J. (1979). *O raciocínio na criança* (V. R. Chaves, Trans.). Rio de Janeiro: Record.

Porter, R. (1988). Aspects of neural development. *International Review of Physiology*, *17*, 105–117.

Posner, M. I., Digirolano, G. J., & Fernandez-Duque, D. (1997). *Cognitive skills. Brain Mechanisms, 6*, 267–290.

Rapin, I. (1989). *Disfunción cerebral en la infancia*. Barcelona: Martinez Rosa.

Rutter, M., Chadwick, O., & Shaffer, D. (1983). Head injury. In M. Rutter (Ed.), *Developmental neuropsychology* (pp. 83–111). New York: Wiley.

Vygotsky, L. S. (1987a). The problem of mental retardation: A tentative working hypothesis. *Soviet Psychology, 26*, 78–85.

Vygotsky, L. S. (1987b). Thinking and speech. New York: Plenum Press.

Vygotsky, L.S. (1989). *A formação social da mente*. (J. L. Camargo, Trans.). São Paulo: Martins Fontes.

Vygotsky, L.S. (1993). *Problems of abnormal psychology and learning disabilities: The fundamentals of defectology*. New York: Plenum Press.

Werstch, J. V. (Ed.) (1981). *The concept of actitity in Soviet psychology*. New York: Sharpe.

Ylvisaker, M. (1989). Cognitive and psychosocial outcome following head injury in children. In J. T. Hoff, T. D. Anderson, & T. M. Cole (Eds.), *Mild to moderate Head injury* (pp. 203–216). Boston: Blackwell Scientific Publications.

V

Planning and Financial Aspects of Neuropsychological Rehabilitation

20

Traumatic Brain Injury Rehabilitation as an Integrated Task of Clinicians and Families

Local and National Experiences

ANNA MAZZUCCHI, RAFFAELLA CATTELANI, SABINA CAVATORTA, MARIO PARMA, ANNA VENERI, AND GIULIANA CONTINI

Historical Review

Within the vast context of rehabilitation, that of the traumatic brain injured (TBI) has taken on a highly and specific relevance, not only because of the extreme seriousness of this pathological condition and its inevitable social implications, but also on account of the enormous amount of cultural and methodological research that it requires. Considering its difficult and intense evolution, it is hardly surprising that, although dating back to recent times (1970s), the history of TBI rehabilitation appears as a theme of particular interest in itself. In this light, the analysis made by Rosenthal (1996) seems particularly noteworthy.

Rosenthal identifies, in the development of TBI rehabilitation, a hierarchical sequence of phases, the first of which was the "modern era" (beginning in 1975), during which priority was given to the improvement of emergency medical services and acute care. This was followed by the "era of enlightenment" (1975–1979), when the need for postacute rehabilitation

ANNA MAZZUCCHI, RAFFAELLA CATTELANI, SABINA CAVATORTA, AND MARIO PARMA • Neuropsychology and Neurorehabilitation Unit, Institute of Neurology, University of Parma, 43100 Parma, Italy.
ANNA VENERI AND GIULIANA CONTINI • Trauma Association of Parma, 43100 Parma, Italy.

International Handbook of Neuropsychological Rehabilitation, edited by Christensen and Uzzell.
Kluwer Academic/ Plenum Publishers, New York, 2000.

was fully acknowledged and the first attempts were made to examine suitable methodologies. Then came the "era of proliferation" (1980–1984), featuring highly specialized centers and the subdivision of specialization in the various cognitive and motor areas, inevitably involving teamwork. After this came the "era of refinement" (1985–1989), in which the various cultural, methodological, and organizational acquisitions of the preceding era of proliferation were further elaborated and honed to the maximum of efficacy. Finally, the "era of accountability and consolidation" (1990–1995) laid emphasis on organizational problems, the verification of results, cost–benefit evaluations, and other issues.

The first interesting fact emerging from Rosenthal's analysis is that the sequence of stages as existing in the United States can be found retrospectively in every other country in which TBI rehabilitation has been able to develop under conditions of a sufficiently advanced health organization. However, it is also interesting to note that, in the European area, the sequence of stages appears to be, so to speak, mismatched in times compared to the United States. Each individual stage took place systematically later in European countries than in the United States, in some countries by a few years, or, as in Italy, by as much as a decade with some stages overlapping. Analyzing the reasons for this would be of interest. However, an analysis of this type would inevitably extend to much more general themes, involving the entire medical and social areas of each country. These notes, adhering to the subject of the history of TBI rehabilitation, are simply an attempt to analyze one aspect. In Italy, experiences at both local and national level have increasingly involved the participation of the victims' families. To this end, we considered that the above-mentioned reference scheme proposed by Rosenthal could be usefully applied in the examination of the Italian context, although, as we have pointed out, the timing was different from that in the United States.

The modern era phase (beginning in the United States around 1975 and in Italy in 1980) was characterized, in general, by an emphasis on emergency medical services, on acute intensive care, and on immediate postacute care. The participation of the patients' families was limited to the agonizingly passive attitude of those waiting for a verdict, even after the start of medical and rehabilitative treatment. Thus, there was no integrated interaction as equals between families and the professional team, but merely a kind of communication between two separate worlds, at times tending to serve more as a means of venting respective frustrations than to encourage collaboration.

In the era of enlightenment that followed (in the United States between 1975 and 1979, in Italy from 1985 to 1989), the families of victims had now long-term experience of the seriousness of the sequelae and of the limits and problems of the rehabilitative process. They began to reflect on their introspective isolation and grief and they often expected much greater results from the professionals than those humanly possible. Thus began a period of painful reflection about their personal grief suffered alone and their passive acceptance of the events, which had overtaken them. Should they leave every action and decision in the hands of the "experts" or face the problem with a community spirit, identifying not only with other patients and their relatives, but also with the team of professionals. The latter should no longer be perceived as judges, coldly pronouncing sentence as to prognoses, therapies, program, and results, but rather as seekers of cooperation, their task being rendered particularly arduous and emotionally draining because of the countless uncertainties, failures,and frustrations. The families were beginning to realize that, in order to emerge from a state of counterproductive "mourning," they had to become in some way protagonists, not just passive spectators wrapped up in their relationship with their own trauma victim. But how should this new role be played? There was certainly no lack of discussion, contrasts of opinion, and temporary desertions. Finally, however, in 1985, the idea prevailed that an association should be formed among the families

(Parma Trauma Association), whose duties were perceived above all as being of a preventive nature. Thus, the epidemiological proportions of the problem were of concern, that is, the reasons for the continuously increasing number of motorcycle and car accidents and the necessity of intensive care needs. As to this latter aspect, the association of the families was decisive at that time in the activation of early intensive care services on the road. Their support led to the speeding up of the introduction of specialized ambulances and helicopters in coordination with the intensive care unit.

Here, it is worth commenting on the position taken by the victims' families at that time. Since theirs was a predominantly organizational contribution, so to speak, concerning social policy or at any rate of an external nature, we should ask ourselves if this was merely a "technical" choice or if it was also influenced by other factors. In those days, there was the distinct feeling of shame, on the one hand, regarding the "private" aspect of personal suffering, born out of the heaviness of care duties and the incessant private suffering on the part of the patients' families. They were afraid to show their feelings and to appeal for help. On the other hand, it would seem that the association of the families, albeit already formed, did not wish to become involved in the rehabilitation teamwork or in the determination of its nature. This was possibly in part because they were anxious to avoid any misunderstanding as to the nature of their role, which they intended as one of support, not of criticism or control. All this served to preserve a certain distance between families and health care teams. As a reaction, the professionals concentrated their attention on the internal dynamics of the families and their increasing difficulties of interacting with them. The reason for this was untreated family stress, total isolation of the family in a hospital setting, and the disruptive consequences of TBI for the family system and for social groups. Consequently, the necessity of providing a support program and other ways of working together with the family became essential.

All this leads to a greater appreciation of the significance of the subsequent phase, which, because of its general characteristics, can be compared to the era of proliferation according to Rosenthal (in the United States between 1980 and 1984, in Italy approximately between 1985 and 1994). During that phase, the Associazione Traumi Parma, which in the meantime had grown in numbers and structure, continued its work. Topics were prevention and improvement in the quality of acute care, including the promotion of informative conferences on local and national television and in the newspapers and the creation of local data banks. But beyond these duties, which had been established from the start, the families now began to overcome their hesitations to take the first steps and to involve themselves directly in the work of the professionals. As they discovered for themselves the problems of the professional team, the families contributed more and more to the technical and methodological development proper, thus appealing for highly specialized centers in one or another field (sensory–motor, cognitive, etc.) and introducing new concepts for team work. It was in this phase that the professional team began to include on a regular basis other medical specialists to treat the infectious, orthopedic, ophthalmological, orthophonic, and other consequences of trauma. This new collegial approach, where applied, was quick to increase the quality of care and the efficacy of the team.

In the era of refinement (in the United States between 1985 and 1989, and in Italy from 1990 up to the present day), the TBI families were to acquire increasing significance and to gain greater awareness of their functions. Thus, the initial role of the Associazione, as a supportive or complementary outsider, gave way to one of an integrated and inseparable part of the entire structure dedicated to the rehabilitation of the persona of the patient and to his or her reinstatement in society. It became a "professional among professionals," taking part in all activities, thus abandoning the notion of "us" and "them," of "us" nonprofessionals who are often obliged to keep silent, even when criticizing the professionals or venting to frustrations were wanted. The completeness of the Associazione's integration into the treatment team is illustrated by the list of functions at this time carried out by the Associazione. Collaboration between family association and postacute and rehabilitation staff mainly consisted, on the part of the family association, of supplying intensive care rehabilitation equipment and grants for staff specialization courses abroad. Collaboration on the part of the rehabilitation centers, together with the family association, consisted of the organization of groups to inform and to support the families of new victims, the preparation of a diary for the families (containing, among other things, a glossary, information on TBI consequences and recovery, a list of professionals, suggestions, opportunities, and a question sheet), participation and organization of national and international associations [such as the European Brain Injury Society (EBIS) and the International Brain Injury Association (IBIA)], and specialized TBI meetings.

The family associations have steadily increased in number in the recent past, although they are still more prevalent in the north of Italy. Direct intervention of TBI family national associations on a local and national scale has been as follows: (1) support for other families regarding medical and rehabilitative questions; (2) legal and bureaucratic needs; (3) the problems of home assistance; (4) information for victims' families about their TBI rights; (5) promotion of coordination between public health services and social services; (6) the publication of papers on TBI "news" (i.e., "Punto di Incontro," "Fase 3"); (7) support of the patients' work and their readmittance to school; (8) organization of group therapy or group support for relatives, siblings, and couples; (9) weekend excursions, cultural visits, and holidays for TBI patients and their families; and (10) promotion of public exhibitions of artistic work done by TBI patients. In particular, the Associazione Traumi Parma has since 1991 supported local planning, thus encouraging, building, equipping, and "defending" the first Italian center entirely devoted to TBI care and rehabilitation (Centro Cardinal Ferrari in Fontanellato, near Parma), which is now finally completed.

Rosenthal's era of accountability and consolidation (1990–1994), in which the general attention was devoted to the improvement of the health care organization for Italy, represents the immediate present and, above all, the future. In this climate of evolution, the Italian family associations founded the Coordinamento Nazionale Associazioni per il Trauma Cranico, consisting of 10 local associations (see Appendix 1) and about 2000 members, having as their principal goals the national data bank on TBI survivors and the coordination of the Italian national association with the international ones (EBIS and IBIA). In short, in the drive to reduce costs, to increase efficiency and efficacy in care and rehabilitation, and to identify new criteria of outcome and "customer satisfaction," the families' aspiration is finally to take part in the dialogue side by side with the professionals.

To conclude, in our experience the evolution of the history of the integration of the families into the rehabilitation of severe TBI patients has not been a predictable one, nor one to be taken for granted. It has been an uphill struggle, not lacking in doubts, hesitations, or obstacles, during which the family associations have passed from a position of purely external assistance to full participation in the rehabilitative process in all its aspects. In other words, there has been a passage from the isolation of personal pain to a sharing in the problems of a whole community of families and in those of an entire community of operators. Furthermore, the recent uniting of the family associations under a national committee and their international involvement are sure signs of their willingness to take a hand in the prevention program and adequate health care solutions for rehabilitation and social reintegration drawn up by national, European, and international communities.

Research Studies on Family Needs and Problems

Research studies on the problems created by a trauma for the victim's family, begun at the Neuropsychology and Neurorehabilitation Unit, Institute of Neurology, University of Parma, were intensified, starting in 1993, in concomitance with the organization of the Congress of the EBIS in Fontanellato, Italy (January 1994). On the occasion of the Congress, which was dedicated specifically to the problems of the victims' families, two of the numerous papers from Italian and European contributors were presented by the authors. The first was dedicated to family experiences in the long-term care of severely head injured patients (Mazzucchi, Cattelani, Gugliotta, Brianti & Janelli, 1994), and the second was concerned with the problems connected with interactions between health care staff and the relatives of head-injured patients (Cattelani, Ferrara, Gugliotta & Mazzucchi, 1994).

A brief summary of the results of these two research studies and of other themes that have been the subject of successive research by our team follows.

Family Experiences in the Long-Term Care of Severely Head-Injured Patients
(Mazzucchi *et al.*, 1994)

In order to identify the needs of victims' families and to suggest appropriate intervention regarding their long-term financial, psychological, and welfare problems, a questionnaire was sent to 161 families of severely head-injured patients who had been referred to the Neurorehabilitation Unit, Institute of Neurology, University of Parma.

The most interesting among the 100 answers (62%) provided by those family members who are carers can be summarized as follows:

1. Significant changes in family structure following the trauma were reported. The families reported an increase in the number of: (1) patients who live alone; (2) patients who had lived alone prior to the accident, but who afterward had to rely on family support; and (3) "only child" patients in the sense that other siblings were required to move away from home.
2. The intrafamily relationships prior to the trauma were reported as "good," "reasonable," or "without problems" in 90% of the cases, but 12% of families reported a definite deterioration in these relationships.
3. The data highlight the severe financial and social burden that is inevitably imposed on the families of severe head injury patients: (1) the money spent can reach tens of millions of lira, and, in extreme cases, can contribute to the financial ruin of the family; (2) more than 40% of the families reported reductions in income by the patients or by the family members; (3) 51% of the cases were still going through the medical–legal process 4.2 years after the accident; and (4) more than 50% of the patients were no longer able to continue prior work or study activities (see Fig. 1).
4. The study demonstrates negative psychological changes and a clear increase in family stress during the posttraumatic period: The most dramatic moment in 42% of the cases was during the intensive care period and in 22% of the cases during the initial news. In spite of a higher frequency of motor and cognitive disabilities than severely disruptive behavior, it was problems experienced by the families that contributed most to increased stress levels. The current emotional state was subjectively defined as "moody" or "guilty" by the majority of the responders. Apart from the economic damage, other limitations are reported as adding to family stress. The most common were the withdrawal from social and cultural activities (50%), no work (25%), and the inability to take a vacation (22%) (see Fig. 2).

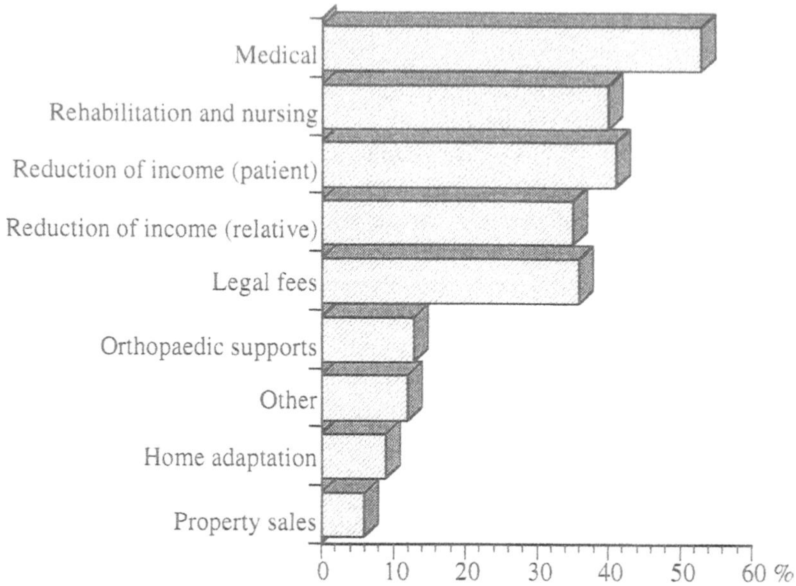

FIGURE 1. General financial burden for the family.

5. The most frequent family complaints were: (1) the indifference of public institutions (51%); (2) general incomprehension or indifference regarding the social and psychological problems of the family (49%); and (3) the lack of rehabilitation centers and trained professionals (43%).

6. The possible factors which families felt contributed to the patient's progress were "the passing of time" and "the thoroughness of the family commitment" for about 40% of the respondents and medical and rehabilitative therapies for only 18%.

Interactions Between Health Care Staff and the Relatives of Head-Injured Patients (Cattelani *et al.*, 1994)

The emotional effects that burden not only the relatives of severe TBI patients but also the health care professionals are well-known and have been commented on in a number of research studies. Less obvious and less well-studied are the emotional effects resulting from the interactions between these two categories involved in the patient's care. Given the obvious stress factors on both sides, misunderstandings and conflicts can easily occur between family members and health care professionals (Shaw & McMahon, 1990; McLaughlin & Carey, 1993). The close relationship between families and professionals over the long course of rehabilitation inevitably creates intense emotions. These emotional reactions have been well described in the field of psychotherapy as "countertransference," similarly to what happens in the psychotherapist–patient relationship. Also, in the professional–relative relationship it is expected that the emotional state of the professional will have as important an impact on treatment as the emotional state of the family members. Discussions on difficult treatment decisions are emotionally draining for both family and professional. Often, the professionals have the paradoxical task of giving satisfactory and reassuring answers to the anxious requests from relatives, while also communicating the usually negative realities of prognosis (McLaughlin & Carey, 1993). The professionals may identify with the family in their grief and outrage over the tragedy of the trauma. Sachs (1991) illustrates three expected and common emotional reactions among brain-injury rehabilitation professionals to the patient and his or her family. He reports both negative and positive effects on treatment of feelings of denial, anger, or exhaustion. He argues that in maintaining a connection with the patient and family the professional goes beyond seeing them as mere recipients of rehabilitation care or as victims, coming to appreciate them as fellow human beings.

A research study carried out at the Neurorehabilitation Unit of the Neurology Institute of Parma was aimed at the subjective assessment of the opinions of three professional health care categories (clinicians, therapists, and nurses) regarding their relationships with relatives of severely head-injured patients. Each professional was required to express the intensity of each of the following components: psychological stress, emotional involvement, feelings of being manipulated, and feelings of being professionally respected and trusted by the patient's family (see the evaluation form used to detect the selected interactive components, reported in Appendix 2).

From the health care worker's point of view as a whole, the results indicate that the interactions reported between staff and relatives were quite positive. None of the professionals from the three categories reported "at risk" levels for the emotional components investigated. The level of psychological stress was generally low, the degree of emotional involvement was "medium" though consistent, and the perceived level of professional respect and trust was generally high. The gender of the professionals revealed no significant effects. However, some qualitative differences were noted:

1. Though more emotionally involved, the physical therapists reported better interactions, particularly with mothers, than the other professionals. This would suggest that

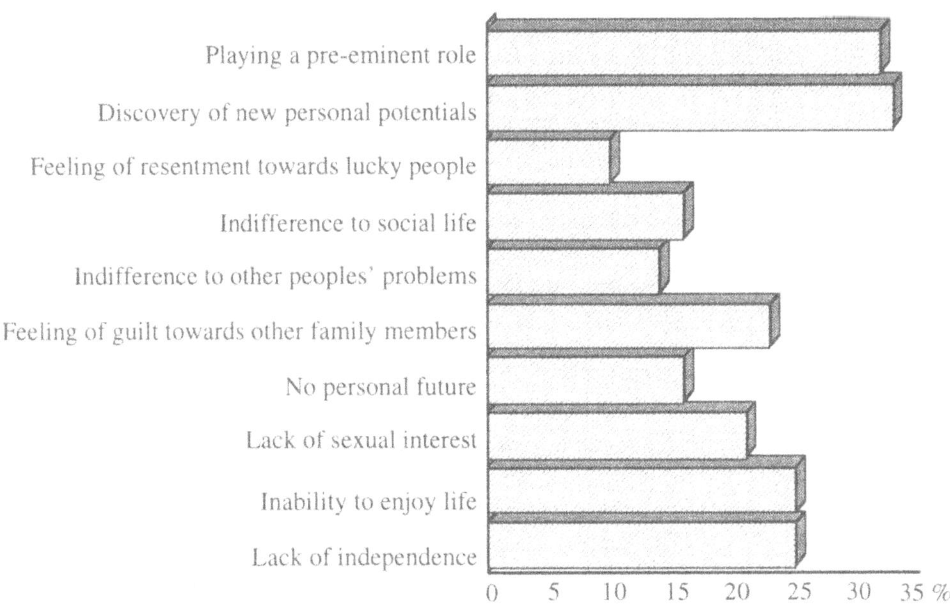

FIGURE 2. The most frequent feelings and moods referred by the relatives.

family members consider motor problems more important and may have greatest expectations of the therapists.

2. Younger health care professionals scored higher levels of psychological stress in coping with the spouses of the clinically more severe patients. This difficulty, however, did not have a negative influence on their interactions with these family members. These patients and their spouses were usually quite young. Hence, it can be supposed that positive interactions were maintained because the younger professionals may identify with subjects of similar age.
3. Nurses appear to have better interactions with fathers of clinically more severe patients, but also with the spouses of patients whose conditions are not particularly severe. In the latter case, the results may relate to the nurse's feelings of being more professionally adequate. For example, the degree of "humble" tasks, such as providing complete personal hygiene, is reduced for patients who are more independent. The better interaction with fathers of more severe patients may relate to the lower frequency of contacts. Usually, it is the mothers who assist in the daily care of the patients, rather than the fathers.

Management of Trauma Effects on the Family System
(Cattelani, Patruno, Cesana, Lombardi, & Mazzucchi, 1997)

The "systemic" model was applied to the TBI families. The observations of the consequences to the victim's family of a severe brain injury, made by predominantly American and English authors (Brooks, Campsie, Symington, Beattie, & McKinlay, 1986; Maitz, 1991; Maitz & Sachs, 1995) appear to result from the idea of a "disintegration" of the family system. The abandoning of the family "code" and values seems to be inevitable. A lack of consensus or agreement of choices of individual members possibly makes it more difficult to maintain family identity. The intrafamily communications would appear to be particularly impaired and chaotic; a decline in or loss of the sense of belonging would seem inevitable in some family members. Adaptability appears to present difficulties to a greater or lesser extent in making decisions adequate to the state of "chronic emergency."

With the aim of using a systemic approach in the evaluation of some of the aforementioned structural characteristics of family functioning, we examined a sample group of parents of a child who had suffered a cranial trauma. The couples had been followed for a lengthy period some years before at the Neurorehabilitation Unit, Neurology Institute of Parma. These couples were now compared with another sample group of parents who had not had such an experience of trauma, on the basis of each family's sociocultural level and of the present age and the sex of the living-in child.

The instrument used for the structural evaluation of the family was the Italian version of the Family Adaptability and Cohesion Scale-III (FACES-III), a self-administered questionnaire that followed the guidelines of the "circumflex model" developed by Olson, Sprenkle, & Russell (1979). The procedure involves placing the families into a matrix generated from crossing two of the variables: adaptability and cohesion.

The circumflex model presumes a better functioning of the types of families placed at the center of the matrix ("balanced") than of those placed at the edges ("extreme"). In addition, we measured the level of social integration of the young adult patients on the Social Adaptability Scale (SAS) (Weissman, 1975)—Italian version. The results obtained from the above-described study can be summarized as follows:

1. No evidence emerges of the tendency toward disintegration of the family system as reported by the English and American authors. The parents of TBI children examined by us report a good degree of family satisfaction, which, if anything, tends to be greater than that reported by control subjects.
2. Regarding "code" of principles, approval of choices, and cohesion, the family structure tends to reinforce the ties between the individual members, sometimes taking on the nature of "rigidity," but never obviously pathological. The authors, however, agree with the reported results of previous studies regarding the other two structural components—adaptability and communication—which would seem to interact in a "chaotic" fashion.
3. The most frequent family problem seems to be social readjustment of the patient in a high percentage of the subjects ("severe maladjustment" at SAS).

The possible reasons for the observations emerging from our inquiry can be summarized along the lines of three hypotheses. First, in comparison with the social models of other countries, it is possible that our families can avail themselves of a more valid social support system; second, the parents followed by us over a long period provide excellent data regarding how parents can learn to cope given informative help and support; and third, the problem of social adjustment of children with cranial trauma does not seem to be comparable to the attitude often detected in families of patients with psychiatric illnesses (Rosenthal & Young, 1988).

When the TBI families take charge of patient care, there must be an adaptation to the particular nature of the case and emotional phase in which the family finds itself. While any "rehabilitation" program inevitably involves teamwork, in these cases it must involve competent and well-coordinated professionals of diverse disciplines, in an approach that could be defined as "transdisciplinary" (Blosser & De Pompei, 1994). A program should operate according to a proactive policy of collaboration and communication with the family from the first phases of the patient's recovery and over a long period of time.

The process of patient recovery in effect can be seen as a series of stages, progressing from the moment of admission to intensive care to the rehabilitation phase, up to his or her readmission into the family. The process of adjustment on the part of the family follows the same course, featuring a series of states of mind and attitudes changing with each phase. Therefore, the family should take charge of caring for the patient as early as possible, but this intervention should be adjusted according to the emotional phase the family is experiencing at a given moment in the delicate and complicated process of acceptance of their changed circumstances. Family willingness to become involved in the care of the patient must be carefully assessed in both emotional and objective terms: In those cases of the most serious posttrauma outcomes, the objective burden carried by the families, and in particular by mothers, often does not permit them the "luxury" of providing the victim with psychological support.

In the chronic phase of the outcome, for each individual case the possibility to "restructure" the system must be carefully evaluated, above all when there is a situation of "compensation" that has been acquired over time with great effort, and thus is indicative of good individual emotional "resources." In TBI families, management should be focused not on problems of identification and differentiation, as in the case of neuroses and psychoses, but on the encouragement and reinforcement of communication and on the sharing of affections and emotions, fantasies, resentments, and aggressiveness.

While on the one hand it is possible to draw suggestions from the existing approaches formulated for the treatment of "dysfunctional" families with chronic ailments of differing nature and in particular of the psychiatric type, on the other hand the adaptation of these models to the TBI families requires further study in order for them to be suitable for assessment and treatment in individual situations.

Sexuality and Couple Relationships after Severe Head Injury (Cavatorta, 1997)

Considering the sizeable number of studies that have been published on several aspects of the complicated phenomenon of trauma, relatively little research has been carried out on changes in sexual relationships after head injury. In view of the epidemiological aspects of brain injury, which mainly concern young adults with a full social and emotional life, this is particularly surprising, because of the importance of sexuality for the individual. Moreover, sexuality is a typical example of a complex function requiring the integration of several components—physical, cognitive, and behavioral—in order to be adequately expressed. Therefore, it is likely to be severely compromised after severe head injury (Elliott & Biever, 1996).

A review of the literature suggests that sexual concerns after head injury have generally been approached in an entirely unilateral way, either from the point of view of the patient or from that of his or her partner. Several workers have focused on changes in sexual behavior generally occurring after damage of the frontal lobes, often resulting in loss of inhibition and in inappropriate sexual responses, or, in contrast, in inertia and diminished libido (Evans, 1981; Zencius, Wesolowski, Burke & Hough, 1990; Kaufman, 1981). In addition, several questionnaires and interviews have been given to patients, in order to assess their level of sexual activity and overall quality of sexual function (Kreutzer & Zasler, 1989; Sandel, Williams, Dellapietra & Derogatis, 1996). Besides, several authors have pointed out the psychosocial impact of head injury on relatives, and above all on partners, reporting that many relationships dissolve within the first year from injury. Divorce rates are remarkably high (about 40% in some studies), the quality of marital relationships faces long-term challenges, and partners often complain of isolation, frustration, and depression (Rosenbaum & Najenson, 1976; Mauss-Clum & Ryan, 1981; Price, 1985; Zasler & Kreutzer, 1991).

We believe that head injury operates as a breakdown factor on both partners, and therefore any analysis has to be directed toward both of them. With this aim, at the Neuropsychological and Neurorehabilitation Unit of Parma a structured interview was given to patients and their partners, in order to widely assess various aspects of the patients' sexual behavior and changes in marital relationships following severe traumatic brain injury. The first three sections are focused on couple relationship, abnormal sexual behavior, and sexual intercourse. The fourth section is limited to males, regarding erection and functional problems. The last section is limited to the partner, regarding his or her own sexual satisfaction and desires and his or her subjective judgment on the patient.

The results of the interview show that in 17 out of the 18 couples (94.4%) conflicts were present, but no divorce or definitive breakdown was registered considering a follow-up of 2 years postinjury. In 29.4% of the cases, problems dated prior to injury. From the pattern of answers (Fig. 3), the majority of the couples sampled complained more about couple relationship problems than about sexual dysfunction. The diminished frequency of intercourse and communication problems were the most frequently reported complaints, while only a few respondents reported erection problems or impaired libido. And, most of all, almost all partners complained of a decrease in sexual satisfaction. Many reported a decreased libido and 66% de-

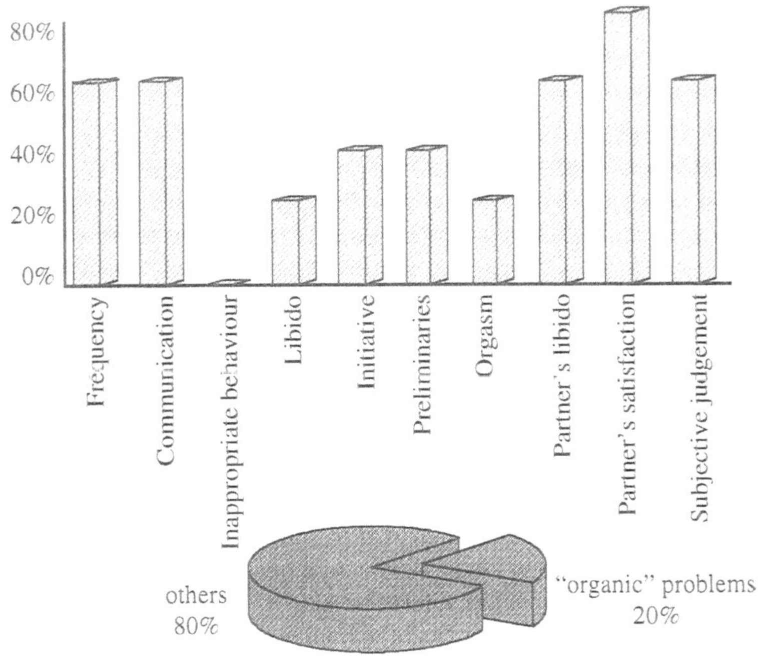

FIGURE 3. Percentages of cases reporting sexual problems.

scribed important changes in the patient ("he/she isn't the same person I took as husband/wife"; "he/she is like a child"). No patient presented abnormal sexual behavior.

In 67% of the cases, there was a qualitative difference in responses obtained from patients compared with their partners. Both reported the same conflicts in their relationship, but the patients were generally more indifferent. If requested to give an explanation for the problems reported, they tended to put the blame on external causes, demonstrating poor self-criticism. Interestingly, we also noticed that couple conflicts were more relevant if the patient was male, because of the greater frustration revealed by the female partner. In order to better define why head injury may interfere with sexuality, the scores obtained at the interview were correlated to the patient's disability. Physical components, such as hemiparesis or hypoaesthesia, did not affect sexuality or relationships, whereas neuropsychological and behavioral components, particularly memory deficits and inertia, did influence couple conflicts.

However, considering the quality of the partners' replies and the neuropsychological profile of the patients, it clearly appears that the sexual and relationship impairment is caused not by individual disabilities, but by the overall "disintegration" of personality and behavior consequent to injury. Because of the mechanical nature of different force vectors applied to the head, TBI is less likely to cause focal lesions and deficits than widespread dysfunction. Such dysfunctions (particularly poor insight and self-criticism, problems in facing and overcoming unusual situations, and difficulties in controlling one's reactions) may be responsible for change in sexuality and relationships.

We think that there should be close collaboration between several clinicians (neurologist, neuropsychologist and physiatrist) to widely assess problems of this nature and to plan compensation strategies that should be included in neuropsychological rehabilitation.

TBI Family Management

Staff Meetings

In order both to improve the information flow among the various professionals and to facilitate their relationship with the family members of the patient, staff meetings concerning the patient are held weekly during the hospital stay. These meetings, which involve neurologists, physiatrists, nurses, therapists, and psychologists and deal with the health, rehabilitation, and social–family problems of the patients, are of both direct and indirect benefit to the family. The information provided by the various staff members to their colleagues is carefully noted, and each staff member is also informed about differing requests and needs of each individual family. Psychologists have the opportunity to learn about the possible difficulties in the interaction between professionals and family, and thus can suggest more efficacious communication strategies, improving collaboration and interaction.

Family Group Sessions

Family group sessions conducted by a psychologist take place weekly from admission to the hospital (Neurology Department) until the discharge from the outpatient neurorehabilitation program (mean length: 4.5 months). In these group sessions, training is provided on how to be flexible in caregiver roles, how to tolerate ambiguities and uncertainties, how to provide, ask for, and receive information from professionals, and how to cope with difficult relations within the health care system. With the collaboration of the Associazione Traumi Parma, we devised the family diary, which is given to the family at the time of the patient's hospital admission. The first part of the diary concerns possible outcomes of cranial traumas, a glossary of the common medical terminology, a list of clinicians responsible for the patient, and a series of weekly sheets in which family members may note their observations of the patient, along with any questions they may want to ask the clinicians. The sheets provide openings for dialogue during weekly sessions, designed to address inquiries and contingent needs, and feature the presence of a voluntary family member representative of the Associazione Traumi. Supplementary meetings for individual families or family members are available where there is difficulty in accepting the outcome and/or particular difficulties in interacting with clinicians.

In relation to the above-mentioned family group sessions, the statistical–descriptive surveys carried out in the period between January 1996 and June 1997 (18 months) provided the preliminary data reported below. There were 36 families with TBI (24 males and 12 females): Patients' mean age for male patients ($M = 24.5$) was significantly different from female patients ($M = 34$). Consequently, the family's role was different.

Family carers were as follows: 18 fathers, of whom 16% attended the group sessions assiduously; 24 mothers, of whom 20% attended the group sessions assiduously; 13 spouses or live-in partners, of whom 38.5% attended the group sessions assiduously.

Looking at the family as a whole: 11 families (30%) refused to participate in the weekly group sessions; 8 families (22%) attended sessions assiduously; 17% participated sporadically; and 30% preferred individual sessions. On discharge from hospital, 53% judged the outcome as "good," 30% as "poor," and 17% neglected the judgment.

In 47% of the cases, no pretrauma family history relating to emotional–behavioral or personality problems of any one member or to social–emotional difficulties of the family system was present. In 39% of the cases, the family experienced difficulties of various kinds (divorces, severe family conflicts, financial problems); in 28% of the cases, difficulties were attributable to personality problems of one member of the family. In 14% of the cases, the patient him- or herself had displayed pretrauma emotional–behavioral problems.

Screening Protocol

In order to collect information revealing the characteristics and facilitating the operative choices of each family, we also established a screening protocol. The findings with the screening protocol are not available, but the purposes can be described. The aim was to identify those families who after some time still found it difficult to accept and adapt to the trauma. The evaluation was made in the course of several sessions with all family members and was usually timed to coincide with the neuropsychological examination 6 months from discharge. It was designed to produce a picture of the aspects summarized below:

1. The present composition of the family and the personal details and role of the individual members.
2. The willingness of other significant individuals not living with the family (relatives, friends, neighbors, voluntary workers, etc.) to provide help.
3. The occurrence of stressing events happening before, at the same time, or after the trauma and the individual family members' emotional reactions.
4. The quantification of needs, in terms of objective and subjective burden (financial burden, health and home assistance, limitations on leisure, educational and social activities, and modifications in affective relations).
5. The compensatory strategies spontaneously enacted by individual family members (passive acceptance, denial, rationalization, sublimation, or requests for social support or for specialist consultations).
6. The levels of cohesion and adaptability found with the above-mentioned questionnaire, FACES III (Olson et al., 1979). On the basis of the picture acquired, it is possible to formulate a "project" of suitable intervention (family therapy, individual psychotherapy, drug therapy, contact with the social services, etc).

Concluding Remarks

The findings reported in this work indicate that in Italy as elsewhere the interaction between professionals and TBI families has progressively intensified. The quality of assistance during the various posttrauma phases was improved at the same pace.

Much remains to be done in terms of quality of assistance and extension of good services to the whole of Italy. Continuous information campaigns an application of insistent pressure on the national health service are needed. The foundations have been laid, especially in terms of the spreading of awareness as to the curative and rehabilitative methods available for enacting appropriate intervention programs in all the structures concerned with assisting brain injured subjects.

Our work, and the work of a few other pioneers, has always been extremely arduous and often frustrating. The task has been sustained, not only by our own personal convictions, but also by our deeply felt and sincere compassion for the suffering and difficulties of the patients and their families. Moreover, we are deeply convinced that working and struggling alongside the families increases our own motivation and alleviates, as far as possible, the feeling of isolation and helplessness that families suffer. It is through a constant and coordinated process of interaction between professionals and TBI families that the most satisfactory results can be achieved.

Appendix 1

Italian TBI Family Associations Supporting the National Committee: Year of Foundation and Address

1985 Associazione Traumi—Parma
at Centro di Rianimazione, Ospedale di Parma
via Gramsci, 14-43100 Parma
tel 39-521-259036; fax 39-521-986700

1987 Itaca—Milano
at Reparto Neurorianimazione Ospedale Niguarda–Cà Granda
p.zza Ospedale Maggiore, 2-20135 Milano
tel 39-2-64442685; fax 39-2-64442908

1989 Genesis—S. Pellegrino Terme-Bergamo
via S. Carlo, 70-24016 S. Pellegrino Terme (BG)
tel 39-345-/21051; fax 39-345-23158

1992 A.R.CO. 92—Roma
via F. Coletti, 35-00191 Roma
tel & fax 39-6-3294665

1993 Brain—Vicenza
contrà Oratori dei Servi, 21-36100 Vicenza
tel 39-444-544528; fax 39-444-927272

1994 Fase 3—Verona
via Fontana del Ferro, 18-37129 Verona
tel 39-45-592251; fax 39-45-594945

1994 Ass.Tra.—Lecco
at Dipartimento Rianimazione, Ospedale di Lecco
via Ghislanzoni, 22-22053 Lecco
tel & fax 39-341-489412

1995 A.A.T.C.—Gorizia
at Servizio di Rianimazione dell'Ospedale di Gorizia
via Vittorio Veneto, 171-34170 Gorizia
tel 39-481-592977

1995 Rinascita-Vita—Genova
P.za della Vittoria, 9 int. 11-16100 Genova
tel. 39-10-582413; fax 39-10-594953

Appendix 2

Self-Evaluation Form

___ Clinician ___ Therapist ___ Nurse ___ Psychologist

Please mark an "X" from 0 to 100 in answer to each of the following questions:

1. How much do you feel PSYCHOLOGICALLY STRESSED by the relationship with this relative:

   not at all ____ very much
   0 100

2. How much do you feel MANIPULATED by this relative:

   not at all ____ very much
   0 100

3. How much do you feel EMOTIONALLY INVOLVED in the relationship with this relative:

   not at all ____ very much
   0 100

4. How much do you feel PROFESSIONALLY RESPECTED by this relative:

   not at all ____ very much
   0 100

5. How much do you think that this relative TRUSTS you:

   not at all ____ very much
   0 100

NOTE: The scale for each emotional component ranges from a minimum of 0 to a maximum of 100 millimeters.

References

Blosser, J., & De Pompei, R. (1994). *Paediatric traumatic brain injury. Proactive intervention*. San Diego, CA: Singular Publishing Group.

Brooks, N., Campsie, L., Symington, C., Beattie, A., & McKinlay, W. (1986). The five-year outcome of severe blunt head injury: A relative's view. *Journal of Neurology, Neurosurgery and Psychiatry, 49*, 764–770.

Cattelani, R., Ferrara, L., Gugliotta, M., & Mazzucchi, A. (1994). Interactions between health care staff and the relatives of head injured patients. *Giornale Italiano di Medicina Riabilitativa, 3*, 210–215.

Cattelani, R., Patruno, M., Cesana, L., Lombardi, F., & Mazzucchi, A. (1998). Effectiveness and limits of the systemic model applied to the therapy of TBI families. In A. Minervino (Ed.) *La psicosomatica del quotidiano: Proceedings of the XVI National Congress of the Italian Psychosomatic Medicine Society* (pp. 170–175). Parma: Tipolitografia Benedettina.

Cavatorta, S., Cattelani, R., Lombardi, F., Ferrara, L., Avanzi, S., & Mazzucchi, A. (1998). Sexual and couple relationship dysfunctions following traumatic brain injury. In A. Minervino (Ed.) *La Psicosomatica del quotidiano:*

Proceedings of the XVI National Congress of the Italian Psychosomatic Medicine Society, (pp. 176–185). Parma: Tipolitografia Benedettina.

Elliott, M. L., & Biever, L. S. (1996). Head injury and sexual dysfunction. *Brain Injury, 10,* 703–717.

Evans, C. D. (1981). *Rehabilitation after severe head injury*. New York: Churchill Livingston.

Kaufman, D. M. (1981). *Neurological aspects of sexual dysfunction. Clinical neurology for psychiatrists*. San Francisco: Grune & Stratton.

Kreutzer, J. S., & Zasler, N. D. (1989). Psychosexual consequences of traumatic brain injury: Methodology and preliminary findings. *Brain Injury, 3,* 177–186.

Maitz, E. (1991). Family systems theory applied to head injury. In J. Williams & T. Kay (Eds.), *Head injury: A family matter* (pp. 65–79). Baltimore: Paul H. Brooks.

Maitz, E. A., & Sachs, P. R. (1995). Treating families of individuals with traumatic brain injury from a family system perspective. *Journal of Head Trauma Rehabilitation, 10,* 1–11.

Mauss-Clum, N., & Ryan, M. (1981). Brain injury and the family. *Journal of Neurosurgical Nursing, 13,* 165–169.

Mazzucchi, A., Cattelani, R., Gugliotta, M., Brianti, R., & Janelli, G. (1994). Family experiences in the long-term care of severely head-injured patients. *Giornale Italiano di Medicina Riabilitativa, 3*(VII), 232–241.

McLaughlin, A. M., & Carey, J. L. (1993). The adversarial alliance: Developing therapeutic relationships between families and the team in brain injury rehabilitation. *Brain Injury, 7,* 45–51.

Olson, D. H., Sprenkle, D., & Russell, C. (1979). Circumflex model of marital and family system: Cohesion and adaptability dimensions, family types and clinical application. *Family Process, 18,* 3–28.

Price, J. R. (1985). Promoting sexual wellness in head-injured patients. *Rehabilitation Nursing, 10,* 12–13.

Rosenbaum, M., & Najenson, T. (1976). Changes in the patterns and symptoms of low mood as reported by wives of severely brain-injured soldiers. *Journal of Consulting and Clinical Psychology, 44,* 881–888.

Rosenthal, M. (1996). 1995 Sheldon Berrol, MD, Senior Lectureship: The ethics and efficacy of traumatic brain injury rehabilitation—Myths, measurements, and meaning. *Journal of Head Trauma Rehabilitation, 11,* 88–95.

Rosenthal, M., & Young, T. (1988). Effective family intervention after traumatic brain injury. *Journal of Head Trauma Rehabilitation, 4,* 42–50.

Sachs, P. R. (1991). *Treating families of brain-injury survivors*. New York: Springer.

Sandel, M. E., Williams, K. S., Dellapietra, L., & Derogatis, L. R. (1996). Sexual functioning following traumatic brain injury. *Brain Injury, 10,* 719–728.

Shaw, L. R., & McMahon, B. T. (1990). Family–staff conflict in the rehabilitation setting: Causes, consequences, and implications. *Brain Injury, 1,* 87–93.

Weissman, M. M. (1975). The assessment of social adjustment. A review of techniques. *Archives of General Psychiatry, 32,* 357–365.

Zasler, N. D., & Kreutzer, J. S. (1991). Family and sexuality after traumatic brain injury. In J. Williams & T. Kay (Eds.), *Head injury: A family matter* (pp. 253–270). Baltimore: Paul H. Brooks.

Zencius, A., Wesolowski, M. D., Burke, W. H., & Hough, S. (1990). Managing hypersexual disorders in brain-injured clients. *Brain Injury, 4,* 175–181.

21

Cognitive Rehabilitation during the Industrialization of Rehabilitation

LEONARD DILLER

Introduction

A maxim is a simple, universally accepted truth. For example, in medicine there is a maxim: "Above all do no harm"; in economics: "There is no free lunch"; in literature: "In the beginning was the word"; and in rehabilitation one might say: "Do what you have to do to optimize the functioning of the patient," with a proviso of "Do not violate the other maxims." If one does no harm, tries to make a citizen with a handicap a productive taxpayer or relieve someone of a burden that hopefully can be translated in economic terms, and writes a clean report to a third-party payer, then all participants will be happy: the patient, the sponsoring agency, and the provider of services. But if one should stray from any one of these maxims, then one of the parties in rehabilitation will be offended and trouble follows.

"Do what you have to do" has a broad moral imperative as well as an uncomfortable generality associated with vague do-goodism and charity, rather than disciplined "scientifically" based procedures. In rehabilitation, in addition to "real" reasons for treatment, one must search for "good" reasons, which are usually tied to regulatory requirements. When modern rehabilitation was launched a half a century ago, in the days before "evidence-based medicine" became a focus of debate, the idea was that a person with a disability faces a life situation dramatically changed by disease or trauma. Changes in sensory, motor, language, or mental status meant that help was needed in walking, grooming, feeding, and toileting and dealing with disruptions in family life, housing, and work. Rehabilitation took upon itself the task of doing all it could, to alleviate the multiple problems confronting each individual. This required a frame or a system that went beyond individual professional disciplines or evidence-based

---

LEONARD DILLER • Rusk Institute of Rehabilitation Medicine, New York University Medical Center, New York, New York 10016.

International Handbook of Neuropsychological Rehabilitation, edited by Christensen and Uzzell.
Kluwer Academic/ Plenum Publishers, New York, 2000.

knowledge. If asked what problems are treated in rehabilitation or what goals are envisioned, answers had to be specific enough to address definable domains, as well as general enough to encompass a larger picture. Although the term enhancing the quality of life was not explicit in those days, it seemed like a good overall fit.

Rehabilitationists approached "quality of life" cautiously. Quality of life indicators are a way to measure aspects of societal functioning. Thus, one could compare the quality of life in different societies, for example, literacy rates in different countries. In ordinary everyday language, the term generally refers to how one is experiencing one's environment with a twofold meaning: the nature of the experiences and the nature of the environment. Psychologists classically focus on the nature of the experience (William James when asked to define quality of life, replied that it depends on the liver). Public policy demands that quality of life be defined by indicators that are objective, observable, and measurable. Examples of such indicators are employment, housing, transportation, educational achievements, and signs of family dysfunction. Indicators drive outlays of public money to improve "quality of life." For a psychologist, in quality of life terms, Shakespeare's Hamlet may be an instance of intrapsychic conflict. For a policy aficionado, Hamlet is a product of a dysfunctional family.

With the success and phenomenal growth has come the industrialization of rehabilitation. With industrialization has come a strong pressure to cut costs. Aiming toward improving QOL poses headaches for stakeholders in rehabilitation. The primary stakeholders who bring varied perspectives are the patient, the provider of services, and the third-party payer. The secondary stakeholders are the regulators and policymakers who look over their shoulders and ride herd over the primary stakeholders. Growing industrialization has led to a situation where patients are divorced from third-party payers who decide eligibility and amount of treatment. Providers are fractionated by reimbursement systems that erode team models and/or standards of professionals delivering services. Picture the dilemma of the case manager who must decide which treatments a person with multiple impairments should receive, if the insurance allows only 60 sessions of all services combined over the lifetime of the patient.

Therefore, it might be useful to look at the stakeholders more closely, to help better understand their situations and arrive at some constructive ways to grapple with larger social and economic forces driving rehabilitation care as we go into the 21st century.

Rehabilitation

A Right or a Privilege

Before dealing with the primary stakeholders, let us look at rehabilitation as the context in which policymakers and regulators operate.

To begin with, society has always been ambivalent with regard to rehabilitation and its role in health care. While acute care has been seen as an "inalienable" right, rehabilitation has alternated between a basic right and a privilege; a quality of life issue. While basic rights are unquestioned and financially supported, quality of life issues are more subject to politics and pressure groups.

The societal pressures that gave rise to modern rehabilitation emerged over concerns with how to deal with wounded war veterans. There were social and political pressures in setting up these programs. Rather than review data on the provider, the costs, and outcomes, a brief introduction to historical forces will be presented (Berkowitz, 1991).

Rehabilitation Teams

Rehabilitation in the United States became an organized endeavor during World War I. To care for the needs of wounded soldiers and veterans, the government set up rehabilitation programs. The organization of the programs became a matter of dispute between medical and vocational branches of the government. Finally, care in the hospitals was placed under the direction of medical leadership, which was originated by the department of orthopedics of Harvard. Care outside of hospitals was under the direction of a vocational arm of the government. Between the two world wars, there was very little interest on the part of organized medicine in rehabilitation, with reports of difficulty in getting articles accepted in scientific and medical journals (Opitz, Folz, Peters, & Gelfman, 1997). In World War II, recognizing a vacuum in medical leadership, a new specialty of physical medicine and rehabilitation emerged (Gelfman, Peters, Opitz, & Folz, 1997). The leaders of this movement developed an alliance with the vocational forces and enabled legislation to help promote and finance medical rehabilitation. Under a banner of the third wave of medical care following diagnosis and treatment, rehabilitation was launched in a rising tide of optimism as a way to help people with residual disabilities and handicaps.

As a program anchored in both medical and vocational delivery systems, medical rehabilitation assembled and configured an expanding array of professional groups. The team approach, although expensive and never exposed to any true experiments, was widely adopted (Diller, 1990; Keith, 1991). A concern with functional ability and an emphasis on activities of daily living and adaptation to the environment were among the unifying themes. This emphasis was one step removed from classical training of the various professions. The members of the team came from professional groups with little validated experience in rehabilitation. For example, physiatrists emerged from an amalgamation of electrocoagulation, hydrotherapy, massage, radiology, and various types of electric stimulation (Opitz *et al.*, 1997); physical therapy had its roots in World War I, when orthopedic surgeons recruited young women (known as rubbin' angels) to assist in massages; occupational therapists had been working with the chronically mentally ill and disabled from the time of the ancient Egyptians; speech therapists in World War I were an academic university discipline interested in drama and elocution; psychologists were largely interested in the development of the new field of psychometric tests; rehabilitation counseling did not exist as a profession, and nursing and social work were viewed peripherally. The team model became one of the defining characteristics of rehabilitation, which was carried over to civilian care.

The Costs and the Payments

Economic constraints translate into a search for efficiency (Reilly, 1997). In industry, this is measured by cost and products. In rehabilitation, costs are translated into reduction of services or length of stay (LOS), a proxy measure of cost for hospital stays and products that are measurable outcomes. Third-party payers with the encouragement of policymakers and regulators have focused primarily on reduction of services and to a lesser extent on measurable outcomes. Service providers having emerged from a tradition that has emphasized processes and outcomes and has focused more on products, or outcomes, while keeping a wary eye on costs over which they have less control. Thus, all disciplines in rehabilitation are scrambling to assemble outcome data to support arguments for the treatments they offer. While costs in rehabilitation have always been a social concern, they now pose an immediate threat.

During the 1980s, to bring health care costs under control, the Health Care Finance Administration, a major government agency responsible for payment of medical insurance, imposed a limit on hospital length of stay, except for certain diagnostic related groupings (DRGs). Rehabilitation centers were considered exempt from DRGs and reduced LOS, and the number of rehabilitation hospitals tripled (Frederickson & Cannon, 1995). Patients could be kept in programs on the basis of need governed more by clinical criteria than arbitrary economic criteria. As a result, the 1980s witnessed a boom in the growth of rehabilitation centers and programs. In the 1990s, the DRG exemption was rescinded. LOS, determined by a third-party payer, became a major determinant of amount of treatment. With no reimbursement for extended treatment, in order to keep beds full, a center must provide many patients with short-term treatments and move patients in and out as rapidly as possible.

Reductions in LOS creates a system where therapists must target their efforts toward the most that could be accomplished by a given discharge date. It reduces the time for mastering skills that may normally require many hours of practice. In effect, the role of the therapist is to prepare the patient for discharge to a home or outpatient program.

Looming on the horizon by the year 2001 (Hoyer, 1998) is the prospect that the government via the Health Care Finance Administration will put into play a third method for payment: capitation, where a third-party payer agrees to pay a network or system of providers a fixed fee to cover all health and medical costs including the cost of rehabilitation. Under such an arrangement the economic resources are pushed to programs of prevention and wellness and away from extended treatments and rehabilitation.

The payment system creates a pattern of incentives, wherein (1) fee for service (1980s) providers treat patients for extended periods of time; (2) fee for case (1990s) providers are paid by the case so that extended treatments are not reimbursed and the incentive is to see as many cases as possible and limit the treatments. This creates a system encouraging rapid turnover of cases where programs empty and fill slots; and (3) capitation (2001) gatekeepers try to curtail extensive or long-term treatment. Although rehabilitationists might argue that one aim of the program is to prevent secondary disability, funds for rehabilitation are clearly not of high priority.

Outcomes

Third-party payers focus on a fixed set of outcome measures to shape the definition of "quality of life" of those who are served. While this strategy appears to be reasonable, rehabilitation is a process like education, where outcomes may be multidimensional and nuanced, with objective scores reflecting only part of the results.

Matthew Arnold, the great 19th-century English essayist, assumed the duties of superintendent of the school system in Scotland. The system was in chaos. Then, there were no standard tests for educational achievement or standard ways of separating slow from fast learners. Teachers were paid by student attendance records and for student mastery of specific basic subjects, for example, reading. Other subjects were taught, but teachers emphasized only those subjects for which they were paid. The system was in chaos because the students were unevenly motivated and discipline was a severe problem. In short, a system of learning with limited targets and a narrow band of outcomes made for unhappy participants. Just as there is more to education than good grades, there is more to be gained in rehabilitation than a narrow band of performance scores. While Matthew Arnold faced chaos, poor morale, and disorganization in education, in a less dramatic way we face an analogous problem in health care. Do outcome criteria fit the needs of the people who go through programs? Do they fit the treatments?

While one cannot survive without reasonable measures of outcome, providers should be concerned about locking in service delivery to existing outcomes. Advances have been made in the development of instruments to assess outcomes (Dittmar & Gresham, 1997), but a provider who tailors services only around existing outcomes does not do justice to treatment potentials.

Impairments are the easiest domain to measure, although the most pertinent measures of cognitive impairments that are sensitive to rehabilitation are far from clear. The measurement of disability has witnessed the greatest advance, but even this domain has huge gaps. For example, the Functional Independence Measure (FIM), the most well-known scale, can be used to predict the amount of supervisory time an inpatient subject will need following discharge from a rehabilitation program (Corrigan, Smith-Knapp, & Granger, 1997). The FIM is not fully sensitive to the range of cognitive, social, and emotional problems that are treated in rehabilitation and become more obvious in outpatient settings. The domain of handicap is under investigation by several research groups. The integration of the different domains of impairment, disability, and handicap has not yet been addressed in systematic ways.

The Stakeholders

Recipients of Rehabilitation Services

Recipients of treatments, who used to be called patients, are now called consumers. Consider some of the repercussions. Consumers are associated with products. Services are put forward as product lines. Neurorehabilitation, for example, is a product line. Products have a fixed, closed-ended quality. Patient care has a broader and individualized connotation. By implication there is a concern with the whole person and the meanings of the treatments. In addition, rehabilitation requires an active engagement in a process rather than a passive consumption of a service or an object. While most people would glide over this distinction as a semantic quibble, consider the different types of issues involved in assessing the concerns of the recipient. From the perspective of the patient, the major concerns are fear, burden on caretakers, costs of services, and the unknown future. While financial sponsors and patients and their families agree on priority rankings for clinical outcomes, there is diagreement with regard to services. Financial sponsors want service that focuses on outcomes, time frames, and prediction, while family members put greater weight on family involvement in decision making, staff experience, staff skills and sensitivity, as well as sponsor involvement (Evans, 1997).

Society in general and health care in particular have seen a rising presence of satisfaction measures and ratings by critics on products and services. What started as ratings of movies, restaurants, and a wide variety of products has spread to ratings of professions including physicians, hospitals, and rehabilitation programs. Hence, along with outcome studies we are on the threshold of a whole generation of satisfaction studies based on consumer models (Seligman, 1996). Yet, the application of satisfaction measures is fraught with methodological problems. Psychotherapy researchers are long familiar with the "hello–goodby" effect, whereby a person at the end of treatment wishes to leave in an upbeat manner. We do not understand much about the relation between satisfaction and initial expectancy, particularly when recovery and treatment are confounded.

Providers and Their Dilemmas

For providers, the pressures in cutting costs include reducing lengths of stay and limiting treatments, lowering standards, comparing providers with each other in terms of cost-benefit indicators, and being forced to treat only what one is paid to do. In view of the fact that there is little empirical evidence for the most basic operations of treatments in rehabilitation, including who treats, how much, how long, how often, and at what points in time, providers are under pressure over every aspect of their programs.

Pressures to lower standards are seen in attempts of the Commission on Accreditation of Rehabilitation Facilities to entertain proposals to dilute mandatory requirements of the team approach. The growth of subacute rehabilitation programs, which imposed less intensive services for inpatients, is also being pushed. Indeed, early studies based on retrospective data (Keith, Wilson, & Guitierrez, 1995) suggest no difference in outcome between acute, that is, intensive rehabilitation programs versus subacute, less intensive programs.

Previously, we have mentioned the entry of different professional groups into rehabilitation. Molding these groups into teams with common goals often results in a diffusion of traditional boundaries between professionals with overlapping skills. Problem situations do not come neatly packaged. For example, cognitive remediation, supportive psychotherapy, dressing activities, and counseling can be delivered by professionals with overlapping skills. The resolution of these issues has not been easy and has given rise to a considerable body of literature on the team approach (Diller, 1990). With the move to look at teams from an economic perspective, there is great concern about reducing the level and diversity present within a team (Keith, 1997) and maintaining the level and coherence of rehabilitation services.

The practitioner also struggles with delivering a treatment that has not been fully validated, or even if fully validated must be adapted to a situation that differs from the one where the validation was conducted. Thus, in cognitive rehabilitation there is a broad literature supporting or failing to support treatment of attention, memory, or problem solving (Wilson, 1997). All the reviews are cognizant of the difficulties in promoting generalization or carry over of what has been taught.

Drawing on the classic gold standard of looking for therapies based on randomized controlled trials, one runs into the problem of whether the patient being treated is the same as the patients who were involved in the clinical trials. In cognitive studies, very few patients present with single deficits such as a pure attention or a pure memory deficit (Diller, Goodgold, & Kay, 1989). In a search for correlates of neglect in hemiplegics who received inpatient rehabilitation over a 4-year period, after we reviewed the medical charts of 643 right-brain-damaged and 700 left brain-damaged patients, a total of 152 right-brain-damaged and 74 left-brain-damaged patients met study criteria and were accessed into the study. In brief, 25% of right-brain-damaged and 10% of left-brain-damaged patients were able to participate in an assessment study. In a sample selected to compare different types of interventions, only 63 right-brain-damaged patients were able to participate in a treatment study. In sum, matched samples who could participate in a treatment study represent only 10% of an impairment entity participating in rehabilitation.

The rising influence of third-party payers has sent a wave of concerns about ethical issues in rehabilitation. While ethical concerns have mushroomed in medicine over the past two decades, application of key ethical principles, for example, beneficence, autonomy, and informed consent, have received only slight attention (Caplan, Callahan, & Haas, 1987). Rehabilitation differs from traditional hospital care because patients are more active in selecting and engaging their therapies, treatment time is more extended and takes longer, there is typically less concern with life and death issues, there is more emphasis on the educational process, and a greater variety of team members conduct hands-on treatment.

The Third-Party Payers

Third-party payers bring a business perspective. They want to provide good value for a product and maintain customer satisfaction and financial viability.

Third-party payers generally emerge from one of two traditions group health plans, which stem from a medical tradition, and workmen's compensation, which stems from a vocational tradition. The medical tradition of insurance when applied to rehabilitation emphasizes recovery from an episode and the development of skills to relieve burdens or avoid danger. Medical insurance may involve a co-pay, with a wide variety of treatments that are covered, so that payment for a given impairment differs even within the same company. Consequently, patients with insurance plans may have to go through a bewildering set of regulations. The matter is made worse when an individual has several insurance plans with regulations that contradict each other. The vocational tradition that is invoked when disability is job-related involves a return to productivity and has a different set of ground rules. Hence, the situation may arise where two patients with the same condition are entitled to different paths of treatment depending on the company sponsoring the treatment.

Payers have a responsibility to provide money for services, but they also have a legal obligation to sources providing the funds. Payers must be in a position to estimate their financial liability and to limit costs. Payers protect their interest by preservice screens for prior approval, resort to a second opinion, ongoing utilization review, and limiting certain services, for example, family treatment. The payer writes policies based on predicting utilization and costs and requires outcome data. The major threats to the payer are consumer dissatisfaction, lawsuits, and competition. From a policy standpoint, a major concern is regulating and monitoring the third-party payers.

Paths Toward Solutions

Short of changes in the system that are beyond the control of providers, there are a number of steps that could be undertaken to help in the current situation. These steps involve what providers can do in terms of their own services as well as interactions with both patients and third-party payers.

Providers must continue to emphasize quality and resist its erosions. If providers are clear on their goals and why they wish to act, they will figure out ways of achieving the results as deLateur (1997) indicates.

While grappling with rapid changes in information management as well economic constraints, efficacy research with all of its difficulties must be a high priority for survival. Third-party payers, in seeking to reduce costs, demand strong evidence for reimbursing procedures.

Databases that provide normative outcome information are slowly being accumulated from different professional groups. These databases sample patients by flow-through institutions or by flow-through individual providers who form voluntary cooperative networks encouraged by professional societies (Evans, 1997; Zarin, Pincus, West, & McIntyre, 1997). The aim is to build an additional set of metrics to examine outcomes. While it is too early to assess the viability of such data, it offers a way in which providers can help themselves.

Providers are developing practice guidelines for the management of specific impairment groups or specific situations. Interdisciplinary guidelines sponsored by government agencies have been developed for poststroke rehabilitation, cardiac rehabilitation, and acute pain. Professional groups are developing more specific guidelines for evidence-based practice.

Clinical pathways are also being developed to sort patients in terms of resources needed for the treatment of a given condition. It is possible to assess with some accuracy stroke patients who present simple as opposed to complex management pictures so that one will be able to place patients on different treatment tracks at the onset of rehabilitation.

While caught up in the wave of outcome studies, there is a great need to search for the underlying mechanisms to understand and improve what takes place in rehabilitation. For example, while there have been important advances in pharmacology during the 1990s—the decade of the brain—the core of rehabilitation still resides in teaching someone to overcome and/or live with impairments. The study of learning has received little systematic inquiry (Baddeley, 1993). What is taught and what is learned in mastering a skill? The infusion of learning theory and cognitive science is a task for the future. Perhaps the 21st century will begin with the decade of behavior, where many of the issues in rehabilitation can receive concentrated application. Outcomes can be improved by applying increased understanding of mechanisms.

Providers can develop more forums for open discussion of ethical issues. In the absence of a more scientific or evidenced basis for decision making, many issues in clinical decision making are resolved without adequate basis in principle. Ethical decision involves a systematic pursuit of clarification of values, rather than the applications of a cookbook of principles. In addition to professional meetings and journals, local meetings can take place via grand rounds. For example, actual cases can be presented where clinicians deal with decision making and the underlying issues are clarified in terms of ethical principles. Several sources for case studies exist (Caplan *et al.*, 1987).

Some Ethical Issues Discussed in Rehabilitation Rounds

Examples of ethical dilemmas that have emerged at grand rounds in our institution and may be common in rehabilitation as opposed to traditional hospitals or mental health settings are:

1. Risk taking in dependent people is a common feature in rehabilitation. Particularly, when improvement is judged in terms of removal of assistance. How is level of assistance judged? Who judges safety? Or supervision which is needed?
2. Is equal access to rehabilitation available given the economics of rehabilitation (Haas, 1988)?
3. With decreased length of stay, how should therapy time be spent?
4. What does a patient agree to upon entering a rehabilitation program? Does informed consent cover multiple treatments?Suppose the patient agrees with only part of a program?
5. Is a team responsible for an unsatisfactory home placement?
6. If insurance runs out, should a team petition an insurer on behalf of a patient?
7. With time limits, how does one deal with a slow learner?
8. How far should a team push a reluctant patient?
9. How are loyalty conflicts dealt with: How does one deal with conflicting allegiances to the patient, the team, the profession, the administration?

10. What are the limits of family responsibility?
11. What if the patient says, "Do not tell my relative"?

Provider–Payer Interactions

Professional groups might attempt to establish communications with third-party payers at broader levels than case-by-case management. For example, professional societies may invite payer representatives to appear in joint symposia, or as invited discussants at symposia. Representatives might be invited to participate as reactors to journal articles (Cervelli, 1987). Professional groups might meet with third-party payers to review sources of databases that are used.

While providers and payers may have competing interests insofar as reimbursement is concerned, in that providers would like greater reimbursement and payers search for less reimbursement, both share a concern about satisfied patients, or consumers. Finally, providers and third-party payers might arrange symposia and programs around ethical issues in managed care. Much cross-education is needed in this arena.

Provider–Patient Interactions

Providers can take a more assertive stance in educating patients about the problems associated in living with a disability and some of the services offered. This education can take place at two levels. One is a public education level to inform people about the nature of rehabilitation, and the other is at a more individual level to inform patients receiving clinical services. At the public level these efforts are best seen as undertakings of professional societies and voluntary health agencies. At the clinical level there can be educational pathways, which engage patients and families as they go through the different phases of rehabilitation. For example, education can begin at the acute hospital, through inpatient rehabilitation hospital and outpatient services. Educating patients about services, expectancies, costs, and outcomes is generally not part of professional training. It is usually seen as part of the job responsibilities that are learned in a given setting. The problem is that service deliverers may be insensitive to the needs for patients and families to know more about their condition and the services that are provided.

Accountability of providers to patients and of patients to providers is not made sufficiently explicit. Providers should educate patients as to their mutual accountability. This may range from providing simple information to providing more elaborate educational approaches for certain population groups, where communication is difficult for cultural or emotional reasons. The way facts are organized and presented requires consideration of the recipients as well as the content of the information.

As previously indicated there is increasing interest in patient surveys. However, few if any of the satisfaction surveys emerge from the perspective of the patient. The new wave of quality of life studies focus on the patient's views of his or her situation. While patient-directed inventories aggregate items into clusters of behavioral symptoms or complaints, the newer studies pay more attention to issues of independent living in the nonmotoric as well as the motoric sphere (Webb, Wrigley, Yoels, & Fine, 1995; Duggan, Djikers, Tate, & Heinrich, 1997). Such studies will lead to better training programs for providers (Wong, 1997). These studies are particularly helpful in showing discrepancies between patients and providers (Fuhrer *et al.*, 1992).

These studies can lead eventually to a better understanding of the situations of people after rehabilitation is completed. This will permit the identification of problems of persons with chronic impairments and the development of a neglected venue for the delivery of rehabilitation services where one can demonstrate good reasons as well as real reasons for interventions. It may be recalled that Flanagan's original methodology consisted of asking people about critical incidents, that is, "Think of the first time you did something important or experienced something important or experienced something that was especially satisfying. What did you do or what happened. Why did this experience seem so satisfying." Results from diverse populations suggest that impairment is only weakly related to quality of life, and that social support, leisure time usage, personal control, and other aspects of handicap are more directly related to quality of life (Webb *et al.,* 1995).

Conclusion

The simple maxims of rehabilitation can be maintained in spite of the industrialization of rehabilitation and the economic threats that are shaking the entire system of health care. Rehabilitation has been most helpful by breaking down actual problems in living into tasks that are often addressed by doable, practical, small steps when major cures seem remote. If we apply this thinking to our present dilemmas, it is possible to reduce the problems and sustain the dynamism of the field.

References

Baddeley, A. D. (1993). A theory of rehabilitation without a model of learning is a vehicle without an engine: A comment on Caramazza and Hillis. *Neuropsychological Rehabilitation, 3,* 235–244.

Berkowitz, E. (1991). The federal government and the emergence of rehabilitation medicine. *The Historian, 43,* 530–544.

Caplan, A. L., Callahan, D., & Haas, J. (1987). Ethical and policy issues in rehabilitation medicine. A Hastings Center Report: Special supplement. *Archives of Physical Medicine and Rehabilitation, 68,* 7–20.

Cervelli, L. (1997). The missing link; structured dialogue between payer and provider communities on the costs and benefits of medical rehabilitation. *Archives of Physical Medicine and Rehabilitation, 78* (Suppl. S3), S36–S38.

Corrigan, J. D., Smith-Knapp, K., & Granger, C. V. (1997). Validity of the Functional Independence Measure for persons with traumatic brain injury. *Archives of Physical Medicine and Rehabilitation, 78,* 828–834.

deLateur, B. J. (1997) Quality of life; a patient centered outcome. The 29th Walter J. Zeiter Lecture. *Archives of Physical Medicine and Rehabilitation, 3,* 78, 237–239.

Diller, L. (1990). Fostering the interdisciplinary team, fostering research in a society in transition. *Archives of Physical Medicine and Rehabilitation, 71,* 275–278.

Diller, L., Goodgold, J., & Kay, T. (1989). *Final report to NIDRR for the Rehabilitation Research and Training Center in Head Trauma and Stroke.* New York: Department of Rehabilitation Medicine New York University Medical Center.

Dittmar, S. S., & Gresham, G. E. (1997). *Functional assessment and outcome measures for the rehabilitation health health professional.* Frederick, MD: Aspen.

Duggan, C. H., Djikers, M., Tate, D., & Heinrich, R. (1997). Quality of life of persons with spinal cord injuries; an analysis based on personal narrative. *Archives of Physical Medicine and Rehabilitation, 78,* 910.

Evans, R. W. (1997). Postacute neurorehabilitation; Roles and responsibilities within a national information system. *Archives of Physical Medicine and Rehabilitation, 78,* (Suppl. 4), S-17–S25.

Frederickson, N., & Cannon, N. L. (1995). The role of the rehabilitation physician in the postacute continuum. *Archives of Physical Medicine and Rehabilitation, 76,* SC-5–

Fuhrer, M. J., Rentala, D. H., Hart, K. A. Clearman, R., & Young, M. E. (1992), Relationship of life satisfaction to impairment, disability, and handicap among persons with spinal cord injury living in the community. *Archives of Physical Medicine and Rehabilitation.* 73, 552–557.

Gelfman, R., Peters, J., Opitz, J. L., & Folz, T. J. (1997). The history of physical medicine and rehabilitation as recorded in the diary of DR Frank Krusen: Part 3. Consolidating the position (1948–1953). *Archives of Physical Medicine and Rehabilitation, 78,* 556–561.

Haas, J. F. (1988). Admission to rehabilitation centers: Selection of patients. *Archives of Physical Medicine and Rehabilitation, 68,* 329–332.

Hoyer, T. (1998). Quoted in "Say goodbye to functional related groups, hello to MDS and RUGS." *Rehabilitation Continuum Report, 7,* 1.

Keith, R. A. (1991). The comprehensive treatment team in rehabilitation. *Archives of Physical Medicine and Rehabilitation, 72,* 269–274.

Keith, R. A. (1997). Treatment strength in rehabilitation. *Archives of Physical Medicine and Rehabilitation, 78,* 1298–1304.

Keith, R. A., Wilson, D. B., & Guitierrez, P. (1995). Acute and subacute rehabilitation for stroke: A comparison. *Archives of Physical Medicine and Rehabilitation, 76,* 495–500.

Malec, J. F., & Basford, J. S. (1996). Postacute brain injury rehabilitation. *Archives of Physical Medicine and Rehabilitation, 77,* 198–207.

Opitz, J. L., Folz, T. J., Peters, J., & Gelfman, R. (1997). The history of physical medicine and rehabilitation as recorded in the diaries of Frank Krusen: Part 1: Gathering momentum (the years before 1942). *Archives of Physical Medicine and Rehabilitation, 78,* 442–445.

Reilly, T. A. (1997). Management dilemmas in rehabilitation today. *Rehabilitation Outlook, 2,* 2–4.

Seligman, M. E. P. (1996). Science as an ally of practice. *American Psychologist, 51,* 1072–1079.

Webb, C. D., Wrigley, M., Yoels, W., & Fine, P. (1995). Explaining quality of life for persons with traumatic brain injuries 2 years after brain injury. *Archives of Physical Medicine and Rehabilitation, 76,* 1113–1118.

Wilson, B. A. (1997). Cognitive rehabilitation: How it is and how it might be. *Journal of International Neuropsychology Society, 3,* 487–496

Wong, E. H. (1997). How to avoid an adversarial alliance with families in acute brain injury rehabilitation: Simple guidelines from clinical observations. *Archives of Physical Medicine and Rehabilitation, 77,* 945–948.

Zarin, D. A., Pincus, H. A., West, J. C., & McIntyre, J. S. (1997). Practiced based research in psychiatry. *American Journal of Psychiatry, 154* (9), 1199–1208.

22

Neurological Rehabilitation in Germany

The Phase Model

PAUL W. SCHÖNLE

Rehabilitation in Germany has its roots in the late 19th century when Bismarck created the social security system. As a consequence, rehabilitation was introduced by the pension funds to avoid premature retirement of the working population (rehabilitation before pension), and rehabilitation became a social right for everyone ensured in the social security system. During World War I, neurological rehabilitation was developed to a high standard service for the brain-injured veterans including specialized centers like that, for example, of Kurt Goldstein's hospital in Frankfurt. After a decline during the years of economic depression it was reorganized during World War II to take care of the many more brain-injured soldiers compared to World War I who survived due to neurosurgery, newly developed in the 1930s, and faster airborne transportation in the fields. With the end of the war, all military hospitals were closed down including the neurological rehabilitation centers.

In 1950, one of the first neurological rehabilitation centers after World War II was founded in Germany on the Swiss boarder, the Schmieder Hospital for Neurological and Psychiatric Rehabilitation, a private institution for the retraining of brain-injured veterans at a level of severity that corresponds to later phase D and E (including motor and cognitive retraining and vocational rehabilitation). Soon after, motorized traffic began to develop gradually and numbers of traumatic brain injury (TBI) cases increased, in parallel more rehabilitation hospitals, mostly private, appeared in resort areas. In the 1970s, phase C started to develop in addition to phases D/E, including more severely disabled patients who were dependent in most activities of daily living. With the advancement of emergency and intensive care medicine, severely brain-damaged patients survived in increasing numbers, including patients with cerebrovascular accidents (CVA) and posthypoxic encephalopathies after

PAUL W. SCHÖNLE • A. R. Lurija-Institute for Rehabilitation Sciences and Health Research, University of Constance, Kliniken Schmieder, D-78473 Allensbach, Germany.

International Handbook of Neuropsychological Rehabilitation, edited by Christensen and Uzzell.
Kluwer Academic/ Plenum Publishers, New York, 2000.

cardiac resuscitation. Therefore, phase B (early intensive care rehabilitation) started to be developed in the end of the 1980s.

Three hundred thousand new cases with TBI and approximately the same number with CVA each year pose major problems to the health care system. To face this problem, comprehensive neurological rehabilitation has been developed over the decades based on the long-standing tradition in the field. It was summarized in the phase model of neurological rehabilitation (PMNR), which attempts to cover the major aspects of rehabilitation from intensive care up to vocational reintegration and long-term care (BAR 1995; BAG, 1994; Ministerium für Arbeit, 1991; Schönle 1990, 1995a, 1996a, b, 1998; VDR 1995). The model was formulated in various publications of expert working groups organized by local government, pension funds, and health insurance companies. It describes neurological rehabilitation in a systematic and detailed way and serves as (1) a conceptual framework to plan neurological rehabilitation and to carry it out and (2) a frame of reference for communication, classification of patients, differential allocation of resources, and quality management.

Basic Aspects of the Phase Model

Neurological rehabilitation in Germany has its scientific basis in neuroscience, including brainpathology (the precursor of neuropsychology as opposed to psychopathology), mostly in the form of localization theory (Kleist), Gestaltpsychology and the holistic approach (Goldstein), experimental psychology (Poppelreuter), and linguistics (Pick) (Poser, Kohler, & Schönle, 1996)

The leitmotiv underlying the conceptualization of neurological rehabilitation is the belief that it is optimal for the patient, if the logic of the brain is the logic of rehabilitation, and if the organizational principals of rehabilitation mirror the organizational and functional principles of the brain in its complexity.

Brain damage, be it due to TBI or CVA or other causes strikes the individual in the center of his or her human existence and changes the social microcosms, especially the family. The functional and organizational principles, the various severity levels of functional disturbances after brain damage, and the differential capabilities of functional systems to recover require planning and realization of neurological rehabilitation, as a treatment concept that is comprehensive but individually designed and geared, if necessary, as a long-term enterprise. Indicative of this rehabilitative complexity is (1) the team approach including the various disciplines (see Fig. 1) and (2) the differentiation of neurological rehabilitation into various phases, which are defined by specific treatment concepts and structural and procedural features (see Fig. 2). These are intrinsic medical factors in contrast to sociolegal, sociopolitical, and economic aspects (extrinsic factors). While the extrinsic factors vary from country to country, the intrinsic remain the same. Both intrinsic and extrinsic factors, however, determine neurological rehabilitation in reality.

In the severest cases of brain damage all functions of the central nervous system are affected—somatic, cognitive, and mental including vital autonomous functions such as the control of the cardiovascular or respiratory systems—resulting in life-threatening conditions and coma. Immediate medical intervention (e.g., operation) and intensive care are required (phase A: acute care). As soon as respiration is stabilized (no more artificial ventilation required) and acute interventions are definitive, early rehabilitation can be started still under intensive care

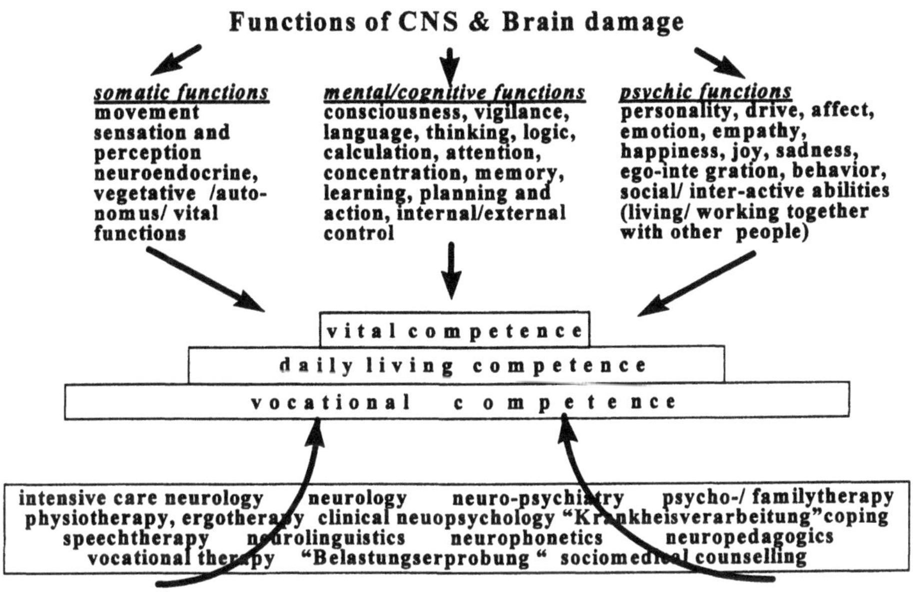

FIGURE 1. The complexity of neurological rehabilitation: Overview on brain functions and integration of various functions into competencies (*vital competency:* integrating life sustaining functions; *daily living competence:* integrating brain functions relevant for dealing with everyday life; *vocational competence:* integrating brain functions relevant for work). Brain damage can result in functional disturbances and disintegration of competencies. Complexity of brain functions requires adequate complexity of the rehabilitation program covering all functional areas and competencies. This can be achieved only by an integrated multidisciplinary rehabilitation team (comprehensive neurological rehabilitation).

monitoring conditions (phase B). Phase B is characterized by a dominating functional impairment in the vital, autonomous domain ("vital competence").

In less severe cases the autonomous vital control systems remain intact from the beginning, but other functions are concerned in various domains and at such levels of severity that patients are dependent in all or almost all activities of daily living (ADL) (e.g., feeding, hygiene). Patients may be unable to move (turn around in bed, stand up, stand, walk, sit down, transfer), to use arms and hands, to chew and swallow, to speak, to use cognition (language, attention, memory, learning, planning, action, executive control). The predominant feature in phase C is the missing ADL competence.

In cases of mild–moderate brain damage neither vital functions nor functions necessary for ADL are affected. Disturbances in the sensorimotor, cognitive, or mental domains are predominant, which may be at a high severity level (e.g., global aphasia) and devastating for social or vocational reintegration (phase D/E*)*. The prominent features in phase D/E are the limitations in the social and vocational competences.

The phases are mainly characterized by the type of functional systems that are predominantly affected, preserved, or in restitution (see Fig. 2). In coma all functions are reduced to a minimum or nil (phase A, intensive care); with recovery from coma, consciousness and control over autonomous functions (cardiovascular–respiratory) return and allow transfer to phase B (early rehabilitation). If only autonomous (i.e., vegetative) functions recover and stabilize, patients are in a vegetative state without mentation–cognition (lower right in Fig 3). Patients can be transferred to phase C when swallowing control is reestablished (no more tracheostoma required) and cognitive functions work at a basic level (attention span, memory span, language communication, some control over actions), even if they are still dependent in ADL due to reduced sensorimotor and/or mental functioning. Patients move on to phase D when ADL competence is re-established.

Transfer from one phase to the next is also mirrored in the development of single functional systems per se, for example, action is nil in deep coma; not even reflex responses can be evoked (no response level). Later, when patients emerge from deep coma, reflex responses appear. Patients who develop further start to show adaptive early learning behavior, for example, in the mulitmodal blink reflex habituation paradigm (Schönle & Schwall, 1993a, b). When stimulated ten times, one stimulus per second [acoustically (hand clap) visually (hand thread), tactily (glabella tap)], patients in comas do not respond (see Fig. 4). Patients emerging and out of coma respond to each stimulus (reflexive response level). Patients who continue to develop start to habituate, that is, they respond only to seven or eight stimuli (adaptive response level); eventually they respond adequately to the stimulus context–situation (context-adequate response level). Finally, they produce self-triggered actions and activities that are situationally adequate (spontaneous behavioral level).

Patients in vegetative state, however, do not follow this development of the functional system "action." They remain on the level of reflexive behavior and respond to each single stim-

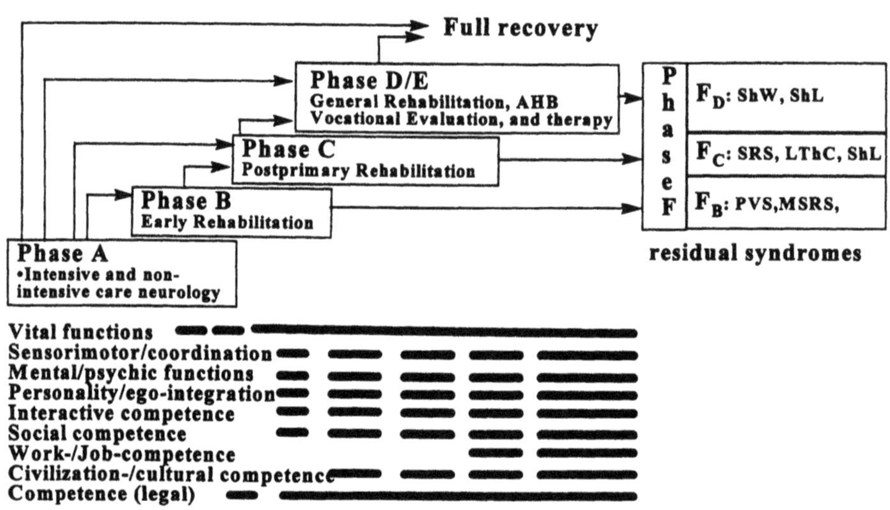

FIGURE 2. A Phase Model of Neurological Rehabilitation. Phases A–F of neurological rehabilitation and underlying impairment of brain functions. After acute brain damage a patient is admitted to acute neurology (A). If all brain functions are impaired as in coma, intensive care is required. When functions return (e.g., vital functions, broken lines) the patient can be transferred to phase B. With further rehabilitation and recovery of functions (full lines), subsequent phases can be passed up to the level of full reintegration. However, patients can also recover only partially (residual syndromes) on various functional levels. They are transferred to phase F on the appropriate level (F_B, F_C, F_D). A patient in persistent vegetative state is transferred to long-term care on the F_B level. Whenever a patient shows positive signs of restitution later in phase B, he or she can be readmitted to a phase B ward (arrows indicate transfer of patients). SRS, severe residual syndromes (highly dependent); MSRS, most severe residual syndromes (totally dependent); PVS, persistent vegetative state; ShW, sheltered work; ShL, sheltered living; LThC, long-term therapy care.

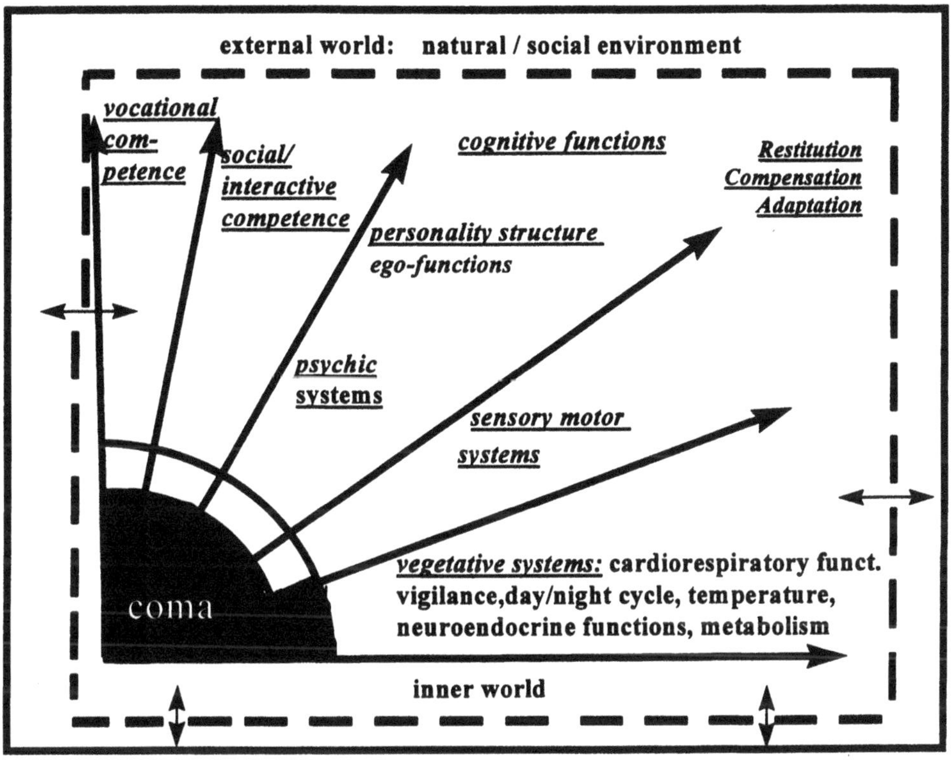

FIGURE 3. Functional impairment in coma and postcomatose recovery; functional systems recover in different domains at different pace (no regular pattern) to a varying degree. If only autonomous (vegetative, vital) functions return, the patient remains in a vegetative state (lower right).

ulus without any sign of habituation. A behavioral feature of vegetative state thus appears to be the inability to monitor incoming stimuli with respect to their ecological significance, that is, to learn that the presented stimuli are not threatening.

It follows directly from the functional systems that are affected by the brain damage what type of acute medical interventions are required in phase A (intensive care vs. normal ward versus outpatient treatment) and what type of rehabilitation measures have to be taken (phase B–E). Some patients do not recover or recover only partially. They remain in a residual syndrome and need long-term care at various levels of disability (phase F) (see right side of Fig. 2).

Phases of Neurological Rehabilitation

Phases are primarily defined by medical criteria but sociolegal and economical aspects also play a role. They are named by letters to avoid conflicts with already existing but inconsistent and underspecified terminologies. The term *early rehabilitation,* for example, is traditionally used for phase B rehabilitation (i.e., rehabilitation under intensive care monitoring conditions). "Early" only refers to the time aspect and confuses nonspecialists who are not

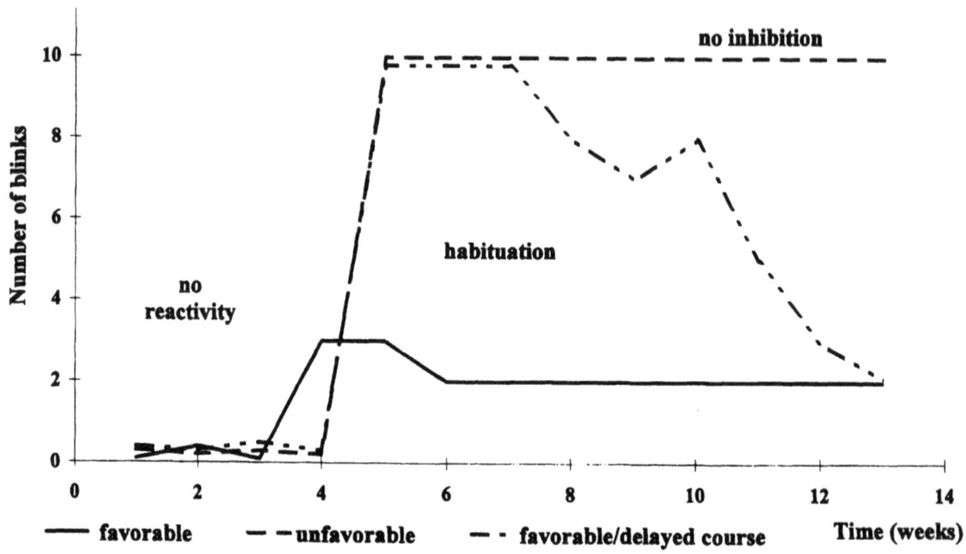

FIGURE 4. Development of blinking behavior after coma. In deep coma, patients do not react by blinking to visual, acoustic, or tactile stimuli in the blink reflex habituation paradigm (ten stimuli are applied [one per second] and number of blinks counted). When patient awakens from coma and returns to normal, he or she starts to habituate early on (e.g., only three or two blink reactions to ten stimuli). A delayed return is characterized by an initial inability to inhibit blink reactions followed by later, gradually emerging habituation (delayed, but favorable course). Patients who remain in a vegetative state are unable to inhibit blinking; they do not habituate (unfavorable course). Blinks are evoked by multimodal stimulation (visual, auditory, tactile); best response modality is taken for evaluation.

familiar with the definition of early rehabilitation. The same is true for "post" in the terms *postprimary* or *postacute* rehabilitation, which are used for phase C.

Phase A

Phase A is the traditional acute neurological or neurosurgical treatment for the vast variety of diseases afflicting the peripheral or central nervous system including CVA, TBI, infections, and tumors. As a consequence, various functional systems are affected either directly by local damage (e.g., aphasia) or indirectly by mass effects (e.g., loss of consciousness, or loss of cardiovascular and respiratory control). In case of coma due to (for example, a massive intracerebral hemorrhage or respiratory or cardiac arrest, patients have to be treated initially on an intensive care unit. Treatment on a normal ward is sufficient if there is no life-threatening situation in the beginning (Fig. 2). When operative interventions and intensive care have been successful, patients can be transferred to a normal ward for further treatment. In many cases full functional recovery (*restitutio ad integrum*) does not occur despite successful medical treatment. Therefore, rehabilitative medicine has to be continued and patients are transferred from acute curative medicine to phases B, C, or D/E according to the rehabilitation needs.

Treatment goals in phase A concentrate on medical diagnosis and treatment of the underlying etiologies and accompanying disorders or injuries (acute curative medical intervention). The objectives are to stabilize and restitute vital autonomous functions (cardiovascular and respiratory), normalize intracranial pressure, provide definitive medical treatment (etiology oriented, e.g., operation, antibiotic medication), minimize impairment of peripheral or central nervous system functions, prevent secondary complications, and give a first preliminary opinion on the rehabilitation potential. First steps in rehabilitation should be taken, including physiotherapy (range of motion, positioning).

The duration of phase A is defined by medical requirements. The transition into the next phase can be possible after a few days or in some cases after weeks.

Whether treatment has to be continued in a rehabilitation unit or not depends on the neurological symptomatology and the accompanying diseases. Some patients (app. 10–20%) need early rehabilitation (phase B); the majority of cases, however, can be transferred to phases C or D/E or can be discharged home. A transition into phase F is an exemption, as every patient has the right to a thorough diagnostic rehabilitation program, including functional therapeutic interventions to evaluate his or her rehabilitative potential. The diagnostic program is directed toward a functional analysis in contrast to acute diagnostics, which are predominantly etiology oriented (functional versus etiological diagnostics and treatment in acute versus rehabilitation medicine).

Phase B

There are certain intake criteria that define the level of functional severity on one hand and the corresponding structural and process qualities of the phase B unit on the other, which is determined by the per day payment through the health insurance companies. Phase B wards must provide structural and process qualities suited to handle life-threatening functional disturbances such as vegetative crises or respiratory insufficiencies. Except for regular intensive care with controlled artificial respiration, patients with high levels of severity can be treated and must be treated on such a ward to justify the high level of per day payment.

As a rule, patients have a history of severe brain damage mostly due to TBI, CVA, hypoxia, and encephalitis. They are comatose or show severe disturbances of consciousness (near-comatose state), vigilance, or awareness, including vegetative state, akinetic mutism, and locked-in syndrome. Additional functions can be severely disturbed, such as chewing and swallowing, which make a tracheotomy and percutaneous enterogastrotomy (PEG) necessary; bladder and bowel functions are not under control. Respiration should be spontaneous and sufficient so that no regular artificial respiration is required. Patients are not able to cooperate or communicate. They are fully dependent except for ventilation and cardiovascular functions. Patients with Guillain–Barré, high-level transsections of the spinal cord, and others who require a high level of care and rehabilitative treatment are also included.

Primary acute interventions have to be completed in the acute hospital, especially in TBI patients who very often have a polytrauma that requires neurosurgery, orthopedic thoracic surgery, and other operations. Intracranial pressure should be normalized and cardiovascular and respiratory functions stable in a supine position and no florid sepsis. Mobilization may not be prevented by accompanying diseases.

The second group of patients who can enter phase B exhibit excessive mental, emotional, and behavioral disturbances following severe brain injury, including posttraumatic dyscontrol syndrome. Patients in severe confusional states endanger others or themselves and need intensive one-to-one care and control. This group is included in phase B to prevent confinement in a psychiatric institution without neurological rehabilitation. These patients are concentrated in a few phase B units that provide special behavioral programs.

Treatment goals focus on improving consciousness and establishing means of communication, interaction, and cooperation. Patients are mobilized regularly. The extent of damage to the peripheral and central nervous system should be limited and secondary complications avoided. A major goal is to define the rehabilitative potential of the patient by a detailed and comprehensive diagnostic program, including repeated clinical examinations and continous behavioral observations (spontaneous and elicited behavior, responses to rehabilitative and pharmacological interventions), long-term monitoring of electrocardiogram (ECG), respiration, electroencephalogram (EEG) (day–night cycles, responsiveness to outer stimuli), event-related potentials, and imaging (computer tomography or magnetic resonance). When serial findings from different methods point in the same direction or converge on one point, prognostic conclusions become possible and future care can be planned and initiated (e.g., transfer to phase F, if there is no rehabilitative potential).

Curative medical tasks in phase B are to continue: (1) the medical treatment of central and peripheral nervous systems (CNS and PNS) problems (e.g., normal pressure hydrocephylus, coma neuropathy, traumatic injuries of peripheral nerves, epilepsy) of accompanying diseases (e.g., infections, diabetes, cardiac failure) and trauma sequelae (e.g., fractures) that began in the acute phase; (2) to follow these problems; (3) to provide intensive care and monitoring; and (4) to deal with intermittent life-threatening situations during mobilization.

Rehabilitative medical tasks focus on functional diagnostics, rehabilitative care, and treatment on the level of impairment and disability. In the sensorimotor domain, motor responses are elicited on various complexity levels. Attempts are made to prevent secondary damage to joints, tendons and muscles. Patients are stimulated in an individually controlled fashion to (1) establish sensory access routes, (2) stabilize periods of consciousness, (3) prolong attentional control and memory continuum, and (4) induce activities and extent action span. Output channels are tested and improved to allow for verbal and nonverbal communication and interaction with the environment. Reestablishment of communication is a primary target to mediate mental status examination and psychotherapeutic treatment as early as possible. Reestablishment of orofacial tract functions are extremely important to avoid aspirations and bronchopneumonia and to allow for decanulization and closure of tracheostomata. When elementary functions are coming back, interventions are embedded in highly automatized behavior preferably in the domain of ADL at a basic level.

Relatives should be integrated into phase B as early and as much as possible on behalf of the patient, since they represent automatized percepts and concepts. For their own sake relatives should be offered counseling and psychotherapy. Therefore, rooming-in is provided for relatives or hotel costs are paid by health insurance companies to allow relatives to live close to their patients.

Duration of phase B is determined on an individual basis. In general, patients can be in phase B rehabilitation up to 6 months. If complications occur (pneumonia, lung embolization), the time period may be extended.

Discharge from phase B becomes necessary when no functional improvement occurs over a time period of 2 months. As long as the patient shows improvement (sensorimotor, mental, cognitive, behavior, etc.), he has a right to remain in phase B. For children, much longer treatment periods may be required and are financed by the health insurance companies.

Transfer criteria to phase C require the patient to be (1) fully conscious, (2) able to communicate and interact with or without aids, (3) able to follow simple commands, (4) at least partially mobilized, that is, he or she can sit in a wheelchair for approximately 4 hours per day, and (5) socially adequate to allow for small-group therapy sessions. The ability to sustain an activity must be sufficient to participate in several therapeutic sessions per day, which extend over 30 minutes each. He or she may be dependent, however, in most ADL. Vegetative functions are stabile, and no more intensive care monitoring is required. Patients with predominantly dyscontrol syndromes or tendencies to run away need to show adequate behavior without aggressive outbursts for integration into a normal ward.

Phase C

In Phase C, patients must be able to participate actively and cooperatively in therapy sessions. As they are still dependent, they need large quantities of rehabilitative nursing, and as they still have medical problems, they require curative medical care. Autonomous functions, however, are stable, and therefore no further intensive care monitoring is necessary. Detailed intake criteria to phase C correspond to transfer criteria from phase B (see above).

The therapy goal in phase C is to reestablish ADL competence by improving drive, motivation, affect, attention, memory, orientation, communication, sensorimotor and coordinate functions up to the level of planning, action, and executive control. Furthermore, the rehabilitative potential needs to be defined and a long-term perspective developed on an individual basis in close cooperation with relatives.

Patients entering phase C need to be evaluated at the level of impairment, disabilities and handicap anew, if coming directly from the acute hospital, or as a follow-up, if coming from phase B, to monitor the course of the functional development. Based on serial reevaluation, prognostic conclusions are extrapolated for relatives and health insurance companies.

Therapy includes activating rehabilitative nursing and functional treatment of the above functional systems with a preponderance of eating, chewing, swallowing, continence, hygiene, dressing, mobility (independent walking or wheelchair use), and speaking. As far as aids are required, for example, for communication or ambulation, they are individually adapted and their use practiced. Supportive psychotherapy and counseling for the patients and his or her relatives are provided throughout rehabilitation. Curative medical tasks include definitive etiologic diagnostics or diagnostic controls and treatment of the underlying and accompanying diseases (also secondary prophylactics) in addition to the above rehabilitative medical activities.

Duration of phase C rehabilitation is up to 6 months, as in phase B. As a rule, 8 weeks are required for evaluation and treatment trials to allow for prognostic conclusions.

Discharge to phase F (continuation of activating long-term nursing) should to be initiated if no functional changes occur over a period of 8 weeks. In special cases rehabilitation can exceed 8 weeks. In children, much longer treatment periods may be necessary.

Transfer criteria to phase D include independence in ADLs, especially hygiene, dressing, toilet use, eating, and mobility.

Phase D

Patients enter phase D either from phase C or directly from the acute hospital (see Fig. 2). Intake criteria are the transfer criteria from phase C. Patients need to be independent in ADLs; minor problems may still be present but need to be handled by the patient him- or herself, such as independent use of a wheelchair, bladder dysfunction, and slowing in various activities. Patients need to be able to continuously learn, to act, and to cooperate. Mental, cognitive dysfunctions, and/or moderate sensorimotor deficits relevant to daily living or vocational competence are predominant.

Rehabilitation goals include the restitution of those central nervous system functions that are a prerequisite to actively participate in a normal social life and to reduce disabilities and handicaps. A major goal is to reestablish basic work abilities As in the other phases, the major tasks are to (1) evaluate the rehabilitation potential continuously, (2) elaborate a long term perspective, (3) detail a rehabilitation plan in close cooperation with the relatives (rehabilitation case management), and (4) initiate the steps of rehabilitation (transfer to phase E or F).

Curative medical diagnostics and therapies should be continued, including for accompanying diseases, and secondary prophylactics need to be initiated. Rehabilitative medical treatment includes repeated evaluation of impairment, disability and handicap levels, and integrated functional therapies performed by the multidisciplinary rehabilitation team (physiotherapy, neuropsychology, ergotherapy, language and speech therapy, neuropedagogics, psychotherapy, family therapy, counseling). Special aids, if necessary, are adapted individually. Patients and relatives participate in seminars in preventive medicine to establish detailed knowledge about diseases and their prevention (health education). Attempts are made to modify behavioral features with negative health effects (health training). Basic functions related to work are evaluated and trained in vocational therapy, such as *Belastungserprobung* (stress tolerance, endurance) and work trials.

Functional therapies are performed either in small groups or on a one-to-one basis, depending on the individual case. At least 20 units of therapeutic interventions are required per week and controlled by insurance companies in the context of an extensive quality management program.

Duration of phase D covers 2 weeks of functional diagnostics and behavioral observation, if patients enter from the acute hospital, and can last up to 6 months especially in cases of severe functional deficits. If return to work is likely to be achieved, longer treatment periods are possible. Phase D rehabilitation can take place in one 6-month period or as an interval therapy, of several inpatient stays in a rehabilitation hospital with or without bridging a day clinic for neurological rehabilitation (i.e., community-based rehabilitation). In face of the complexity of brain functions and their disturbance, neurological rehabilitation is thought to require long periods of time for restitution, compensation, adaptation, coping, and adjustment: It is not a one-step type of treatment.

Discharge from phase D is required if no functional gains can be achieved over a period of 8 weeks, or when rehabilitation goals are reached. Patients return to work, if medical–vocational therapy is successful, or go on to phase E for further vocational training (to return to the previous job or to move into a new job). Specialized centers are available for vocational training (*Berufsförderungswerke*). If patients do not return to work and go on pension, special measures for social reintegration are available.

Phase E

Phase E represents vocational rehabilitation and follows, when a patient has successfully gone through the phases B–D of intensive medical rehabilitation. There is no more need for curative or rehabilitative medical interventions. All somatic, mental, cognitive, and behavioral functions have been reestablished, so that the patient can get intensive vocational training (specific knowledge and skill) in specialized centers (*Berufsförderungswerke*) and return to work under special programs. They include stepwise vocational reintegration, with increasing work time over a period of 6 months, which is paid by the health insurance companies.

Phase F

The level of functional disturbances, disabilities, and handicaps in phase F corresponds to the phases B, C, or D level, respectively, at which the patient plateaued, F_B, F_C, F_D. Patients in phase F need permanent support, care, and/or nursing. Most patients are dependent on others either partially or completely (e.g., in the vegetative state syndrome). Patients should enter phase F only if adequate rehabilitation has preceded and no tendencies of functional improvement were noticeable.

The goals of phase F are to (1) keep the patient on a performance level reached during rehabilitation, (2) delay functional decay in chronic progressive diseases, and (3) prevent secondary complications. Functional therapies can be continued, but are applied less frequently and are not as comprehensive as in the rehabilitation phase. Social support, counseling, organizational help, and technical aids are provided in the community, including sheltered living and work. Nursing is provided by ambulatory services and paid by nursing insurance companies. Relatives play a major role in this phase and require continuon counseling and support. Duration of phase F is in most cases for a life time. If functional improvement occurs patients may be readmitted to phases B, C, or D.

Who Pays for Neurological Rehabilitation?

Payment for the different phases varies with respect to basic investment and per day payment and depends on the status of medical care of the phase. There are two basic categories of medical care: curative (acute medicine) and rehabilitative (rehabilitation medicine). Phases A and B belong to the curative; acute medical sector and phases C, D, and E belong to the rehabilitation medicine sector, which is subdivided into medical rehabilitation (phases C and D) and vocational rehabilitation (phase E). Phase F is a special sector.

In the acute medical sector the basic investment for the infrastructure, that is, hospital building, equipment, beds, and so forth is provided by the social ministry of the local state, including the follow-up investment for maintenance of the infrastructure. The cost for administrating the hospital, staff, medication, and other consumptive goods are provided by the health insurance companies on a day-by-day payment basis (dual financing system). Therefore, phases A and B are financed in the dual way, as they are part of the acute medical sector. Phases C and D are part of medical rehabilitation and are paid by the pension funds, if return to work is a likely prognosis. If vocational reintegration is not likely, health insurance companies bear the cost of rehabilitation. Phase E is only paid by pension funds or in some cases by the public unemployment insurance office. If no institution is in charge to provide rehabilitation, the local community pays. The dominant principle is that whatever source of payment covering the damage has to provide means to prevent, reduce, or overcome the damage. Pension funds must pay the pension in case a person can no work and must provide the means for rehabilitation and reemployment. Thus pensions are saved and additional money flows into the funds when the patient is back to work. The same holds true for nursing. Rehabilitation is provided to prevent, reduce, or overcome dependency. In case of work accidents, workers' compensation funds pay for the entire chain of rehabilitation. Allocation to the early phases B, C, and D is controlled by instruments such as the FBI [*Frühreha–Barthel Index* (early rehabilitation Barthel index)] (Schönle, 1995b; Schönle & Schwall, 1995).

Current Developments

Historically, neurological rehabilitation was mostly an inpatient type of rehabilitation that developed away from the population centers in resort areas with no industry (i.e., to become a "white" industry). In the last decade major efforts have been made to complement the system and to establish out-patient community-based facilities for phase D. To further improve community-based rehabilitation, neurologists in their practices need to be trained in neurological rehabilitation to establish local neurorehabilitation teams to continue or to replace/supplement inpatient rehabilitation in phase D, while patients in phases B and C will be continued to be treated as inpatients to keep costs in an affordable range (Schönle, 1997).

References

BAG Bundesarbeitsgemeinschaft medizinisch-beruflicher Rehabilitations-Zentren Phase II. (1994 December). Empfehlungen der Arbeitsgemeinschaft Neurologisch-neurochirurgische Frührehabilitation. [Recommendations of the working group on neurological–neurosurgical early rehabilitation.] Bonn.

BAR (Bundesarbeitsgemeinschaft für Rehabilitation). (1995). Empfehlungen zur Neurologischen Rehabilitation von Patienten mit schweren und schwersten Hirnschädigungen in den Phasen B und C. [Recommendation for neurological rehabilitation of patients with several brain damage in phase B and C.] Frankfurt.

Ministerium für Arbeit, Gesundheit und Sozialordnung, Baden-Württemberg. (1991). Das Apallische Syndrome. [The apallic syndrome.] Stuttgart.

Poser, U., Kohler, J. A., & Schönle, P. W. (1996). Historical review of neuropsychological rehabilitation in Germany. *Neuropsychological Rehabilitation, 6,* 257–278.

Schönle, P. W. (1990). Die Einordnung der Frührehabilitation in den Ablauf der Neurologischen Rehabilitation: ein explizites Gesamt-Phasenmodell. [Early rehabilitation in neurological rehabilitation: An explicit phase model.] Allensbach: Kliniken Schmieder.

Schönle, P. W. (1995a). Möglichkeiten und Bedingungen der Rehabilitation bei und nach apallischen Syndrom—von der Akutphase bis zur Wiederherstellung in der Familie. [Possibilities and conditions of rehabilitation of patients in the apallic syndrome from the acute phase till reintegration in the family.] In K. D. Voß, W. Blumenthal, F. Mehrhoff, & M. Schmollinger (Eds.), *Aktuelle Entwicklung in der Rehabilitation am Beispiel neurologischer Behinderungen* [Current developments in rehabilitation and the case of patients with neurological handicaps.] (pp. 261–274). Ulm: Universitätsverlag.

Schönle P. W. (1995b). Der Frühreha-Bartelindex (FBI)—eine früh-rehabilitationsorientierte Erweiterung des Barthelindex. [The Early-Rehab-Barthel Index—an early-rehab extension of the Bartol index.] Rehabilitation, 34, 69–73.

Schönle, P. W. (1996a). Personale Anforderungsprofile in den frühen Phasen der Neurologischen Rehabilitation. [staff requirement in the early phases of neurological rehabilitation.] *Neurology and Rehabilitation, 3,* 165–175.

Schönle, P. W. (1996b). Rehabilitation bei Patienten mit Schädelhirntraumen. [Rehabilitation of patients with traumatic brain injury.] *Nervenheilkunde, 15,* 200–205.

Schönle, P. W. (1997). Ambulante Neurologische Rehabilitation. [Outpatient neurological rehabilitation.] *Neurologie und Rehabilitation, 2,* 87–95.

Schönle, P.W. (1998). Phasen der neurologisch-neurochirurgischen Rehabilitation und ihre Entwicklung aus der rehabilitativen Praxis einer deutschen Klinik [Phases of neurological–neurosurgical rehabilitation and its development in a German hospital.] (pp 98–119). Schorndorf: Weber Verlag.

Schönle, P. W., & Schwall, D. (1995). Die KRS—eine Skala zum Monitoring der protrahierten Komaremission in der Frührehabilitation. [KRS-coma-remission Scale-monitoring prolonged coma remission in early rehabilitation.] *Neurologie und Rehabilitation, 2,* 87–96.

Schönle, P. W., & Schwall, D. (1993a). Habituation des Blinkreflexes —Prognostisches Kriterium für Patienten im apallischen Durchgangssyndrom. [Habituation of the blink reflex as a prognostic factor in apallic syndrome patients. In K. Schimrigk, A. Haaß, & G. Hamann (Eds.), *Verhandlungen der Deutschen Gesellschaft für Neurologie 7* [Transactions of the German Neurological Society] (pp. 387–393). Berlin: Springer-Verlag.

Schönle, P. W., & Schwall, D. (1993b). Habituation des Blinkreflexes als Zeichen früher Lernvorgänge bei apallischen Patienten. [Habituation of the blink reflex as an indicator of early learning in the apallic patient.] In K. von Wild (Ed.), *Spektrum der Neurorehabilitation,* [*Spectrum of Rehabilitation*] (pp. 158–163). München: W. Zuckschwerdt Verlag.

VDR (Verband Deutscher Rentenversicherungsträger). [Union of German Pension Funds]. (1995). Phaseneinteilung in der neurologischen Rehabilitation. [Phases in neurological rehabilitation.] *Rehabilitation 34,* 119–127.

23

Central Case Management and Postacute Rehabilitation in Denmark

MUGGE PINNER

Introduction

The purpose of this chapter is to provide an overview of the developments that have taken place in Denmark in adult postacute rehabilitation during the past 13 years. Denmark has $5^1/_2$ million inhabitants spread more or less equally across Fyn, Jutland, and Zealand. Rather good coverage of neurosurgical and neurological services exists and a few traditional physical rehabilitation hospitals are available. Refer to Fig. 1 for an overview of the distribution of physical rehabilitation hospitals, neurosurgical and neurological units.

Postacute neuropsychological rehabilitation programs, however, were lacking up until 1985, when the Center for Rehabilitation of Brain Injury (CRBI) in Copenhagen, and a few months later, the Center of Development and Rehabilitation, Vejlefjord, located further west in Jutland was established. In subsequent years, services within postacute neuropsychological rehabilitation remained somewhat limited, although a number of time-limited projects were initiated for the treatment of patients and their families.

In 1991, the Association of County Councils in Denmark reviewed the status of postacute rehabilitation in Denmark. The rehabilitation activities in the various counties were described. Inherent difficulties were noted, such as lack of knowledge concerning the incidence of moderate to severe traumatic brain injury and consequently difficulties in identifying the number of centers necessary for the treatment of moderate traumatic brain injury. Geographic access problems were described and financing difficulties were presented, namely, that in some instances treatment was paid for by the county and/or hospitals (as part of the health system), whereas in other instances treatment was paid for only by the municipalities (as part of the

MUGGE PINNER • Center for Rehabilitation of Brain Injury, University of Copenhagen, 2300 Copenhagen S, Denmark

International Handbook of Neuropsychological Rehabilitation, edited by Christensen and Uzzell. Kluwer Academic/ Plenum Publishers, New York, 2000.

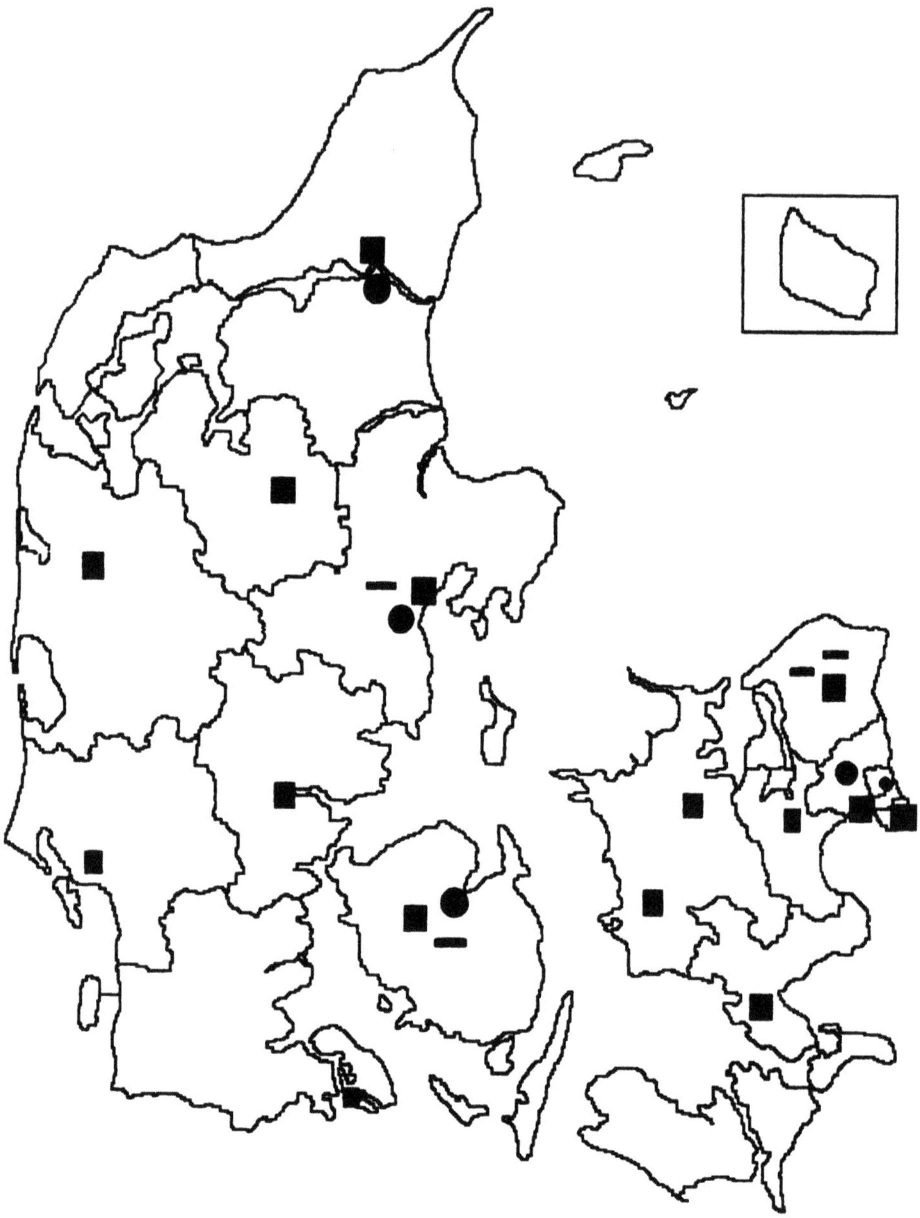

FIGURE 1. Distribution of services. (■) Neurology units; (●) Neurosurgery units; (—) Rehabilitation hospitals.

social system) and therefore was dependent on the patient's economic status. Unfortunately, very few recommendations were made to the counties as a result of these findings.

At approximately the same time, the first outcome results from the two neuropsychological centers were published: The Center for Rehabilitation of Brain Injury, Copenhagen, described a 70% return to work, further education, or voluntary work activities. Living conditions and patients use of leisure time activities were at the same level after treatment as at preinjury (Christensen *et al.*, 1992). Case studies were also published (e.g., Christensen,

Randrup Jensen, & Risberg, 1990), indicating the process of treatment. The Center of Development and Rehabilitation, Vejlefjord, published a report that showed small but significant improvements in cognitive function after rehabilitation (based on neuropsychological test results) and improvements in general well-being as measured by a self-made questionnaire (Engelbrecht *et al.,* 1989). In addition, the County and Municipalities Research Institute showed that rehabilitation at the CRBI is cost- efficient after 3 to 5 years (Larsen, Mehlbye, & Gørtz, 1991).

In 1997, the National Board of Health (1997) (which is part of the Ministry of Health) published a report entitled, "The rehabilitation of traumatic brain injury and corresponding disorders." The incidence of traumatic brain injury (TBI) was officially presented for the first time (based on the Nationwide Patient Register), indicating that there are about 12,000 new TBI patients hospitalized per year. Most of these patients are diagnosed as minor head injury (MHI), and it was estimated that there are about 700 new cases of moderate to severe head injury [the severity level of the latter being defined as patients who have been hospitalized for at least 14 days and survived for more than a year (National Board of Health Report, 1997)].

Briefly stated, the conclusion of the report was that the current situation in Denmark could be defined as lacking resources when compared internationally and the following recommendations were made, namely:

1. To establish a uniform trauma intervention system throughout Denmark.
2. To establish a few highly specialized neurorehabilitation units for coma treatment.
3. To establish neuroconsultation/coordination teams (NCT) in every county.
4. To make available postacute neuropsychological rehabilitation as needed.
5. To address the specific living, educational, and vocational facilities needed for TBI.
6. To establish specialized facilities for children with TBI.

The current status of the above-mentioned recommendations is as follows: with reference to the first recommendation, that is, requesting that an uniform trauma intervention system should be created throughout Denmark, a Danish/Nordic Neurotrauma Task Force group has been established to determine the best manner in which this type of system can be established. Regarding the second recommendation concerning coma treatment and stimulation, one specialized unit is being established in Jutland in connection with a physical rehabilitation hospital, and one to two more are being considered.

Developments regarding recommendations three and four will be discussed under the next two headings. Concerning recommendation five, different living, educational, and vocational projects are being established. Examples include, brain-injured persons living together in facilities with part-time staff, special education schools being provided for adults, and a work integration project that makes use of a work colleague as a support person to the brain-injured person returning to work. Regarding the final issue, that is, establishing specialized facilities for children, a task force group from the Resource Center for Brain Injury is currently in the process of making recommendations for the development of such facilities.

The Neuroconsultant Team

The first NCT was established in the beginning of the 1990s, and may be described as a central case management system in each of the 14 counties. While the structural organization of the NCTs differs a little from one county to another, they share many elements as well as being county based and funded. Some have representatives from local institutions, such as directors of local rehabilitation centers or specialized nursing homes for brain-injured patients, while others also include administrators from the counties and municipalities. All consist of professionals within the field of brain injury (some are employed full-time and others work part-time, or as consultants). Each team has a neuropsychologist and most teams also have a occupational therapists, a physiotherapist, a social worker, and a special education teacher, with physicians acting as consultants. The team usually varies in number from three to seven full-time staff. Nine out of the 14 counties in Demark now have NCTs and more are planned. See Fig. 2 for the geographic distribution of these teams.

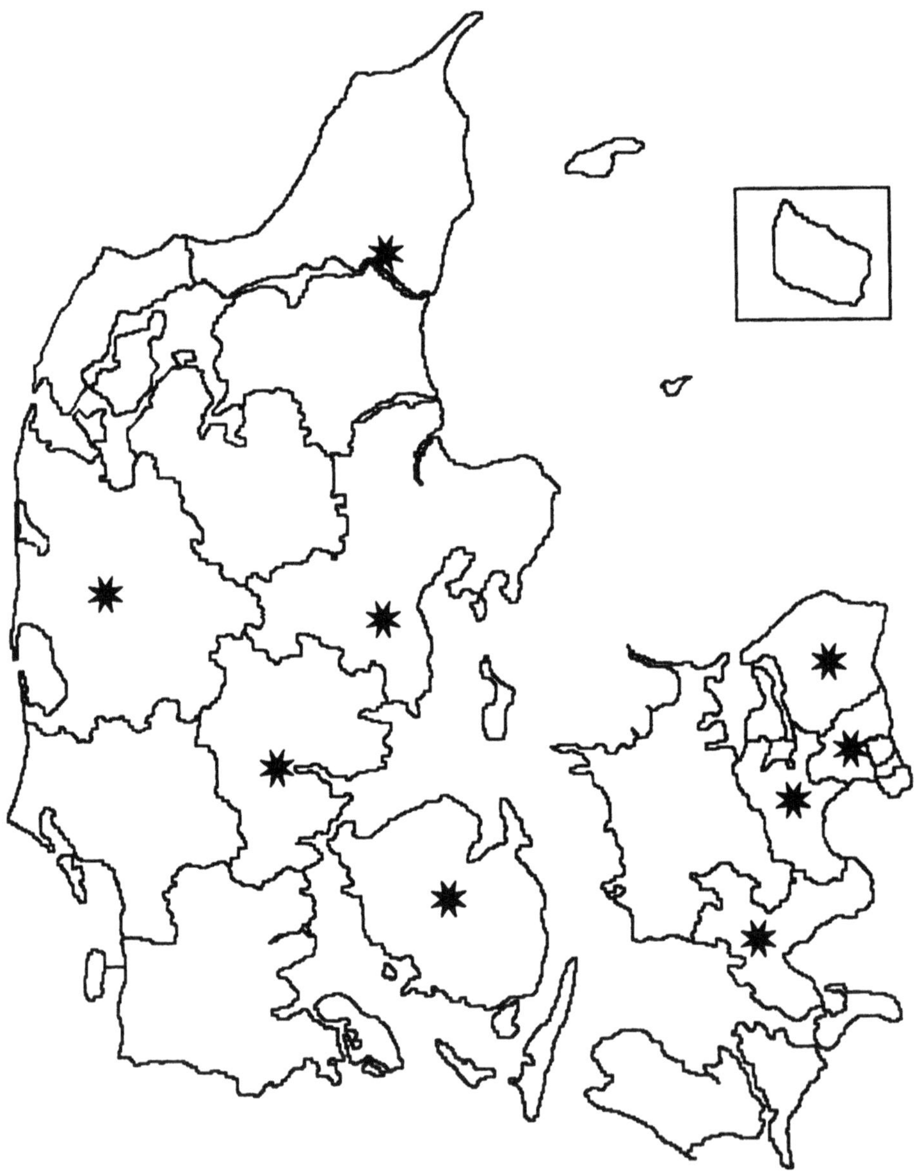

FIGURE 2. Location of the neuroconsultation teams.

The objectives of the NCTs are multifaceted:

1. The primary function of the NCT is to ensure that rehabilitation plans are coordinated across the various intervention sites and over time that is, that no brain injury patient gets lost in the system, especially after discharge from initial hospitalization.
2. The NCT makes individualized rehabilitation plans and ensures that these plans are fulfilled by close monitoring of the process.
3. The NCT has the right to refer patients to the appropriate institutions in some counties, whereas in others this is the domain of the institutions themselves.
4. The NCT provides information, education, consultation, and supervision services to professionals working with head injury patients in the county.
5. The NCT assists in clarifying the need for new initiatives in the county they represent and assist in the establishment and evaluation of new projects/facilities, such as day program centers, education, work integration projects, and so forth.

The Seven Neuropsychological Centers

In Denmark, there are currently seven neuropsychological rehabilitation centers situated across the country (see Fig. 3) that seem to meet the needs of moderately brain-injured adults reasonably well. Additional services, however, are needed for the mild and more severely brain injured as well as for brain-injured children, in general.

The centers are all publicly funded, but the funding differs. Two are county funded through health and hospital financing (i.e., the centers in Sønderborg and Roskilde). One is county funded through the educational department (the center in Aalborg). Two centers are half funded from the county social department and half from local municipality sources (the centers in Aarhus and Odense). The remaining two centers (i.e., in Copenhagen and Vejlefjord) are financed half by the county health department (via the state) as specialized hospitals and half by municipality sources.

Furthermore, the organization of the centers are different. Two centers offer inpatient programs, while the others offer outpatient programs. The patients treated may suffer from TBI, cerebral vascular accidents (CVA), and brain injury due to anoxia and infections. One center admits brain injuries due to exposure to toxic solvents or substance abuse and another also takes patients with psychiatric diagnoses. Most of the patients are moderately brain injured, but one center also takes those with mild head injury. The total number of patients who can receive neuropsychological rehabilitation is approximately 300 per year (see Table 1).

The patients are treated by a variety of professional groups, usually neuropsychologists, physiotherapists, occupational therapists, social workers, special education teachers, and medical personal. The staff structure, however, does differ from one center to the other (see Table 2).

While all the centers have neuropsychologists and physiotherapists, the ratio per patient varies, and only some have occupational therapists, speech pathologists, social workers and special education teachers. Most centers use physicians as consultants and those that offer an inpatient program also have nurses. Treatment takes place in groups and individually, ranging from 11 to 18 weeks. While all the centers admit patients in groups that start and complete the program at the same time, most of the centers also offer individual treatment to additional patients. The weekly treatment elements in the various programs are described in Table 3.

As can be seen, the treatment elements vary a little from one center to the other. All offer physiotherapy or physical training (from 1 hour per week up to 5 hours weekly) and cognitive training, individually (up to 3 hours weekly) and in groups (2 to 4 hours per week).

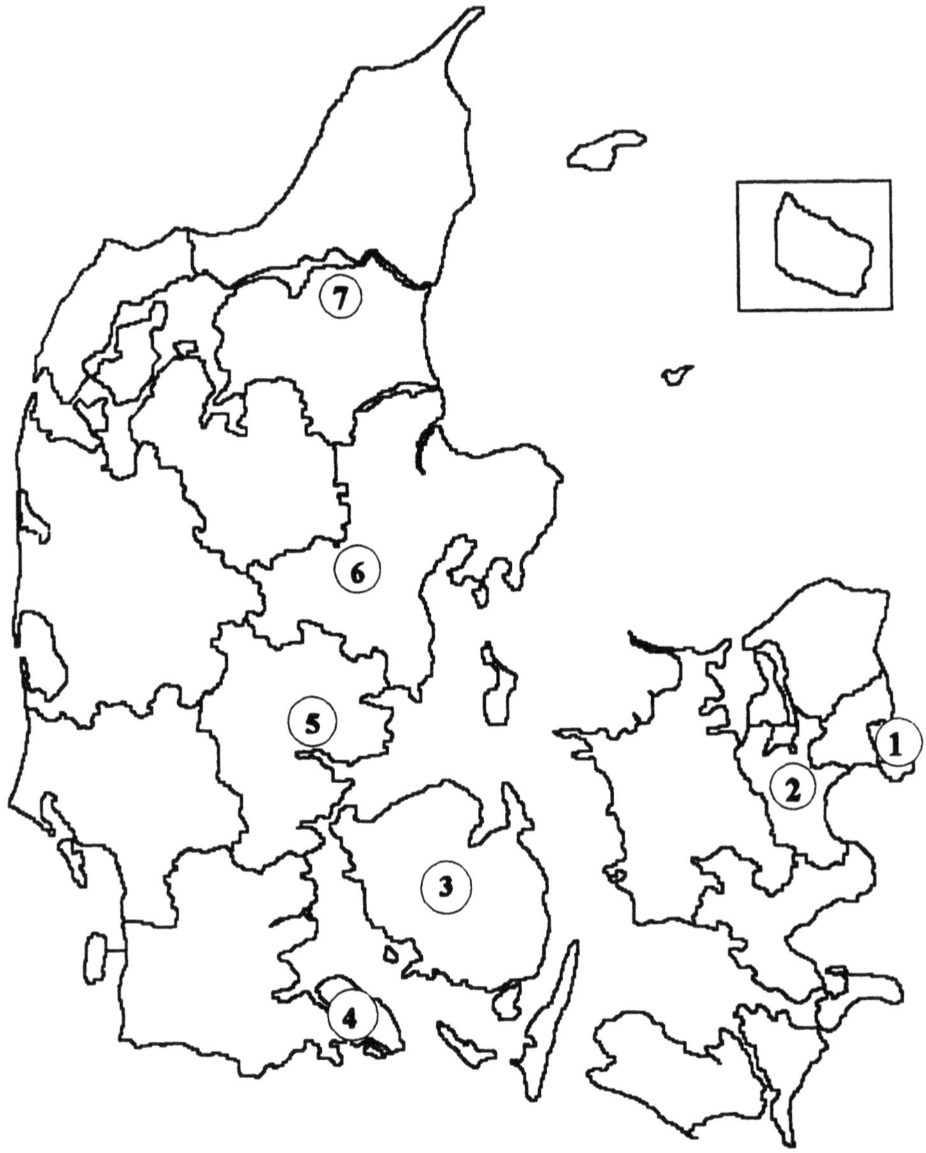

FIGURE 3. Location of neuropsychological rehabilitation centers. 1. Center for Rehabilitation of Brain Injury, Copenhagen. 2. Sct. Hans Hospital, Roskilde. 3. Brain Injury Rehabilitation-Center, Odense. 4. Department of Neuropsychology N50, Sønderborg. 5. Center of Development and Rehabilitation, Vejlefjord. 6. The Rehab-Center of Head Injury, Aarhus. 7. Brain Injury Rehabilitation Center, Aalborg.

Psychotherapy is offered individually (up to 2 times per week) and in groups (1–2 times per week) by most of the centers. However, most but not all the centers offer speech and language therapy (up to 5 hours weekly). All except one center have groups for relatives once or twice a month, and occupational therapy is provided as needed at most centers. Almost all the centers provide some kind of follow-up and work integration, but this may range from a few meetings after treatment to as much as 24 months of follow-up and work replacement.

TABLE 1. Description of the Seven Neuropsychological Centers

	Center[a]							
	Copenhagen	Vejlefjord	Sønderborg	Odense	Aarhus	Roskilde	Aalborg	Total
Funding source	Hospital county/national municipal	Hospital county/national municipal	Hospital county	Social county municipal	Social county municipal	Hospital county	Educational county	
In/outpatients	Out	In	Both	Out	Out	In	Out	
Treatment courses per year	2	4	2	3	2	3	2	
Total patients in groups per year	30	76	8	18	22	36	16	206
Individual patients	20	10		30	15	12		87
Total per year								293

[a]Copenhagen, Center for Rehabilitation of Brain Injury; Vejlefjord, Vejlefjord Center of Development and Rehabilitation: Sønderborg, Department of Neuropsychology N50; Odense, Brain Injury Rehabilitation Center; Aarhus, the Rehab-Center for Brain Injury; Roskilde, Sct. Hans Hospital; Aalborg, Brain Injury Rehabilitation Center.

TABLE 2. Staff Structure

Staff	Copenhagen	Vejlefjord	Sønderborg	Odense	Aarhus	Roskilde	Aalborg
	Center[a]						
Director	Neuro-psychologist	MD/ administrator	Neuro-psychologist	Social worker	Neuro-psychologist	Clinical psychologist	Speech pathologist
Neuropsychologist	10	6.5	1.5	2	7	2	1.75
Physiotherapist	2.5	3	0.5	1	1	0.5	0.5
Occupational therapist		3	2	2	1	1	
Special education teacher	1	2			1	1	2
Social worker		2			1	0.5	0.5
Speech pathologist	1	1	Consultant		Consultant		Consultant
Nurse		5				6.5	
Medical doctor	Consultant	Consultant	Consultant	Consultant	Consultant	1	Consultant

[a]Copenhagen, Center for Rehabilitation of Brain Injury; Vejlefjord, Vejlefjord Center of Development and Rehabilitation; Odense, Brain Injury Rehabilitation Center; Sønderborg, Department of Neuropsychology N50; Aarhus, the Rehab-Center for Brain Injury; Roskilde, Sct. Hans Hospital; Aalborg, Brain Injury Rehabilitation Center.

Thus, while the seven centers may be regarded as differing in certain ways, they do have similarities in program structure and theoretical principles. Common theoretical principles are as follows: (1) rehabilitation is based on a thorough, qualitative, neuropsychological evaluation; (2) a therapeutic milieu is encouraged, where a collaborative, educational environment is created between staff and participants; (3) the role of primary therapist is emphasized, that is, one therapist is allocated as the contact person to the participant throughout the treatment process; (4) interdisciplinary team work, where staff are specialized not only within their fields but also jointly, adhere to neuropsychological principles for treatment; (5) program participants are encouraged to shift from the patient role to greater independence and are expected to take personal responsibility for both the rehabilitation process and their lives, in general; and (6) program participants and their significant others are regarded as central to the treatment process. These principles have been significantly influenced by the work of Ben-Yishay (see, for example, Ben-Yishay, 1996; Ben-Yishay & Gold, 1990), Prigatano (see, for example, Prigatano *et. al.*, 1986), Goldstein (see, for example, Goldstein, 1942), and Luria (see, for example, Luria, 1963, 1966, Christensen, 1975; Christensen, Malmros, & Townes, 1987).

In the past 2 years, the centers have started collaborating closely, such that currently contact is maintained on a regular basis, that is, the directors meet on a regular basis, and all the staff meet annually. In addition, the various professional groups meet in each of their groups respectively several times a year as, for example, physiotherapists and occupational therapists.

The seven centers have also created a conjoint research group: One of the first goals of the group is to create a database of demographic data, injury data, evaluations from each professional group, and so forth, from the seven centers. Another project is to make extended program descriptions of each center, by describing theoretical principles and treatment activities and documenting interventions as specifically as possible.

In addition to this collaboration, the various centers are also involved in specific research projects such as work integration methods (Kristensen, Kristensen, & Jespersen, 1997; Siert & Teasdale, 1997; Jespersen, Kristensen, & Pinner, 1997). The centers in Vejlefjord and Copenhagen (and others) are planning to study fatigue–tiredness after TBI and several centers are

TABLE 3. Frequency of Treatment[a]

Treatment elements	Center[b]						
	Copenhagen	Vejlefjord	Sønderborg	Odense	Aarhus	Roskilde	Aalborg
Cognitive (individual)	1–2	1–3	1–2		2	If needed	2.5
Cognitive (group)	3	3	4	2	3	2	2–3
Psychotherapy (individual)	2	1–2	1	If needed	2	If needed	1
Psychotherapy (group)	1	2	2	1	2	2	2
Family therapy (group)	Yes	Yes	Yes	Yes	Yes	Yes	Yes
Speech therapy	1–3	1–5	(2)		1–3		Yes
Physical therapy	3	3–5	3	1	2–3	4	2
Special education	1–2	1			1–3	3	Yes
Occupational therapy	Yes	Yes	Yes	Yes	Yes	Yes	Yes
Follow up (in months)	6–24	5 times in 12 months	18	Varies	12	24	
Individual and/or group work reentry	Yes	Yes	Yes	Yes	Yes	Yes	Yes

[a] Per week, unless otherwise specified.

[b] Copenhagen, Center for Rehabilitation of Brain Injury; Odense, Brain Injury Rehabilitation Center; Sønderborg, Department of Neuropsychology N50; Odense, Brain Injury Rehabilitation Center; Aarhus, the Rehab-Center for Brain Injury; Roskilde, Sct. Hans Hospital; Vejlefjord, Vejlefjord Center of Development and Rehabilitation; Aalborg, Brain Injury Rehabilitation Center.

interested in ecological training principles. Two centers (in Aalborg and Odense) have conducted some research regarding awareness (see, for example, Kristensen, 1996), while the center in Roskilde is involved in quality measurements of tests and treatment. The center in Odense has tried different treatment elements especially when working with mild head injury. Publications from several centers are expected in the near future.

The center in Copenhagen is highly involved in further education of staff and international collaboration and to date, has been the most active of all the centers in research activities as, for example, in conducting outcome studies (e.g., Teasdale & Christensen, 1994; Teasdale, Skovdal Hansen, Gade, & Christensen, 1997a); in developing a rating scale with international collaboration (e.g., Teasdale *et al.*, 1997b) and specifically the theoretical applications of Luria's approach (e.g., Christensen & Caetano, 1997; Christensen & Caetano, in press).

Conclusion

While the above may be viewed as developments in the right direction, there is a long way ahead for the rehabilitation of brain injury in Denmark. As Denmark does not have a tradition of , or laws for, accreditation of rehabilitation programs or staff (except for doctors and psychologists), this issue must be addressed by all the rehabilitation centers in the future to ensure that quality of treatment is of high standard, consistent, and cost-effective. An equally important concern is that of research, which must address the complexity of brain injury with various, appropriate methods. In addition, research collaboration must take place in relationship to professionals working in the fields of neuroscience (neurophysiologists, neurologists, etc.) not only in Denmark, but within Europe and abroad. Such developments are necessary for ensuring optimal services to brain injured individuals in the future.

References

Ben-Yishay, Y. (1996). Reflections on the evolution of the therapeutic milieu concept. *Neuropsychological Rehabilitation, 6*, 327–343.

Ben-Yishay, Y. & Gold, J. (1990). Therapeutic milieu approach to neuropsychological rehabilitation. In R. L. Wood (Ed.) *Neurobehavioral sequelae of traumatic brain injury* (pp. 194–218) New York: Taylor & Francis.

Christensen, A. L. (1975). *Luria's neuropsychological investigation. Manual and test materials* (1st ed.). New York: Spectrum.

Christensen, A-L., & Caetano, C. (1997). Alexander Romanovitch Luria (1902–1977): Contributions to neuropsychological rehabilitation. *Neuropsychological Rehabilitation, 6*, 279–303.

Christensen, A-L., & Caetano, C. (In press). Scandinavian neuropsychological evaluation as influenced by A. R. Luria. *Neuropsychological Review, Special Issue.*

Christensen, A. L., Malmros, R., & Townes, B. D. (1987). Rehabilitation planned in accordance with the Luria neuropsychological investigation: A case history of a patient with left sided aneurysm. *Neuropsychology, 1*, 45–48.

Christensen, A-L., Randrup Jensen, L. R., & Risberg, J. (1990). Luria's neuropsychological and neurolinguistic theory. *Journal of Neurolinguistics, 4*, 137–154.

Christensen, A-L., Pinner, E. M., Moller Pedersen, P., Teasdale, T. W., & Trexler, L. E. (1992). Psychosocial outcome following individualized neuropsychological rehabilitation of brain damage. *Acta Neurologica Scandinavica, 85*, 32–38.

Engelbrecht, J., Bræmer, J., Jensen, J. C. L., Laursen, O., Mamsen, P., & Nielsen, H. (1989). *Genoptrænings-behandling af hjerneskadede på Vejlefjord. En effektundersøgelse*. Rapport nr. 2. [Rehabilitation of brain injury at Vejlefjord. An outcome study] Vejlefjord, Denmark: Center of Development and Rehabiltation, Stouby.

Goldstein, K. (1942). *Aftereffects of brain injuries in war: Their evaluation and treatment* (1st ed.). London: Heinemann.

Jespersen, M., Kristensen, J., & Pinner, E. M. (1997). *Arbejdsintegration af hjerneskadede. Evaluering af et 4-årigtforsøg ved Hjerneskadecentret, Revalideringsklinikken, Århus Amt.* [Work integration after brain injury. An evaluation of a four-year study by the Rehab-Center for Brain Injury, Rehabilitation Clinic and Århus Munincipality] Århus, Dennark: The Rehab-Center for Brain Injury.

Kristensen, O. S. (1996). *Hverdagsliv og selverkendelse—en kvalitativforløbsundersøgelse af udviklingen i selverkendelsen hos deltagere i et genoptræningsforløbfor hjerneskadede på Taleinstituttet i Aalborg.* [Daily living and self-awareness—a qualitative investigation of self-awareness in participants of the rehabilitation program for brain injury at the speech institute in Aalborg] Aalborg, Denmark: Brain Injury Rehabilitation Center, Speech Institute.

Kristensen, O. S., Kristensen, J., & Jespersen, M. (1997). *Hjerneskade og arbejde: Hvilke tiltag kan medvirke til en vellykket arbejdsintegration?* [Brain injury and work: Which factors contribute to succesful work integration?] Conference Report 3. Nordic Conference on Work Integration for Acquired Brain Injury, Denmark.

Larsen, A., Mehlbye, J., & Gørtz, M. (1991). *Kan genoptræning betale sig? En analyse af de sociale og økonomiske aspekter ved genoptræning af hjerneskadede-*. [Does rehabilitation pay? An anaysis of the social and economic aspects of brain injury rehabilitation] Copenhagen: AKF Forlaget.

Luria, A. R. (1963). *Restoration of function after brain injury* (Basil Haigh, Trans.). London: Pergamon Press. (Original work published 1948)

Luria, A. R. (1966). *Higher cortical functions in man* (1st ed.). London: Tavistock.

National Board of Health. (1997). *Behandling af traumatiske hjerneskader og tilgrænsende lidelser.* [Treatment of traumatic brain injury and corresponding disorders] Copenhagen: Ministry of Health, Printing Office.

Prigatano, G. P., Fordyce, D. J., Zeiner, H. K., Roucche, J. R., Pepping, M., & Wood, B. C. (1986). *Neuropsychological rehabilitation after brain injury.* Baltimore: Johns Hopkins University Press.

Siert, L. & Teasdale, T. W. (1997). Rehabilitation for employment and leisure activities. In J. León-Carrion (Ed.), *Neuropsychological rehabilitation—Fundamentals, innovations and directions* (pp. 469–82). Florida: GR/St. Lucie Press.

Teasdale, T. W., & Christensen, A-L. (1994). Psychosocial outcome in denmark. In A.-L. Christensen & B. Uzzell (Eds.), *Brain injury and neuropsychological rehabilitation: International perspectives* (pp. 235–244). Hilldale, NJ: Lawrence Erlbaum.

Teasdale, T. W., Skovdal Hansen, H., Gade, A., & Christensen, A-L. (1997a). Neuropsychological test scores before and after brain-injury rehabilitation in relation to return to employment. *Neuropsychological Rehabilitation, 7,* 23–42.

Teasdale, T. W., Christensen, A-L., Willmes, K., Deloche, G., Braga, L. W., Stachowiak, F. J., Vendrell, J. M., Castro-Caldas, A., Laaksonen, R., & Leclercq, M. (1997b). Subjective experience in brain injured patients and their close relatives: A European brain injury questionnaire. *Brain Injury, 11,* 543–563.

VI

State of the Art at the End of the 1990s Decade of the Brain

24

Neuropsychological Rehabilitation

B. P. UZZELL

Conceptualizations and Definitions

Neuropsychological rehabilitation is as baffling to some as the brain damage itself. Its purpose is unclear to many lay persons and professionals who lack familiarity with treatments for brain damage. Neuropsychological rehabilitation is often conceptualized as cognitive exercises to improve mental functioning after an insult to the brain. While this is true in part, neuropsychological rehabilitation is much more. It is learning, relearning, and compensating for skills in reading, spelling, writing, arithmetic, remembering, attending, organizing, executing, or performing daily tasks. And it is much more. Neuropsychological rehabilitation addresses affective and social difficulties. Treatment is necessary when areas in the brain controlling emotions are effected by a brain insult, or during reactions after brain damage.

An individual with a brain insult has wants, needs, and desires and lives in a society. Motivations do not necessarily end when brain damage is sustained; they remain with the individual and are intertwined with the social environment in which he or she lives. Neuropsychological rehabilitation addresses many facets of a brain-damaged individual, treating him or her with appropriate techniques and strategies for cognitive, emotional, and societal skills while increasing awareness and understanding of the new self. Treatment of cognitive functioning has been directed toward disabilities, not impairments.

The distinction between disabilities and impairments is often overlooked. Disabilities are particular problems caused by impairments, such as difficulty completing a task. On the other hand, impairments are identified as damage to mental and physical structures (Wilson, 1997). Emotions are most often guided by release of inhibitory brain systems due to brain damage and individual reactions to cognitive disabilities. Results are most often maladaptive for the individual and his or her existence in society, requiring modifications with the current, best-known treatment: neuropsychological rehabilitation.

B. P. UZZELL • Memorial Neurological Association, Houston, Texas 77074.

International Handbook of Neuropsychological Rehabilitation, edited by Christensen and Uzzell.
Kluwer Academic/ Plenum Publishers, New York, 2000.

Typically, inpatient and outpatient neuropsychological rehabilitation is a comprehensive, time- and resource-intensive process in which decisions are made by a clinical team. The services rendered through individualized programs cease when treatment goals have been achieved. In some programs, annual follow-ups are continued for 5 years following termination of intensive treatment. Additional individualized neuropsychological rehabilitation is often provided privately on a one-on-one outpatient basis following in- or outpatient team treatment as needed. Moreover, private neuropsychological rehabilitation is provided in cases where brain impairment is mild (Uzzell, 1999), and the funding source may consider team treatment programs not financially justifiable. Present consensus of treatment supports a model of neuropsychological rehabilitation that is humanistic and neuropsychologically not medically based once a patient's medical condition has stabilized.

When a patient, family member, or service payers discover the availability of neuropsychological rehabilitation for the first time, the question usually asked: "Is it needed?" The answer is "yes," if the brain-damaged individual is to have a satisfactory quality of life and contribute to his or her own well-being, to the family, and to society at large. Certainly, in the current managed care environment in the United States, this question is often raised, but it is also raised in other parts of the world with socialized medicine environment. Most social systems have limits of privately or government-sponsored funding.

The vast number of individuals living with brain damage in the world answers the international question of whether there is a need for neuropsychological rehabilitation with a resounding, "yes!" Considering the number of disorders that can affect the brain (e.g., trauma, vascular disorders, tumors, infections, inflammations, toxic, deficiency, metabolic disorders, demyelinating diseases, degenerative diseases, congenital malformations and perinatal disorders, etc), there is indeed a need for neuropsychological rehabilitation, if patients are to return to productive and/or quality lifestyles.

As one father of a brain-injured son told me many years ago in relation to neuropsychological rehabilitation for his son, "The choice of life without neuropsychological rehabilitation is no choice at all. If there is a remote possibility it is going to help my son, I want it." Whether available or not, most patients and knowledgeable families demand it. Because of resource limitations, it is necessary to examine why, what, and how neuropsychological rehabilitation is being conducted, not only to improve scientific methods, but to examine costs and cost containment. The true answers to these questions come from professionals experienced in the field, patients who have participated in neuropsychological rehabilitation in the past and their relatives. But before launching into this discussion, a brief review of the origins of neuropsychological rehabilitation, mainly during the past two centuries, will illustrate its evolving nature and provide an indication of how it might change during approaching millennium.

Historical Perspective

From a historical perspective, the first recorded case of treatment of cognitive losses was believed to be treatment of an aphasic patient reported by Broca in 1865 (Berker, Berker, & Smith, 1986). Cognitive and personality changes after brain damage was most noticeable as exemplified in the now-famous crowbar-penetrating case of Phineas P. Gage described by Harlow in 1848 and 1868. Although mere survival of Mr. Gage was initially fascinating to scientists at the time, full appreciation of personality changes was not realized until Harlow's second, follow-up report of Mr. Gage's activities during the 13 years after the accident until his death (Steegman, 1962). The case still stimulates conceptualizations of frontal lobe functioning (Stuss, Gow, & Hetherington, 1992) and highlights an area that is treatable with neuropsychological rehabilitation.

While medications and psychotherapy treatments have been prescribed historically, records of comprehensive programs entirely devoted to treating brain damage are sparse. They have appeared mainly after a war during which time many young men had acquired brain damage. The pioneering programs spearheaded by Walter Poppelreuter and Kurt Goldstein, in Germany after World War I, are examples of early innovative new methods and approaches. While Poppelreuter was practical, Goldstein was theoretical, providing the rationale for selecting restorative or compensatory therapy. Although the concepts of these programs were different, it is amazing that either of these programs were ever begun at all in the prevailing atmosphere at the time of localizing and mapping brain functions. Walter Poppelreuter, in 1917, was aware of such thinking when he said "as long as the brain damaged patient is still alive, the question of localization of the brain injury is of no practical interest and only of limited use as a diagnostic tool" (Posner, Kohler, & Schönle, 1996, p. 258). This statement reflects the practical philosophy that is central to neuropsychological rehabilitation in assisting a patient in everyday life, once brain damage has been identified and localized. The question then, and now, is what practically can be done for complex brain functions of abstraction and memory that are not easily localized.

Modern day programs in the United States began with cognitive rehabilitation with stroke patients (Diller, 1976). Likewise, in 1973, Yehuda Ben-Yishay created a holistic neuropsychological rehabilitation program in Israel to serve the head injured survivors from the Yom Kippur War. In developing this holistic program, Ben-Yishay, influenced by teachings and writings of Kurt Goldstein, concluded that cognitive, psychological, and functional aspects are treated together, not separately. This model moves a patient through a hierarchy of stages, with each stage requiring a level of mastery before proceeding to the next level. The stages include engagement, awareness, mastery, control, acceptance, and identity (Ben-Yishay *et al.*, 1985).

Each member of the human race encapsulates a duality of the biological and the neuropsychosocial. First, a person is a biological being, with recognizable anatomical descriptors and physiological drives and needs. The other part of the duality is represented by the term, *neuropsychosocial,* created here to encompass both cognitive and psychosocial needs, wants, and functioning. A person has neuropsychosocial needs for adequate recall and cognitive capacity, self-worthiness, social interaction, acceptance, and love. On some occasions either a strong biological or a neuropsychosocial emphasis may predominate, but most of the time the duality works together, creating a unique individual. These dual aspects are not lost with brain damage, but remain part of one's being. The purpose of this chapter is look at the past in relation to the future of neuropsychological rehabilitation. To do this, the following abbreviated account of duality in neuropsychological rehabilitation during this past century has been addressed, in order to understand how biological and neuropsychosocial aspects might evolve in the future.

Biological Aspects

Generally, professionals in the field of rehabilitation are not always cognizant of activities in acute care and their influence on rehabilitation. While it does take more time to become informed about acute care when treating chronic conditions in rehabilitation, such knowledge vastly improves understanding of chronic conditions and treatment plans for chronic care. The author's past personal experience as a neuropsychologist working in both departments of neurosurgery and rehabilitation facilitated transfer of knowledge accumulated about patients' acute condition to rehabilitation professionals, providing better understanding and treatment of those patients in a rehabilitation setting.

Improvements in acute care management have resulted in an increased survival rate among the head injured, and consequently increased the need for rehabilitation. During the 1970s, changes in neurosurgical management throughout the world (Jennett *et al.,* 1977), in prehospital emergency care (Mangiardi, 1986; Baxt & Moody, 1987), and in increased use of motor vehicle restraining devices (Daffner, Deeb, Lupetin, & Rothfus, 1988) resulted in a dramatic growth in the number of traumatic head injury survivors. This increased survival rate was the impetus for creating more neuropsychological rehabilitation programs, just as the increased volume of head injuries after past wars spurred its development.

Over the years, knowledge about the biological aspects has been accumulating and evolving. It is well known that insults to the brain do not all come from the initial injury, but from secondary effects, such as brain swelling and edema (Miller, Sweet, Narayan, & Becker, 1978). Severe brain edema may interfere with neuronal transmission triggering a chain of events at the synapse (Castejon, 1998).

Neurosurgeons, in treating acute head injuries, are faced with the problem of brain swelling and edema, which correlate highly with intracranial hypertension. Suitable neurosurgical treatments for intracranial hypertension, including pharmaceuticals, cerebrospinal fluid drainage, hyperventilation, and hypothermia, are not always successful, and intracranial pressure can remain high (>20 mmHg). In those cases with intracranial hypertension who survive, neuropsychological functioning has been found to be more disruptive than injuries without such secondary effects (Uzzell, Obrist, Dolinskas, & Langfitt, 1986; Uzzell, Dolinskas, & Wiser, 1990).While brain insults cannot be prevented from occurring, particularly in a modern society with fast-moving automobiles, secondary effects can be reduced. Ongoing acute care research is focusing on ways to reduce secondary injuries, thereby reducing severity of injuries entering rehabilitation.

Prevention of secondary injuries requires better understanding of pathological alterations in endogenous neurochemical systems at the microscopic or cellular level. Not only will the search continue for neurotransmitter synthesis, release, and re-uptake mechanisms, but also in synthesis and release of endogenous neuroprotective compounds (e.g., antioxidants), release of endogenous "autodestructive" compounds, factors associated with inflammation, and nerve growth factors. Timing of the precise cascade of neurochemical events is poorly understood (McIntosh, 1994), but hopefully, not for long. During the next decade researchers will search for understanding, so that optimal timing of pharmacological treatment may be applied to reverse or impede negative events. Understanding the mechanisms underlying traumatic brain injury and repair will come eventually from merging the findings of neurochemical alterations in the whole brain with data from intensive behavioral testing (Stein, Glasier, & Hoffman, 1994).

The microscopic story of "too much of a good thing" has already been realized with intracellular calcium. While moderate intracellular calcium levels can result in modified outgrowth, too much calcium can decrease neurite outgrowth, prune dendrites, and ultimately result in death of individual neurons (Kater, Mattson, & Guthrie, 1989). Evidence has been found for a destabilizing peptide (ß-amyloid) of neuronal calcium regulation that renders neurons more vulnerable to environmental stimuli, thereby elevating intracellular calcium levels (Mattson *et al.,* 1992). Other evidence suggest that calcium levels can be controlled pharmaceutically. The calcium channel blocker, nimodipine, effective in maintaining synaptic contacts during the aging process, may also be effective in rehabilitation (DeJong, Buwalda, Schuurman, & Luiten, 1992). Continued ongoing study of intracellular calcium activity may contribute to identifying appropriate treatment for brain-damaged individuals.

For years scientists have studied regeneration of nerve fibers and found some processes to be maladaptive. All systems in the brain do not regenerate at the same rate. Age is factor in regeneration, with ease of the regeneration process slowing in adulthood. Throughout the lifespan, the brain is changing (Johnson & Almli, 1978). The infant brain has been simultaneously characterized as more plastic and with greater vulnerability to pathological conditions (nutritional, hormonal, and environmental deficiencies) than the mature brain. Pediatric patients tend to have a significantly lower mortality rate in comparison to adults (Luerssen, Klauber, & Marshall, 1988), while older survivors have reduced potential for recovery with increased rates of severe disability (Teasdale, Skene, Spiegelhalter, & Murray, 1982). The age of the child determines the type of head injury that may be sustained and the selection of the most appropriate radiological technique to reveal the trauma (Zimmerman & Bilaniuk, 1994). To maximize recovery in the pediatric brain, the focus continues to be on what is known about brain plasticity and its influence.

From the work of the famous Spanish anatomist and Nobel laureate, Santiago Ramon y Cajal, at the beginning of the 20th century, neuronal regeneration has been thought to be absent in the adult brain. Unable to find proof of regenerative repair in adult brains, he became convinced it did not occur. He hoped future scientists would work on ways to prevent degeneration and make it possible for new pathways to develop. Later investigations have established regeneration in adult brains (Stein, Brailowsky, & Will, 1995). Now the challenge is to discern factors associated with both positive and maladaptive regeneration after brain insults.

Scientists continue to look for ways to see inside a living brain and to view brain activity during thinking. In the mid-1970s, a clearer window to brain morphology was provided when a three-dimensional technique, computed tomography (CT), first appeared. Within the next 10 years, another three-dimensional technique, structural magnetic resonance imaging (sMRI), provided additional static information about the brain. Although both these techniques advanced understanding of brain morphology, neither technique provided information on the functional activitiy of the brain during actual thought processes. The first cortical activation studies were performed with the two-dimensional xenon-133 technique developed in the 1960s and 1970s. Measuring regional cerebral blood flow changes permitted inferences about cortical metabolic activity during various mental activities (Obrist & Wilkinson, 1990). Results from this two-dimensional technique correlated with clinical recovery from brain injuries (Terayama, Meyer, & Kawamura, 1991), with language dysfunctioning after stroke (Knopman, Rubens, Selnes, Klassen, & Meyer, 1984) and with cognitive activation after the neuropsychological rehabilitation process (Risberg & Jensen, 1994). The recently developed xenon-CT technique has provided additional information about subcortical blood flow and its relationship to long-term cognitive recovery (Terayama, Meyer, Kawamura, & Weathers, 1991).

Another functional, three-dimensional technique is positron emission tomography (PET), which directly measures regional metabolism in the brain (Heiss, Herholz, Pawlik, Wagner, & Wienhard, 1986). Application of PET to rehabilitation is not yet well realized, perhaps due to its limited availability and cost; nevertheless, reports are beginning to appear (Carlomagno *et al.*, 1997). Findings from another more available functional technique—single photon emission computed tomography (SPECT)—have shown significant increases in cerebral blood flow after cognitive treatment in mild, moderate and severe injuries 18–23 months postinjury (Laatsch, Jobe, Sychra, Lin, & Blend, 1997) and in cerebrovascular accidents (Deutsch *et al.*, 1998).

As we approach the 21st century, newly available brain-imaging techniques may be used to evaluate neuropsychological rehabilitation. These include: (1) diffusion-weighted MRI (DWI) to detect subtle changes in the diffusion of water molecules; (2) perfusion MRI (pMRI) to evaluate blood volume, blood transit time, and blood flow as relative measures; and (3) functional MRI (fMRI) to measure changes in tissue perfusion based on changes in blood oxygenation. Results from these newer techniques afford opportunities to better understand the process of neuropsychological rehabilitation, particularly from pre- and posttreatment measurements and during cortical activation.

Clinical neurological examinations, biochemical mechanisms at the cellular level, and neuroimaging during this century have provided knowledge about brain functioning. More work is required to grasp all the necessary biological aspects. For instance, prolonged vegetative posttraumatic state (Arts, Van Dongen, Van Hof-Van Duin, & Lammens, 1985) remains a puzzling phenomenon. Those patients who do emerge from prolonged coma follow consecutive steps representing restoration of increasingly complex neurological functions (Bricolo, Turazzi, & Feriotti, 1980). But we do not know, for example, the appropriate pharmaceuticals to apply at selected steps to accelerate mental recovery while decreasing limb contractures. Further understanding of the basic biological processes should provide solutions to such challenges.

Neuropsychosocial Aspects

Neuropsychosocial aspects represent cognitive and psychosocial functioning and their interrelationships. An individual who has sustained brain damage of varying degrees of severity requires treatment of the whole individual and attention to both cognitive and psychosocial functioning. It is almost impossible to clearly separate the two, although at times cognitive dysfunctioning may be more evident than psychosocial, and vice versa. A further step needs to be taken here to include biological aspects, which truly cannot be separated from cognition and psychosocial functioning. The biological aspects are the physical underpinnings from which cognition and emotion–motivations develop. Whether an individual has brain damage or not, his or her being is a combination of biological and neuropsychosocial functioning. Admittedly, the artificial separation makes it easier to conceptualize past and future developments. In keeping with this thought, attention is primarily directed to neuropsychosocial aspects.

The question becomes how to proceed with neuropsychological rehabilitation given the complexity of an individual with the biological, cognitive, and psychosocial aspects, all of which are disrupted with brain damage. Wilson (1997) has enumerated and critiqued four neuropsychological rehabilitation methods (cognitive rehabilitation, cognitive–neuropsychological-theoretical, combined learning theory–cognitive psychology–neuropsychology, and holistic). Of these, the holistic approach has been acclaimed as the most successful, although its success is not irrefutable. The holistic model recognizes that cognition and emotion interact in a complicated way, requiring simultaneous considerations of emotional and motivational disturbances during rehabilitation of cognitive deficits (Prigatano, 1997). On a simplistic level, a sensitive observer who has viewed cognitive disturbances soon after brain damage will be struck by the interconnectiveness of cognition and emotion. In some instances, increased emotional responses will be more apparent as the individual tries to function cognitively in the preinjury manner. On other occasions, the paucity of emotions is revealing. For any model of neuropsychological rehabilitation to be successful, it must address not only cognitive and emotional functioning but also biological and psychosocial aspects. Although not always formally stated, implicit in the holistic model are elements of biological aspects. As stages of a hierarchy are transversed in this model, biological substructure becomes modified and changes with treatments evident in ongoing social group or milieu setting.

Three major areas of cognitive dysfunctioning after brain damage are memory, language skills, and visuospatial relationships. The cardinal cognitive symptom after brain insults has been memory, which is most bothersome to survivors. Small items in everyday activities are forgotten, for example, where car keys were placed on returning home, mailing bill payments, and times for appointments or meetings. Many survivors initially believe after the brain insult some type of medication will restore short-term memory functioning to its previous uninjured state. When this does not happen, they often become depressed. Medications enhancing memory functioning are linked to the cholinergic system (Stein & Strickland, 1998). Nootropics are pharmaceutical drugs thought to improve learning and memory by favorably enhancing brain metabolism and cerebral circulation and by protecting the brain from physical and chemical damage (Kolakowsky & Parente, 1997). Here, case studies abound with numerous selective substances, and a review of these are beyond the scope of this discussion. However, two recent studies convey somewhat the ongoing research in this area. For example, acetylcholine-esterase inhibitor, donepezil, (Taverni, Seliger, & Lichtman, 1998) and amantadine plus L-dopa/carbidopa (Kraus & Maki, 1997) have been reported successful in treating attention, thereby improving recall. More critical double-blind studies with many types of memory disorders and brain insults are necessary to gain substantive results. We have just begun to "scratch the surface" in this area.

Memory disorders vary on several dimensions: ranging from mild to severe, acute to chronic, auditory–verbal versus visual, semantic versus episodic, procedural versus semantic, long-term versus short-term, and storage versus retrieval. Often these are not specified. Yet common remediation techniques applied are drills and practice, organization augmentors, visual imagery, vanishing cues (Glisky, Schacter, & Tulving, 1986), peg systems, errorless learning (Wilson & Evans, 1996), programs based on residual learning abilities (Leng & Copello, 1990), and prosthetic devices (Tate, 1997) or orthotic devices (Bergman, 1991; Bergman & Kemmerer, 1991). All these techniques have limitations, and selection of any one technique requires clinical judgment of a professional for each individual case to be rehabilitated. The complexity of memory disorders needs refinement. Just what kinds of memory (semantic vs. episodic or combination thereof, etc.) are being successfully rehabilitated with what kind of technique at what stage of biological, emotional, and psychosocial recovery needs to be revealed through memory research. However, practically, the focus has been on acquisition of domain-specific knowledge: knowledge pertaining to a particular task, subject, or function important to a patient in his or her everyday life (Schacter & Glisky, 1986). Furthermore, even when memory rehabilitation techniques are successful, they do not show long-lasting effects (Milders, Berg, & Deelman, 1995). The psychosocial benefit of recalling better during an earlier stage of recovery, however, was not disclosed in this study.

Learning theory principles of stimulus generalization do not always apply to the brain damaged, so what is learned in one situation does not generalize to other similar situations, although attempts are being made to promote generalization during attention and memory interventions (Sohlberg & Raskin, 1996). Response maintenance and generalization are more likely to occur if the opportunity for response practice and reinforcement are provided after training and under different generalization dimensions (Lloyd & Cuvo, 1994). The ecological factor is important. Most brain-damaged individuals want to complete activities of daily living without interferences from memory losses. They want to remember the location of car keys or to remove a cooking pot from the stove, for example. They are less interested in recalling a word list or letters in words that do not relate to their daily life.

The relationship between memory and language functioning is not easily conceptualized in some brain disorders. Conventional language assessment models examine language expression and reception in terms of phonological, semantic, and syntactical characteristics at no greater complexity than a sentence (Friedland & Miller, 1998). Many head-injured patients perform within normal limits on conventional aphasia batteries, although a significant proportion of severely head-injured, nonaphasic patients have residual deficiencies in confrontation naming, word-finding, or verbal association areas (McDonald, 1992). The question has been whether these deficits represent memory losses, slowed processing speed, or a linguistic problem. For instance, the inability to immediately recall a name of a longtime friend could relate to either memory, linguistic, or processing decrements. Sometimes this is difficult to determine, but it is important for professionals to note the patient's perspective, not just superficially, but truly realize the emotional impact of cognitive losses when an item of importance is not readily accessible.

The most likely model for verbal communication competence is interplay between linguistic and cognitive processes (Hinchliffe, Murdoch, Chenery, Baglioni, & Harding-Clark, 1998). The obviousness of expressive language deficits after brain insults is devastating to an individual. It interplays with emotions, resulting in further deficits as frustration and confusion diminish communication satisfaction (Snow, Douglas, & Ponsford, 1997). Both expressive and receptive language losses decrease psychosocial functioning. The person can isolate him- or herself and remain alone most of the time. Evidence shows disruptions in conversations can persist long term (Snow, Douglas, & Ponsford, 1998). Using conversational analysis that does not rely on formal language assessments offers opportunities for completion of an individualized treatment plan and, if coupled with emotional and motivational plan, has a greater potential for success.

Another major area of cognitive rehabilitation relates to visuospatial dysfunctioning, which can be devastating as the individual becomes imperceptive to the "unseen world." Visual field defects in head trauma survivors indicate cognitive losses of greater severity (Uzzell, Obrist, Dolinskas, Langfitt, & Wiser, 1987; Uzzell, Dolinskas, & Langfitt, 1988). Visual field neglects and other visuospatial dysfunctioning produce confusion about space and inabilities to read or write, operate power tools, assemble items such as bicycles or furniture, walk in the park alone, or numerous other activities. Safety becomes an issue with visuospatial dysfunctioning, as impending danger goes unnoticed, such as approaching vehicles while crossing a busy street or walking too close to a burning stove. For most adults visuospatial dysfunctioning means the end of driving a motor vehicle, and thus the end of personal independence. Fortunately, rehabilitation techniques of visuospatial losses developed during the late 1970s and early 1980s have been successful (Diller & Weinberg, 1977; Calvanio, Levine, & Petrone, 1993).

Much attention in neuropsychological rehabilitation is given to psychosocial components involving interactions between the brain-injured person and others. Distinctions are made between feelings, motivations, and emotions. Among the many definitions, feelings are conceptualized as sometime primitive perceptions of internal bodily states, while motivation is considered to be complex feeling states that parallel hierarchical goal behavior. Emotions are complex feeling states that parallel an interruption of ongoing goal-seeking behaviors (Prigatano *et al.*, 1986). Theories of emotions are tied to the limbic system (LaBar & LeDoux, 1997), but the influence does not stop here, as the limbic system is intimately connected to other parts of the brain (Derryberry & Tucker, 1992). In normal persons or patients with unilateral brain damage, a general dominance of the right hemisphere for various aspects of emotional behaviors prevails (Borod, 1992; Gainotti, 1997), although bilateral brain damage yields less brain specificity. Left hemisphere with its high incidence of aphasic disturbances increases agitation (Prigatano, 1992).

A commonly held belief is the uniqueness of personality of each individual, although species-specific similarities exist among each of us as human beings. Personality represents the sum of influences of life experiences, particularly early life experiences, as well as the influences of cognitive and biological processes. Personality changes are noted in both adults and children after brain injuries, although certain behaviors (e.g., occasionally socially inappropriate remarks) are tolerated more in children than in adults.

Personality disorders after brain injury have been classified into three broad categories in order to assist professionals in understanding and treating the disorders (Prigatano *et al.*, 1986). This first category contains typical reactionary problems, such as anxiety, depression, irritability, and mistrust. Some patients perceive losses as devastating, causing them to curtail social activities, since they may feel unable to remember sequential statements in ongoing conversations or names of acquaintances. The net result translates into feelings of inadequacy, self-disparagement, and lowering of self-esteem. The second type of personality disorder relates to neuropsychologically mediated problems. Here, the individual may be unaware of deficits and react impulsively. The third personality disorder relates to typical characterological styles. The patient may have selected characteristics, such as obsessiveness. These are treatable during neuropsychological rehabilitation with individual and group psychotherapy adapted for the brain injured (Prigatano *et al.*, 1986; Davis, Turner, Rolider & Cartwright, 1994; Alderman, Fry, & Youngson, 1995; Chittum, Johnson, Chittum, Guercio & McMorrow, 1996).

Personality changes after brain damage generates most complaints of family members, and these are not ignored in neuropsychological rehabilitation. Family members generally remain longer in the lives of brain-injured individuals than do professionals. Divorces do occur and older family members may die, but some family members usually stay involved. Comprehensive neuropsychological rehabilitation programs involve the family, not only in their educational services, but utilize the input of family members in establishing goals and services. The involvement of family members in neuropsychological rehabilitation is important not only because it assists the family in understanding the problems of the brain injured, but also management techniques of these problems at home or in social situations.

Transmutations in the 21st Century

As the 20th century closes, neuropsychological rehabilitation is best exemplified as a holistic outpatient treatment program that treats cognitive, emotional, psychosocial, and physical functions and their interrelationships in individuals who have sustained brain insults. Functioning of a holistic program is more than the sum of its parts. The program begins at a time of medical stability, requires a hierarchy of mastery stages, meets personal needs and goals, and maintains a humanistic orientation. The program developed during the 20th century (although some may call this as a reawakening rather than a development) and is now practiced on at least four continents: Australia, Europe, and North and South America.

Rosenthal (1996) described the development of traumatic brain injury rehabilitation in the United States in several eras: enlightenment (1975–1979), proliferation (1980–1984), refinement (1985–1989), accountability (1990–1994), and consolidation (1995–1999). If these apply to holistic neuropsychological rehabilitation in this century, then what is the era at the beginning of the 21st century? There are several choices, but the era of transmutation is chosen. The reason for this selection is because of anticipated changes, transformations, or metamorphosis that will be made to create a new and successful holistic program during the 2000–2004 era. Let us now review some of these anticipated transmutations.

The first transmutation to consider is how concepts of neuropsychological rehabilitation will evolve. No longer will it to be thought of as a poor stepchild of neuropsychology as a discipline, but on equal footing with assessment, which has been the main function of neuropsychology. This conceptualization change will initiate a chain of events. The first link in the chain—the amount of time a neuropsychologist will spend dispensing treatment—will increase over the amount of time spent in assessment. Already this is happening in the United States, with the percentage of treatment time rivaling the percentage of assessment time for neuropsychologists (Putman & Deluca, 1990).

The second link in the chain results from increased need for academic institutions to prepare their students by offering more neuropsychological rehabilitation graduate-level courses so graduating neuropsychologists are better prepared to serve the public. A recent proposed recommendation for specific rehabilitation training guidelines include issues of disability, ecological validity of tests, vocational evaluation/training, academic programs for students with disabilities, independent living resources, specific cognitive–behavioral interventions, resources for individuals with disabilities, and government assistance programs for individuals with disabilities (Johnstone & Farmer, 1997). Undoubtedly, these and other training guidelines will be considered and some adopted during the 21st century, changing neuropsychological rehabilitation by giving it equal parity with assessment and producing better-trained neuropsychologists for the field. The recent credentialing practice of neuropsychologists in the United States for rehabilitation emphasizes requirements for neuropsychological rehabilitation training (Bergquist & Malec, 1997).

The third link in the chain is changing the graduate assessment curriculum for neuropsychologists to include more ecological, functional assessment techniques or functional modification of existing techniques for assessment for neuropsychological rehabilitation. This will require development of neuropsychological instruments/tests that are sensitive to functional activities so that inferences from them will be appropriate to everyday life activities. While the validity and reliability of neuropsychological tests have been established, their robustness in predicting future functioning in community life has not been sufficiently documented in the literature (Acker, 1986). Efforts to remedy this situation are emerging (McPherson, Berry, & Pentland, 1997). The need to identify aspects of neuropsychological assessment with specific predictors and variance of rehabilitation success at different stages of the rehabilitation process (Bergquist *et al.*, 1994) may then be fulfilled. While Luria's neuropsychological investigation techniques have dominated the neuropsychological rehabilitation field in many parts of the world, it is taught less frequently in US graduate level courses, but this may change as the need to educate and prepare neuropsychologists for neuropsychological rehabilitation increases. Creativity will be fostered in developing sensitive neuropsychological assessment techniques for functional activities in environments of ever-present cost curtailment that shrinks neuropsychological rehabilitation service time.

Measurement growths will also change the concept of neuropsychological rehabilitation in the future. Greater accountability to patients, their families and third-party payers (both private or public) and the need to convince skeptics of the validity of treatment will take place through increased use of measurement approaches suitable for neuropsychological rehabilitation. Amid concerns about the validity of neuropsychological rehabilitation (High, Boake, & Lehmkuhl, 1995), outcome studies are already beginning to appear (Christensen, Pinner, Moller-Pedersen, Teasdale, & Trexler, 1992; Franklin, 1997). Expect to see more of these in the future as the individualized nature of neuropsychological rehabilitation is revealed through single case designs (Wilson, 1987) selected among five single case design possibilities (Sohlberg & Mateer, 1989) and specialized corrections for missing data (Watson, Horn, Wilson, Shiel, & McLellan, 1997).

The second transmutation will be the variety of rehabilitation settings in which a neuropsychologist can be found. If neuropsychologists pick up the gauntlet for a role their training has prepared them, then the public will benefit. Certainly there are challenges for the roles neuropsychologists assume in rehabilitation (Nelson & Adams, 1997). The holistic model with a humanistic approach to treatment, rather than a mechanical one, has survived well in this century under the direction of pioneering neuropsychologists with involvement of other disciplines. These programs with continue under the direction of neuropsychologists. The medical model of rehabilitation that prevails in many rehabilitation facilities today often harbors interdisciplinary antagonism. This does not mean that the neuropsychologist cannot be involved in the medical model, but it does mean changing conceptualizations. Other disciplines are involved and needed in rehabilitation, but it is the knowledgeable neuropsychologist who has the overview of the effects of damage to the brain itself and neuropsychosocial functioning in medically stable patients. The domain of cognitive rehabilitation belongs to no profession and can be provided by professionals from different disciplines whose background and training differ. Such redundancy, when coordinated, can be beneficial to brain-damaged patients. The role of the neuropsychologist is not meant to usurp or alienate medicine or other disciplines but to bring the overview of patient treatment into a program in many different ways: ecological assessment, cognitive retraining, and behavioral treatment and management. The skilled neuropsychologist knows this and also knows how to acquire knowledge and understanding from members of other disciplines on the rehabilitation team.

Expect the role of the neuropsychologist to be further transformed by participating in treatment early during the acute care recovery phase. Again, academic training guidelines need to include training in this area, as well as clinical practicums and experience to prepare the neuropsychologist for this task. If secondary injuries become controlled as planned, then patients entering the neuropsychological rehabilitation in the acute phase may be less severely injured than those treated in the past. It is important for a neuropsychologist to become involved in the acute phase as early as possible not only because this increases chances for greater rehabilitation success, but also because it reduces the likelihood of patients developing maladaptive behaviors. The net result is reductions in later treatment costs and psychological distress of patients. Expect to see transformations of neuropsychological rehabilitation in the 21st century as neuropsychologists begin working in a variety of rehabilitation settings .

A third transmutation of neuropsychological rehabilitation comes from the biological aspects with the development of new pharmaceuticals or old drugs applied in new ways and revelations revealed by neuroimaging from the next generations of scanners. Both positive and negative aspects of these techniques are present. It is well known that prescribed medicines that control one set of symptoms can be counterindicated for recovery. Preferred pharmaceutical efficacies provide constant improvement of symptoms for long periods of time, but these are not always found in clinical practice. The pharmaceutical treatments most desired by patients and their families are ones that improve cognitive daily functioning, but these are most elusive, although donepezil hydrochloride and tacrine hydrochloride have been beneficial in some cases. Negative side effects limit effectiveness of these and other drugs. Natural substances, such as, *gingko biloba,* have been sought and used to improve memory with mixed outcomes until multiple controlled investigations are completed. While the benefits of the pharmacological treatments may enhance or facilitate neuropsychological rehabilitation for longer periods of time, the quest for the "magic pill" so desired by every patient to decrease memory losses, increase processing speed, and make simultaneous processing possible may be in the offing in the 21st century. Beneficial nerve growth and interneuronal connections are so desired that this path of research will continue to be pursued. Experimentation with the growth hormone is in progress, but other substances undoubtedly will be found and tried, including even human brain tissue implants, before the 21st century closes. Strides made in understanding biological aspects will subsequently metamorphose neuropsychological rehabilitation.

Improved functional neuroimaging with better spatial resolution and prolonged durations of cognitive activation will transform neuropsychological rehabilitation through verification of cognitive improvements after treatment and by discriminating treatment effectiveness and preferences. The duration of treatment effects over time will also be noted with repeated neuroimaging studies during treatment and nontreatment times. Certainly those treatments deemed not useful with this technique will be discontinued, thereby changing neuropsychological rehabilitation. In short, functional neuroimaging will have a greater role in determining neuropsychological rehabilitation effectiveness in the future.

A fourth transmutation concerns cognitive retraining or remediation techniques, which will focus on training for independence rather than attempting to retrain or train for compensation of a selected function, such as memory. Independence training requires a more global focus of cognitive rehabilitation, utilizing carefully selected cognitive technique or combination of techniques required to assist an individual in becoming more independent. The level of independence in each case can be assessed and treated individually for ecological validity (Hart & Hayden, 1986). Assessment techniques used to evaluate the success of cognitive retraining are already focusing on ecological validity (Ho & Bennett, 1997; Kibby, Schmitter-Edgecombe, & Long, 1998). Evaluation of individual cognitive techniques that show promise in improving skills (Thomas-Stonell, Johnson, Schuller, & Jutai, 1994) will continue, but since the goal is to assist the brain-damaged person toward an independent lifestyle, a combination of cognitive techniques plus prosthetic and/or orthotic devices will be utilized.

Associated with training for independence are problems characterized as "personality." In the future this area requires much investigation of three main affective disturbances: (1) early agitation and long-term consequences; (2) lack of motivation (aspontaneity); and (3) lack of self-awareness (Prigatano, 1992). Added to these disturbances is a call for investigation to better understand the influence of preexisting affective disturbances (Max *et al.*, 1997). Not all affective disturbances occur in any one patient or in one kind of brain insults, such as head injury. In terms of self-awareness, the call for investigations seems to have been heard (Chittum *et al.*, 1996; Sbordone, Seyranian, & Ruff, 1998; Sherer, Bergloff, Boake, High, & Levin, 1998), but more needs to be learned. Medications do not increase self-awareness, but often reduce agitation and increase spontaneity, and their long-term use requires more investigation. One therapy that might transmute neuropsychological rehabilitation is physical activity, which improves mood, depression, anxiety, self-concepts, and personality (McDonald & Hodgdon, 1991; Gordon *et al.*, 1998) and possibly mentation. While physical therapy generally has been a part of neuropsychological rehabilitation in the past, it has not necessarily been viewed as a technique for improving affective or cognitive functioning. Application of results from these investigations during the 21st century will enable clinicians to assist patients toward a more independent state.

A fifth transformation considered here are specialized neuropsychological rehabilitation programs anticipated to develop in the future. In the past, two major diseases—cerebrovascular accidents and trauma head injuries—have dominated specialized programs due to the sheer numbers of individuals affected by these disorders. These programs will likely continue as long as the number of individuals affected remains high. What will be new in the 21st century will be specialized programs based on age with subprograms (i.e., specialized program segments) based on gender, bilingualism, and substance abuse. Neuropsychological rehabilitation of children, adolescents, adults, and the elderly require different approaches and methods. Pediatric neuropsychological rehabilitation is expected to generate a considerable amount of activity, and its prominence will transmute neuropsychological rehabilitation in the 21st century. Holistic neuropsychological rehabilitation rather than only language intervention or learning disability treatment with children (Warren & Reichle, 1992; Gerber, 1993) is anticipated. Programs that focus on the greater plasticity in children than adults may maximize recovery. One suggestion has been to use computer-generated virtual environments tailored to the precise sensory and motor capacities of the brain-injured child (Rose, Johnson, & Attree, 1997). Unlike the real world, virtual environments can be constructed to offset partial sensory loss and contingent on whatever response repertoire the participant has available. Virtual reality has the potential to become a very powerful tool not only for children but for adults in the 21st century. Its usage will certainly transform neuropsychological rehabilitation.

As the population ages and lives longer, the numbers of the elderly increases. While older persons have a more difficult time surviving brain damage insults, many of them do. Programs tailored to the needs of the older individual have developed and continue to grow. Older adults progress at different rates during rehabilitation, and psychosocial problems predict losses of independence (McNeill & Lichtenberg, 1998). Goals mainly address quality of life at a slower pace. The transmutation in these programs will occur with developments of methods that rapidly return the older individual to his or her previous lifestyle.

Subprograms that are gender-, bilingual, and substance abuse-specific will play a role in modifying parts of neuropsychological rehabilitation. Cognitive neuropsychologists tell us that women recover language skills more rapidly than males of the same age, suggesting considerations for modification of remediation programs. Language recovery for the bilingual patient is different than that of the monolingual patient. The influence of culture on thoughts and reactions cannot be ignored and will transmute neuropsychological rehabilitation. Cross-cultural analyses will add much to what is required for rehabilitation of the bilingual patient. Both gender and bilingual specificity recovery patterns of other functions, such as visuospatial and memory skills, also require attention. Indications of two distinct types of recovery following alcohol use (Kelly,1995; Uzzell, 1998) requires sensitivity in developing subprogramming to address these distinctions.

The sixth transmutation of neuropsychological rehabilitation comes from families and caregivers who have had an active part in neuropsychological rehabilitation programs. They provide input to professionals about their loved ones (Teasdale *et al.*, 1997), despite being distressed by the symptoms (Knight, Devereux, & Godfrey, 1998). In addition to their many past influences, they are transforming neuropsychological rehabilitation through training they receive to provide cognitive intervention in naturalistic settings (Sohlberg, Glang, & Todis, 1998). This transmutation is the beginning of neuropsychological rehabilitation in the home. More changes are sure to follow.

This review has selectively focused on the ways neuropsychological rehabilitation has evolved during the 20th century and will continue to evolve during the millennium and the 21st century. Professionals, patients, and their families from the past, present, and future have contributed to what neuropsychological rehabilitation is and what it will continue to be worldwide. By virtue of its origins, neuropsychological rehabilitation will remain humanistic in the future. Many challenges still remain to be unraveled to increase our knowledge about biological and neuropsychosocial aspects following brain damage.

References

Acker, M. B. (1986). Relationships between test scores and everyday life functioning. In B. P. Uzzell & Y. Gross (Eds.), *Clinical neuropsychology of intervention* (pp. 85–117). Boston: Martinus Nijhoff Publishing.

Alderman, N., Fry, R. K., & Youngson, H. A. (1995). Improvement of self-monitoring skills, reduction of behaviour disturbance and dysexecutive syndrome: Comparison of response cost and a new programme of self-monitoring training. *Neuropsychological Rehabilitation, 5,* 193–221.

Arts, W. F. M., Van Dongen, H. R., Van Hof-Van Duin, J., & Lammens, G. (1985). Unexpected improvement after prolonged posttraumatic vegetative state. *Journal of Neurology, Neurosurgery, and Psychiatry, 48,* 1300–1303.

Baxt, W. G., & Moody, P. (1987). The impact of advanced prehospital emergency care on the mortality of severely brain-injured patients. *The Journal of Trauma, 27,* 365–369.

Ben-Yishay, Y., Rattok, J., Lakin, P., Piasetsky, E. G., Ross, B., Silver, S., Zide, E., & Ezrachi, P. (1985). Neuropsychologic rehabilitation: quest for a holistic approach. *Seminars in Neurology, 5,* 252–259.

Bergman, M. (1991). Computer-enhanced self-sufficiency: Part 1. Creation and implementation of a textwriter for an individual with traumatic brain injury. *Neuropsychology, 5,*17–23.

Bergman, M., & Kemmerer, A. G. (1991). Computer-enhanced self-sufficiency: Part 2. Uses and subjective benefits of a text writer for an individual with traumatic brain injury. *Neuropsychology, 5,* 25–28.

Bergquist, T. F., & Malec, J. F. (1997). Psychology: Current practice and training issues in treatment of cognitive dysfunction. *NeuroRehabilitation, 8,* 49–56.

Bergquist, T. F., Boll, T. J., Corrigan, J. D., Harley, J. P., Malec, J. F., Millis, S. R., & Schmidt, M. F. (1994). Neuropsychological rehabilitation: Proceedings of a consensus conference. *Journal of Head Trauma Rehabilitation, 9,* 50–61.

Berker, E. A., Berker, A. H., & Smith, A. (1986). Translation of Broca's 1865 report: Lcalization of speech in the third left frontal convolution. *Archives of Neurology, 43,* 1065–1072.

Borod, J. C. (1992). Interhemispheric and intrahemispheric control of emotion: A focus on unilateral brain damage. *Journal of Consulting and Clinical Psychology, 60,* 339–348.

Bricolo, A., Turazzi, S., & Feriotti, G. (1980). Prolonged posttraumatic unconsciousness: Therapeutic assets and liabilities. *Journal of Neurosurgery, 52,* 625–634.

Calvanio, R., Levine, D., & Petrone, P. (1993). Elements of cognitive rehabilitation after right hemisphere stroke. *Behavioral Neurology, 11,* 25–57.

Carlomagno, S., Eeckhout, P. V., Blasi, V., Belin, P., Samson, Y., & Deloche, G. (1997). The impact of functional neuroimaging methods on the development of a theory for cognitive remediation. *Neuropsychological Rehabilitation, 7,* 311–326.

Castejon, O. J. (1998). Morphological astrocytic changes in complicated human brain trauma. A light and electron microscopic study. *Brain Injury, 12,* 409–427.

Chittum, W. R., Johnson, K., Chittum, J. M., Guercio, J. M., & McMorrow, M. J. (1996). Road to awareness: An individualized training package for increasing knowledge and comprehension of personal deficits in persons with acquired brain injury. *Brain Injury, 10,* 763–776.

Christensen, A.-L., Pinner, E. M., Moller-Pedersen, P., Teasdale, T. W., & Trexler, L. (1992). Psychosocial outcome following individualized neuropsychological rehabilitation of brain damage. *Acta Neurologica Scandinavica, 85,* 32–38.

Daffner, R. H., Deeb, Z. L., Lupetin, A. R., & Rothfus, W. E. (1988). Patterns of high-speed impact injuries in motor vehicle occupants. *The Journal of Trauma, 28,* 498–501.

Davis, J. R., Turner, W., Rolider, A., & Cartwright, T. (1994). Natural and structured baselines in the treatment of aggression following brain injury. *Brain Injury, 8,* 589–597.

DeJong, G. I., Buwalda. B., Schuurman, T., & Luiten, P. G. M. (1992). Synaptic plasticity in the dentate gyrus of aged rates is altered after chronic nimodipine application. *Brain Research, 596,* 345–348.

Derryberry, D., & Tucker, D. M. (1992). Neural mechanisms of emotion. *Journal of Clinical and Consulting Psychology, 60,* 329–338.

Deutsch, G., Mountz, J. M., Twieg, D. B., Southwood, M. H., San Pedro, E. C., & Liu, H. G. (1998). Xenon SPECT, fMRI and FDG evidence for reorganization post stroke. *NeuroImage, 7,* S–498.

Diller, L. L. (1976). A model for cognitive retraining in rehabilitation. *Clinical Psychologist, 29,* 13–14.

Diller, L. L., & Weinberg, J. (1977). Hemi-attention in rehabilitation: The evolution of a rational remediation program. *Advances in Neurology, 18,* 63–92.

Franklin, S. (1997). Designing single case treatment studies for aphasic patients. *Neuropsychological Rehabilitation, 7,* 401–418.

Friedland, D., & Miller, N. (1998). Conversation analysis of communication breakdown after closed head injury. *Brain Injury, 12,* 1–14.

Gainotti, G. (1997). Emotional disorders in relation to unilateral brain damage. In T. E. Feinberg & M. J. Farah (Eds.), *Behavioral neurology and neuropsychology* (pp. 691–698). New York: McGraw-Hill.
Gerber, A. (1993). *Language-related learning disabilities.* Baltimore: Paul H. Brookes.
Glisky, E. L., Schacter, D. L., & Tulving, E. (1986). Learning and retention of computer-related vocabulary in amnesic patients: method of vanishing cues. *Journal of Clinical and Experimental Neuropsychology, 8,* 292–312.
Gordon, W. A., Sliwinski, M., Echo, J., Mcloughlin, M., Sheerer, M., & Meili, T. E. (1998).The benefits of exercise in individuals with traumatic brain injury: A retrospective study. *Journal of Head Trauma Rehabilitation, 13,* 58–67.
Hart, T., & Hayden, M. E. (1986). The ecological validity of neuropsychological assessment and remediation. In B. P. Uzzell & Y. Gross (Eds.). *Clinical neuropsychology of intervention* (pp. 21–50). Boston: Martinus Nijhoff.
Heiss, W.-D., Herholz, K., Pawlik, G., Wagner, R., & Wienhard, K. (1986). Positron emission tomography in neuropsychology. *Neuropsychologia, 24,* 141–149.
High, W. M., Boake, C., & Lehmkuhl, L. D. (1995). Critical analysis of studies evaluating the effectiveness of rehabilitation after traumatic brain injury. *Journal of Head Trauma Rehabilitation, 10,* 14–26.
Hinchliffe, F. J., Murdoch, B. E., Chenery, H. J., Baglioni, A. J., Jr., & Harding-Clark, J. (1998). Cognitive–linguistic subgroups in closed head injury. *Brain Injury, 12,* 369–398.
Ho, M. R., & Bennett, T. L. (1997). Efficacy of neuropsychological rehabilitation for mild–moderate traumatic brain injury. *Archives of Clinical Neuropsychology, 12,* 1–11.
Jennett, B., Teasdale, G., Galbraith, S., Pickard, J., Grant, H., Braakman, R., Avezaat, C., Maas, A., Minderhoud, J., Vecht, J., Heiden, J., Small, R., Caton, W., & Kurze. T. (1977). Severe head injuries in three countries. *Journal of Neurology, Neurosurgery, and Psychiatry, 40,* 291–298.
Johnson, D., & Almli, C. R. (1978). Age, brain damage and performance. In S. Finger (Ed.), *Recovery from brain damage: Research and theory* (pp.115–134), New York: Plenum Press.
Johnstone, B., & Farmer, J. E. (1997). Preparing neuropsychologists for the future: The need for additional training guidelines. *Archives of Clinical Neuropsychology, 12,* 523–530.
Kater, S. B., Mattson, M. P., & Guthrie, P. B. (1989). Calcium-induced neuronal degeneration: A normal growth cone regulating signal gone awry (?). *Annals of the New York Academy of Sciences, 568,* 252–261.
Kelly, D. F. (1995). Alcohol and head injury: An issue revisited. *Journal of Neurotrauma, 12,* 883–890.
Kibby, M. Y., Schmitter-Edgecombe, M., & Long, C. J. (1998). Ecological validity of neuropsychological tests: Focus on the California verbal learning test and the Wisconsin card sorting test. *Archives of Clinical Neuropsychology, 13,* 523–534.
Knight, R. G., Devereux, R., & Godfrey, H. P. D. (1998). Caring for a family member with with a traumatic brain injury. *Brain Injury, 6,* 443–454.
Knopman, D. S., Rubens, A. B., Selnes, O. A., Klassen, A. C., & Meyer, M. W. (1984). Mechanisms of recovery from aphasia: Evidence from serial Xenon 133 cerebral blood flow studies. *Annals of Neurology, 15,* 530–535.
Kolakowsky, S. A., & Parente, R. (1997). Nootropics, nutrients and other cognitive enhancing substances for use in cognitive rehabilitation. *The Journal of Cognitive Rehabilitation, 15,* 12–24.
Kraus, M. F., & Maki, P. (1997).The combined use of amantadine and L-dopa/carbidopa in the treatment of chronic brain injury. *Brain Injury, 11,* 455–460.
Laatsch, L., Jobe, T., Sychra, J., Lin, Q., & Blend, M. (1997). Impact of cognitive rehabilitation therapy on neuropsychological impairments as measured by brain perfusion SPECT: Longitudinal study. *Brain Injury, 11,* 851–863.
LaBar, K. S., & LeDoux, J. E. (1997). Emotion and the brain: An overview. In T. E. Feinberg & M. J. Farah (Eds.), *Behavioral neurology and neuropsychology* (pp.675–689). NewYork: McGraw-Hill.
Leng, N. R. C., & Copello, A. G. (1990). Rehabilitation of memory after brain injury: is there an effective technique. *Clinical Rehabilitation, 4,* 63–69.
Lloyd, L. F., & Cuvo, A. J. (1994). Maintenance and generalization of behaviours after treatment of persons with traumatic brain injury. *Brain Injury, 8,* 529–540.
Luerssen, T. G., Klauber, M. R., & Marshall, L. F. (1988). Outcome from head injury related to patient's age. *Journal of Neurosurgery, 68,* 400–416.
Mangiardi, J. R. (1986). Head injury. *Hospital Physician, 22,* 20–32.
Mattson, M. P., Cheng, B., Davis, D., Bryant, K., Lieberburg, I., & Rydel, R. E. (1992). ß-Amyloid peptides destabilize calcium homeostasis and render human cortical neurons vulnerable to excitotoxicity. *Journal of Neuroscience, 12,* 376–389.
Max, J. E., Lindgren, S. D., Knutson, C., Pearson, C. S., Thrig, D., & Welborn, A. (1997). Child and adolescent traumatic brain injury: Psychiatric findings from a paediatric outpatient speciality clinic. *Brain Injury, 11,* 699–711.
McDonald, D. G., & Hodgdon, J. A. (1991). *Psychological effects of aerobic fitness training: Research and theory.* New York: Springer-Verlag.

McDonald, S. (1992). Communication disorders following closed head injury: New approaches to assessment and rehabilitation. *Brain Injury, 6,* 283–292.

McIntosh, T. K. (1994). Neurochemical sequelae of traumatic brain injury: Therapeutic implications. *Cerebrovascular and Brain Metabolism Reviews, 6,* 109–162.

McNeill, S. E., & Lichtenberg, P. A. (1998). Predictors for functional outcome in older rehabilitation patients. *Rehabilitation Psychology, 43,* 248–257.

McPherson, K., Berry, A., & Pentland, B. (1997). Relationships between cognitive impairments and functional performance after brain injury, as measured by the functional assessment measure. *Neuropsychological Rehabilitation, 7,* 241–257.

Milders, M. V., Berg, I. J., & Deelman, D. G. (1995). Four-year follow-up of a controlled memory training study in closed head injured patients. *Neuropsychological Rehabilitation, 5,* 233–238.

Miller, J. D., Sweet, R. C., Narayan, R., & Becker, D. P. (1978). Early insults to the injured brain. *Journal of American Medical Association, 240,* 439–442.

Nelson, L. D., & Adams, K. M. (1997). Challenges for neuropsychology in treatment and rehabilitation of brain-injured patients. *Psychological Assessment, 9,* 368–373.

Obrist, W. D., & Wilkinson, W. E. (1990). Regional cerebral blood flow measurement in humans by xenon-133 clearance. *Cerebrovascular and Brain Metabolism Reviews, 2,* 283–327.

Posner, U., Kohler, J. A., & Schonle, P. W. (1996). Historical review of neuropsychological rehabilitation in Germany. *Neuropsychological Rehabilitation, 6,* 257–278.

Prigatano, G. P. (1992). Personality disturbances associated with traumatic brain injury. *Journal of Clinical and Consulting Psychology, 60,* 360–368.

Prigatano, G. P. (1997). Learning from our successes and failures: Reflections and comments on "Cognitive rehabilitation: How it is and how it might be." *Journal of International Neuropsychological Society, 3,* 497–499.

Prigatano, G. P., Fordyce, D. J., Zeiner, H. K., Roueche, J. R., Pepping, M., & Wood, B. C. (1986). *Neuropsychological rehabilitation after brain injury.* Baltimore: John Hopkins Press.

Putnam, S. H., & DeLuca, J. W. (1990). The TCN professional practice survey: Part 1: General practices of neuropsychologists in primary employment and private practice settings. *The Clinical Neuropsychologist, 4,* 199–243.

Risberg, J., & Jensen, L. R. (1994). The valued of regional cerebral blood flow measurements in neuropsychological rehabilitation. In A.-L. Christensen & B.P. Uzzell (Eds.), *Brain injury and neuropsychological rehabilitation: International perspectives* (pp. 71–83). Hillsdale, NJ: Lawrence Erlbaum.

Rose, F. D., Johnson, D. A., & Attree, E. A. (1997). Rehabilitation of the head-injured child: Basic research and new technology. *Pediatric Rehabilitation, 1,* 3–7.

Rosenthal, M. (1996). 1995 Sheldon Berrol, MD senior lectureship: The ethics and efficacy of traumatic brain injury rehabilitation—Myths, measurements and meaning. *Journal of Head Trauma Rehabilitation, 11,* 88–95.

Sbordone, R. J., Seyranian, G. D., & Ruff, R. M. (1998). Are subjective complaints of traumatically brain injured patients reliable? *Brain Injury, 6,* 505–515.

Schacter, D. L., & Glisky, E. T. (1986). Memory remediation: Restoration, alleviation, and the acquisition of domain-specific knowledge. In B.P. Uzzell & Y. Gross (Eds.), *Clinical neuropsychology of intervention* (pp. 257–282). Boston: Martinus Nijhofft.

Sherer, M., Bergloff, P., Boake, C., High, W., & Levin, E. (1998). The awareness questionnaire: Factor structure and internal consistency. *Brain Injury, 12,* 63–68.

Snow, P., Douglas, J., & Ponsford, J. (1997). Conversational assessment following traumatic brain injury: A comparison across two control groups. *Brain Injury, 11,* 409–429.

Snow, P., Douglas, J., & Ponsford, J. (1998). Conversational discourse abilities following severe traumatic brain injury: A follow-up study. *Brain Injury, 12,* 911–935.

Sohlberg, Mc. M., & Mateer, C. A. (1989). *Introduction to cognitive rehabilitation: Theory and practice.* New York: Guilford Press.

Sohlberg, Mc. M., & Raskin, S. A. (1996). Principles of generalization applied to attention and memory interventions. *Journal of Head Trauma Rehabilitation, 11,* 85–78.

Sohlberg, Mc. M., Glang, A., & Todis, B. (1998). Improvement during baseline: Three case studies encouraging collaboration research when evaluating caregiver training. *Brain Injury, 12,* 333–346.

Steegman, A. T. (1962). Dr. Harlow's famous case: The "impossible" accident of Phineas P. Gage. *Surgery, 52,* 952–958.

Stein, D. G., Glasier, M. M., & Hoffman, S. W. (1994). Pharmacologic treatments for brain-injury repair: Progress and prognosis. In A.-L. Christensen & B. P. Uzzell (Eds.), *Brain injury and neuropsychological rehabilitation: International perspectives* (pp.17–39). Hillsdale, NJ: Lawrence Erlbaum.

Stein, D. G., Brailowsky, S., & Will, B. (1995). *Brain repair.* New York: Oxford University Press.

Stein, R. A., & Strickland, T. L. (1998). A review of the neuropsychological effects of use prescription medications. *Archives of Clinical Neuropsychology, 13,* 259–284.

Stuss, D. T., Gow, C. A., & Hetherington. (1992). "No longer Gage": Frontal lobe dysfunction and emotional changes. *Journal of Clinical and Consulting Psychology, 60,* 349–359.

Tate, R. L. (1997). Beyond one-bun, two-shoe: Recent advances in the psychological rehabilitation of memory disorders after acquired brain injury. *Brain Injury, 11,* 907–918.

Taverni, J. P., Seliger, G., & Lichtman, S. W. (1998). Donepezil mediated memory improvement in traumatic brain injury during post acute rehabilitation. *Brain Injury, 12,* 77–80.

Teasdale, G., Skene, A., Spiegelhalter, D., & Murray, L. (1982). Age, severity and outcome of head injury. In R. G. Grossman & P. L. Gildenberg (Eds.), *Head injury: Basic and clinical aspects* (pp. 213–220), New York: Raven Press.

Teasdale, T. W., Christensen, A.-L., Willmes, K., Deloche, G., Braga, L., Stachowiak, F., Vendrell, J. M., Castro-Caldas, A., Laaksonen, R. K., & Lecclercq, M. (1997). Subjective experience in brain-injured patients and their close relatives: A European brain injury questionnaire study. *Brain Injury, 11,* 543–563.

Terayama, Y., Meyer, J. S., & Kawamura, J. (1991). Cognitive recovery correlates with long-term increases of cerebral perfusion after head injury. *Surgical Neurology, 36,* 335–342.

Terayama, Y., Meyer, J. S., Kawamura, J., & Weathers, S. (1991). Role of thalamus and white matter in cognitive outcome after head injury. *Journal of Cerebral Blood Flow and Metabolism, 11,* 852–860.

Thomas-Stonell, N., Johnson, P., Schuller, R., & Jutai, J. (1994). Evaluation of a computer-based program for remediation of cognitive–communication skills. *Journal of Head Trauma Rehabilitation, 9,* 25–37.

Uzzell, B. P. (1998). Inconsistent effects of alcohol on head injury outcome. Presentation at American Neuropsychiatric Association.

Uzzell, B. P. (1999). Mild head injury: much ado about something. In N. R. Varney & R. Roberts (Eds.), *Evaluation and treatment of mild TBI* (pp. 1–13). Mahwah, NJ: Lawrence Erlbaum.

Uzzell, B. P., Obrist, W. D., Dolinskas, C. A., & Langfitt, T. W. (1986). Relationship of acute CBF and ICP findings to neuropsychological outcome in severe head injury. *Journal of Neurosurgery, 65,* 630–635.

Uzzell, B. P., Obrist, W. D., Dolinskas, C. A., Langfitt, T. W., & Wiser, R. F. (1987). Relation of visual field defects to neuropsychological outcome after closed head injury. *Acta Neurochirurgica, 86,* 18–27.

Uzzell, B. P., Dolinskas, C. A., & Langfitt, T. W. (1988). Visual field defects in relation to head injury severity: A neuropsychological study. *Archives of Neurology, 2,* 19–27.

Uzzell, B. P., Dolinskas, C. A., & Wiser, R. F. (1990). Relation between intracranial pressure, computed tomographic lesion and neuropsychological outcome. *Advances in Neurology, 52,* 269–274.

Warren, S. F., & Reichle, J. (1992). *Causes and effects in communication and language intervention.* Baltimore: Paul H. Brookes.

Watson, M. J., Horn, S., Wilson, B. A,. Shiel, A., & McLellan, L. (1997). The application of a paired comparisons technique to identify sequence of recovery after severe head injury. *Neuropsychological Rehabilitation, 4,* 441–458.

Wilson, B.A. (1987). Single-case experimental designs in neuropsychological rehabilitation. *Journal of Clinical and Experimental Neuropsychology, 9,* 527–544.

Wilson, B. A. (1997). Cognitive rehabilitation: How it is and how it might be. *Journal of the International Neuropsychological Society, 3,* 487–496.

Wilson, B. A., & Evans, J. J. (1996). Error-free learning in the rehabilitation of people with impairments. *Journal of Head Trauma Rehabilitation, 11,* 54–64.

Zimmerman, R. A., & Bilaniuk, L. T. (1994). Pediatric head trauma. *Neuroimaging Clinics of North America, 4,* 349–366.

Index

References with page numbers followed by italicized *t* and *f* refer to tables and figures, respectively.

www.ingramcontent.com/pod-product-compliance
Ingram Content Group UK Ltd.
Pitfield, Milton Keynes, MK11 3LW, UK
UKHW051451290926
15471UKWH00008B/1143

* 9 7 8 1 4 7 5 7 5 5 7 0 1 *